Praise for
DR. JORDAN D. METZL

"All athletes know the frustration of not being able to play due to injury. Decrease your time on the sidelines with these nuggets of wisdom about dealing with injuries large and small."

JULIE FOUDY, former captain, U.S. Women's Soccer team, 2-time Olympic Gold Medalist

"Dr. Jordan Metzl has done it again! A clearly written, beautifully illustrated guide for athletes of all ages and levels."

LYLE J. MICHELI, M.D., professor of orthopedic surgery at Harvard Medical School and author of the *Healthy Runner's Handbook*

"For those of you who are true competitors on and off the field, Dr. Metzl puts you ahead of the game. His knowledge, experience, and forward-thinking methods not only prevent injury, but give you the tools to be the most healthy, athletic, confident YOU possible."

JESSICA MENDOZA, Olympic Gold Medalist, U.S. Softball Team, and ESPN analyst for Major League Baseball

"An amazing resource for athletes of all levels, from professional to high school, young to old. There is great advice here for everyone."

RILEY J. WILLIAMS, M.D., team physician, New York Red Bulls Soccer Club

"The importance of optimal fitness for injury prevention, rehabilitation, and performance cannot be overstated. Since an informed athlete will be a more successful and healthier athlete, the highly practical information about injury prevention, recognition, and management in this book will help athletes of all ages and ability levels to 'stay in the game.'"

SCOTT RODEO, M.D., team physician, U.S. Swim Team and U.S. Olympic Team

"A great tool for professionals to use with their athletes to keep them positive and motivated to achieve their goals despite injury. I found the book exceptionally inspirational and will use it to help educate our dancers."

ELAINE WINSLOW-REDMOND, A.T.C., head athletic trainer, Radio City Rockettes

"I am always pushing my body to the edge and riding the fine line between maximizing performance and overtraining/injury. Dr. Metzl's advice about striving for balanced and full-body strength and the Iron Strength workouts he teaches have become a critical part of my training and instrumental in keeping injuries at bay. Whether you're an elite athlete, fitness enthusiast, or those looking to lead a more active lifestyle, all will find this book is an absolute must for staying strong and healthy."

SARAH PIAMPIANO, professional triathlete

"Dr. Metzl has written a book that will help athletes. The information is clear, concise, and easy to digest. I will recommend this book to my patients as a resource to help them learn about injury and recovery. Well done!"

ROBERT G. MARX, M.D., professor of orthopedic surgery and public health, Weill Cornell Medical College

"Dr. Metzl offers a unique perspective as doctor, patient, and fitness coach to the athlete who is, or in the future may be, injured. His combined approach of staying active, addressing the injury, and providing guidelines on return to play is very helpful."

BRIAN HALPERN, M.D., author of the *Knee Crisis Handbook*

"A great resource for the competitive athlete, as well as the weekend warrior. As an athlete and sports medicine physician, Dr. Metzl has a unique perspective, and the result is a book that is both practical and accurate."

ROBERT SALLIS, M.D., past president, the American College of Sports Medicine

"As Dr. Metzl writes, the care and maintenance of the athletic body will decrease injury, help performance, and make training and competition more productive and enjoyable."

DAVID W. ALTCHEK, M.D., head team physician, New York Mets

The Athlete's Book of HOME REMEDIES

1,001 Doctor-Approved Health Fixes & Injury-Prevention Secrets for a Leaner, Fitter, More Athletic Body!

BY JORDAN D. METZL, M.D.

(29 Marathons & 9 Ironmans)

with MIKE ZIMMERMAN

RODALE.

Dedication

This book is dedicated to the millions of athletes who wake up each morning at 5:30, with no fanfare, and drag themselves out of bed to keep fit. Whatever your level or ability, may the information in this book help you pursue your goals. The most important thing you can do every day is keep moving forward.

TABLE *of* CONTENTS

Acknowledgments

The following people were instrumental in turning the dream of this project into a reality. First of all, my parents, Drs. Marilyn and Kurt Metzl, created an environment in our home that encouraged fitness, learning, and goal setting. All of these attributes have helped me in every stage of my life and career. My brothers—Drs. Jonathan, Jamie and Joshua—and sister-in-law Alexandra Metzl have all been training partners, often pushing me harder and encouraging me to do more than I ever would have done by myself.

My patients, now more than 20,000 in number, from professional athletes to those just starting on their first day of fitness, each teach me something different. I am so appreciative for the chance to assist them as they strive for their own goals. Hospital for Special Surgery in New York City has allowed me the chance to practice sports medicine in the most incredible atmosphere of learning, growth, and support. I am so appreciative of my good fortune to have landed there.

Special thanks to my mentors along the way, Drs. Lyle Micheli, Kurt Spindler, and Russell Warren, each of whom has helped shape my knowledge and passion for the practice of sports medicine. Dejuanna Richardson, my strength-training guru at Asphalt Green in New York, has taught me everything I know about strength and conditioning. And thanks to my good friend and office manager Meghan Macalpine, and also to Equinox Health Clubs, both of whom have been so helpful in coordinating my strength and conditioning programs where I teach athletes about injury prevention.

Lastly, I'd like to thank the crew at Rodale: Stephen Perrine, Mike Zimmerman, Debbie McHugh, George Karabotsos, Elizabeth Neal, Erin Williams, Chris Krogermeier, Nancy Elgin, and Sona Vogel, who helped transform this idea into one amazing book.

ATHLETE, HEAL THYSELF

You hurt. Maybe it's just a nagging pain, something in your knee. Maybe it's a serious pain—borderline agony—in your lower back. You want to know what's wrong, of course. But there's something else: You're an athlete. You might be a weekend warrior, or you might be a serious competitor, but either way, you just love to be out there doing it. You love the adrenaline. You love your chosen sport. And you want, more than anything, to get back in the game. How long will this pain keep you out? What can you do to help yourself right now? Do you need a doctor's care?

This book will answer all of your questions. You see, I'm a doctor. I'm also an athlete.

Am I a doctor first, or an athlete first? Neither. I'm both at all times, and those two identities constantly feed off each other. If I'm on mile 24 of the marathon stage of an Ironman, you can bet that the doctor in me is assessing how I feel. You can also bet that the athlete in me is disregarding my own advice and fighting for the finish line, damn the consequences. And when I evaluate a patient with knee pain, the athlete in me is reminding me of what it feels like to be out of the game and how important it is to get that patient back to full form.

Becoming a doctor was probably my fate. My dad is a pediatrician, my mom is a psychologist, and two of my three siblings became medical doctors (the other guy has a PhD but gives medical advice freely). Helping people is in my DNA. When I was a kid I used to do rounds with my dad, carrying a little plastic doctor bag. Little did I know that my little candy pills would one day be replaced by antiinflammatories.

I also love sports. In high school, it was soccer and baseball. In college, I played even more soccer while doing pre-med. Then I did my first triathlon on a mountain bike in Columbia, Missouri, as a third-year medical student, and it was the most fun thing I'd ever done. As I swam in a semi-polluted lake, I kept thinking, *This is awesome, I want to keep doing this.*

Flash forward a few years and I was diving headlong into Ironman-level races where you swim 2.4 miles, bike 112 miles, and finish with a 26.2-mile marathon. During my first Ironman, I carried a microphone for CBS's *The Early Show* as its medical correspondent, thinking that if I was going to die, there at least should be a record of it. It was insane, I loved it. I've now done nine of those, and each was a killer in its own way. The Hawaiian Ironman is the hottest 12 hours you'll ever spend anywhere. I felt like a cooked lobster and couldn't have been happier.

So, you see why the combination of medicine and athletics seems so natural to me. People like you and me who play games or run races get injuries, from simple strains to broken bones. Having that athletic background fed my medical training, and vice versa.

Now I'm a sports medicine physician at New York City's Hospital for Special Surgery, the number-one hospital for orthopedics. Every day I go to work and realize how lucky I am to help people achieve their goals. My practice has more than 20,000 patients, and I treat athletes of all ages and ability levels, from kids to adults, football players to dancers. (I'm also the sports medicine physician for the Radio City Rockettes.)

I focus on nonsurgical sports medicine. That means I try to keep people moving and find alternatives to surgery whenever possible.

Sometimes surgery is both necessary and helpful, but not always. If there's a way to get an athlete back in the game without surgery, I try to find it.

That's where this book comes from. It's the combination of what I do professionally and personally—15 years as a doctor, 30 years as an athlete. It all comes together here.

I want you to stay healthy, and if you do get injured, I want to help you get back to whatever activity it is that you love as quickly and safely as possible. One of our greatest gifts as humans is our ability to move. Anyone who lives an active lifestyle—whether it's as a serious competitor or a weekend warrior who just likes to drip a good sweat for fun—knows what I'm talking about. We weren't built for couches and cubicles. We need to move. And when that ability is compromised by pain, you need solutions at your fingertips. I want to get you moving again.

I'll be honest, sometimes you'll need a doctor. I'll tell you when—and you'd better go. But many times you'll be able to use these home-based treatments to fix yourself and get back to what you love doing. Knowledge empowers you.

I've always said, "If you're an athlete, see an athlete." An athlete-doctor, athlete-nutritionist, athlete–physical therapist, etc. I have a whole network of athletes for my patients. Athletes understand athletes. Use this book to help yourself.

The athlete will see you now.

Your Body:

Why It Breaks Down and How You Can Prevent Injury

During my first year of med school, I was playing soccer for a club team at the University of Missouri. It was just a practice, but it was a beautiful day to be out and moving. I was playing striker up front, and as the goalie cleared the ball, I twisted to get it and felt this popping sensation and incredible pain in my knee. I dropped, screaming, "I tore my ACL, I tore my ACL!"

That would be the anterior cruciate ligament in my right knee. I knew it right away. And knowing it right away devastated me. Why? It wasn't just the pain in my knee. I knew that my sports career had just taken a horrible turn. Psychologically, that cut me deep. See, when I was in school, I exercised

every day. No joke, I found that I definitely was a better student—better focused, better motivated, better energized—when I exercised every day. Research has certainly proven that mind-body connection since then, but more than 15 years ago, I knew it so well that soccer was literally a big part of my schooling.

So yes, my knee was hurt, but my mind was totally thrown off its game. I'd never been hurt like this before. I didn't know how to process it. I didn't know how *not* to play sports. I'd defined myself as an athlete for virtually my entire life. But this was the first time that athletics had been taken away from me.

Looking back, I see that I actually went through the classic stages of death and dying: denial, depression, acceptance, and so on. I had to realize that my knee would never again work the way it had before. I had this black pit inside me when that was taken away from me. I was *that* dialed in to my sports (and still am!).

Obviously, the hospital trip that day confirmed my self-diagnosis. I didn't have surgery to fix it right away; a funny thing about this kind of injury is that after a couple of weeks you feel pretty normal. In the beginning, I was hopeful. Maybe it wouldn't be so bad, maybe it would heal on its own. But then every time I twisted my knee even a little bit, I felt it give out. The joint was totally unstable.

But I was stubborn. I kept going. I swam and biked. Then one day I was playing basketball with my brothers and I went up for a layup and my knee gave out. I hobbled off the court realizing I had to have it fixed.

A hundred questions flew through my head, and they all sounded a lot like "Will I be able to perform the way I could before surgery?"

The process was tremendously painful. Back then, ACL surgery and recovery hurt more than the injury did. That's improved a whole lot since, but back then...ouch.

What I didn't know at the time was that there are a whole host of preventive exercises I could've been doing. Later in life, when I got into plyometrics and strength training as both a doctor and an athlete, I realized that my knee felt better when I kept the muscles around it strong.

When my hips, glutes, and legs were strong, my knee hurt less.

It's amazing: I can control almost all of my pain with strength.

This is crucial, because a) strength can prevent an injury like this in the first place, and b) if you do have a joint injury like a torn ACL, whether you have it repaired or not, you have a 60 percent chance of developing osteoarthritis later in life (I have a little bit myself). But strength and conditioning work in such a way that I can reduce the symptoms of the injury. How? Muscle supports and stabilizes a joint. Think about that next time you want to skip a workout or skimp on rehabbing what's hurting.

My knee is better now, of course, and I train every day for various endurance races and athletic events. But I never forget how awful that injury felt not just literally in my knee, but also in my mind.

That experience has helped me take care of people with injuries. The joy of movement is why I do what I do. I understand the difficulty that goes along with an injury not just physically, but also emotionally. When you're active and that's taken away from you, it's traumatic. That's one of the biggest reasons I went into medicine, and why I wrote this book. If you're in pain and don't know why, or even if you know exactly why, my goal is to help you figure out what to do about it. I want you back in the game ASAP.

SURGERY OR NO SURGERY?

There's a lot of gray area related to surgery for athletes. This book will let you know where those gray areas exist—meniscus tears in the knee, for example—and what questions you should ask your doctor. In this book's discussion of each injury, you'll see sections called "When to Call a Doctor" and "Do You Need Surgery?" There you'll find out how doctors typically treat a given injury and what could make you a surgical candidate. Sometimes surgery is necessary and gives you a terrific outcome. But it's also useful to know when you may have effective nonsurgical options.

Why We Get Hurt

I'm a huge fan of exercising every day. I encourage everyone to do it. Get out there, sweat it up, have a blast. Of course, using your body means it could break down. A lot of things can cause an injury and we have a lot of body parts that can be hurt. Here are the three primary things that cause an injury.

• STRESS. Not "holy cow, is my boss nuts!" stress. I mean putting stress on a body part—muscle, ligament, joint, etc.—that is unprepared for it or can't handle it. This is very common in former school athletes or couch potatoes who haven't done anything for a few years and go too fast, too soon. It can also happen to well-conditioned athletes who simply move the wrong way at the wrong time. When I blew out

my knee, it was because I stressed my ACL in a way it didn't agree with. These kinds of injuries can be severe and even shocking. You think, *Whoa, I'm really hurt here,* though I guarantee you use much stronger language.

That physical stress can then lead to emotional stress—the devastation of realizing your game has just been taken away from you. That is a psychological sports injury, and its own effect shouldn't be underestimated.

• IMBALANCE. Simply put, your body isn't properly trained for the activity you're doing. It happens to someone who runs nothing but half-marathons for 5 years and then suddenly decides a 100-meter sprint is a good idea. Well, distance running trains your hamstrings in the exact opposite way that's required for a sprint. Guess who's limping home? The most important exercise advice I can give you is to train your entire body. Switch up your activities and hit all the muscle groups, even if you play only one sport. On top of being a doctor, I now teach plyometric strength classes that involve functional body motion. I'm a huge fan of this—it trains your body for real-world movement. Back when I was rehabbing my knee, I'd sit in the gym and do leg extensions, hamstring curls—these isolated movements that have no basis in reality. Now I never use those machines. I do balance work, single-leg work, and plyometric exercises like lunges

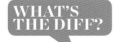

WHAT'S
THE DIFF?

Strain and sprain

Strain: An injury to a muscle or tendon. Depending on the severity, a strain can involve a simple overstretching of the tissue or a tear (partial or complete). They're graded in severity from 1 to 3.

Sprain: An injury to a ligament. This can also include overstretching or a tear.

The Athlete's Top 10 "Prime Directives"

1 An injury does not grant you a vacation from exercise. Work out the body parts that don't aggravate your injury so you retain your fitness.

2 You can control pain with strength. Strong muscles support and stabilize a vulnerable joint.

3 If a joint is swollen, see a doctor.

4 A strong butt is the key to a happy life. Healthy glutes mean healthy hips, back, and hamstrings.

5 Have two massages a month for healthier muscles.

6 Sleep is the most important activity of your day.

7 Exercise every day. Exercise is medicine. It will keep you healthy and happy.

8 Train your entire body for real-world movement, even if you play only one sport. Isolated, single-muscle exercises have no basis in reality.

9 Single-leg exercises—squats, hops, lunges—build incredible strength and stability in your ankles, knees, and hips.

10 And never, ever forget to...have fun!

THE IMPORTANCE OF MASSAGE

I'm a huge believer in having a massage twice a month and even more often when you are training hard. This goes for athletes of all types. A good massage is one more way to help keep your muscles supple and less prone to injury.

and squat jumps, real-world movements that hit a lot of muscles at the same time and keep the body in balance. It's so easy for sport-specific folks to train only for that sport. And yes, obviously, training for your sport is critical. But if you neglect body parts that then throw your muscles out of balance, you're just asking for the pain.

• OVERUSE. This one is common sense and yet still so common. If you work your body too hard, it will break down. It's like any other machine that needs maintenance and restoration. I think a deep drive for excellence and performance is huge for any athlete—it's what fuels you. But if you don't temper it by listening to your body and knowing your limitations, you'll never know when to back off. And then, again, guess who's limping home?

Now, all that said, you could do everything right and still be injured for any number of reasons. It happens to the best of us. But the more you know and understand about how your body works, the better you'll be able to see how injuries can happen. The benefits to that are twofold:

• The next time you train, you'll visualize and feel how your body is performing at that moment. That makes bad training habits easier to break.

• As your understanding of proper form and better technique grows, so will your athletic performance. Who doesn't want to get better?

So, what do you need to know? Let's start with one of the most important body systems—yet it's typically the least known to the average amateur exerciser/athlete. Understand how it works and you'll understand how important total-body fitness is to staying on the field.

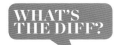

Tendon, ligament, and cartilage

Tendon: Connective tissue that attaches muscle to bone.

Ligament: Connective tissue that attaches bone to bone.

Cartilage: Connective tissue that cushions bones between and around joints. It can also act as a support structure to give a body part its shape, such as in the nose and ear.

An Athlete's Trade Secret: The Kinetic Chain

So what's the big secret? It's what sports doctors, trainers, and researchers know and use to train better athletes. It's called the kinetic chain. It's basically your entire body from the top of your neck down to your toenails, one big interconnected chain of muscles, ligaments, tendons, bones, and so on.

"What's the big deal?" you ask. Naturally, looking at the human body when it's just standing there doesn't tell you anything. Health classes and gym memberships have filled your brain with a lot of colorful anatomical terms like biceps, quads, and everyone's favorite cosmetic goal, abs. This has sent millions of people off to work individual muscles, thinking that a big biceps or a defined quad is the ultimate goal. Meanwhile, vital complementary muscles like the triceps and hamstrings go neglected. And when these folks actually move their bodies in an athletic way, they get hurt. "But why?" they ask. "I work out!"

Put simply, they've never been educated about the importance of training the kinetic chain in a balanced way. Yes, you have biceps, abs, and quads. But they're useless if you don't understand how they function as part of the kinetic chain. It's time to put them all together into one system and watch them work.

KINETIC MEANS MOVEMENT

When an at-rest human body takes a step forward, then jukes to the side, then jumps, instead of seeing individual muscles like biceps, quads, and abs, you see a fluid, functional combination of all three, as well as every other muscle, bone, and connective tissue in the body. That's the kinetic chain: Each body part is a link, and each link depends on the others for normal, healthy performance.

Kinetic means motion or movement. So we're talking about a chain of movement. It's the words to that old anatomy song, "your shin bone's connected to your knee bone," but on an epic level.

Now, because we have a chain, what happens around the weak links?

Yep, you guessed it: injury.

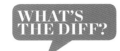

WHAT'S THE DIFF?

Bulging disk, herniated disk, and slipped disk

Bulging: A benign bulging of a spinal disk outside of its normal space, usually with no symptoms or pain. It's a common side effect of aging.

Herniated: A crack in the outer layer of a disk's cartilage has allowed the inner cartilage to emerge. It can cause pain, but sometimes doesn't.

Slipped: Another term for herniated.

Here's a closer look at how the kinetic chain works.

First, as I said, everything is interrelated. Patients come in all the time with injuries caused by other injuries, like a patient with plantar fasciitis who now says her knee hurts or her lower back hurts. When one piece hurts, people focus on that one piece and it throws off the whole way they move. Example: Baseball fans hear all the time about how a major league pitcher hurt his shoulder because his knee was already hurt. To protect the knee or alleviate pain, he changed his pitching motion (which no pitcher should ever do) and stressed his shoulder in a way it wasn't trained for.

For us, let's start with your feet. They're the foundation of almost all movement. Everyone uses them all day long. The foot is an amazing, dynamic structure, a collection of 26 bones, 33 joints, 19 muscles and tendons, and 107 ligaments. Why so many moving parts? Your feet don't just have to support your body weight, they also need to propel it in different directions, sometimes with explosive force. Foot stability is essential to healthy movement.

One training method that delivers great results in this area is barefoot running, which intrinsically trains all the muscles in the foot. Think about that: When was the last time you did strength training for your foot muscles? Those muscles are responsible for supporting all the bones in the foot, and people can develop weak foot muscles from simply wearing supportive shoes all the time. Look at Africa, where more people run without shoes than with them. They develop some of the best runners on the planet. (I'll talk in more detail about barefoot training in a moment.)

Now let's move up the chain. There's a strong connection between foot mechanics and knee position, so when you run, your leg and knee can be affected by how your foot strikes the ground. Some people pronate, which means that their feet roll to the inner side as they strike. Other people supinate, which means that their feet roll to the outer side as they strike. Some fortunate and/or well-trained athletes have a neutral footstrike, which is the healthiest for the rest of your body.

How does this apply to you?

If your foot rolls inward, you put a lot more stress on the inside part of the shin. So shin splints are often

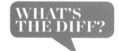

WHAT'S THE DIFF?

Ankle sprain and high ankle sprain

Ankle sprain: An injury to the ligaments in the ankle. The most common sprain comes from "twisting" or "rolling" your ankle.

High ankle sprain: A sprain of the syndesmotic ligaments, which connect the tibia and fibula in the lower leg. It's called a high sprain because it happens above the ankle, in the lower leg, and takes longer to heal.

related to having a foot that rolls inward too much.

Also, the most common knee pain we see in the office, patellar-femoral knee pain (pain under the kneecap), often happens because the foot rolls inward too much. But here's another kinetic chain reaction: This knee pain can also be caused by weak muscles in the hips and pelvis. That's right, you can have a knee injury caused by either your footstrike or your hip strength. The knee has the distinction of being sandwiched between the ground and the hip. That's the kinetic chain in action.

MOVING UP THE CHAIN

Hopefully, you're beginning to make some connections about how your body works. Muscle function is very much related to joint function, and vice versa. The best thing you can do is train your entire body, strengthen all your muscles so your kinetic chain works better. Throughout the book I talk about simple yet incredible bodyweight exercises like burpees, squat thrusts, squat jumps, lunges, and more that you can do at high repetitions and high intensities, and at any age (see the workout chapter). That goes for anyone doing anything, whether you want to run a marathon or win with a local fast-pitch league.

There's more. As we move up the chain, we come to one of the most frequently injured parts of the body, the back. Back pain can be caused by a specific back injury, such as a her-

LET'S TALK ABOUT RICE

RICE is a common acronym in sports medicine that stands for rest, ice, compression, and elevation. The conventional wisdom for a lot of sports injuries, especially strains and sprains, is to rest the body, ice the injured area a few times a day in the first 48 hours, apply compression to prevent swelling (an elastic bandage is a classic example), and elevate the body part above your heart to decrease bloodflow and lessen swelling.

Most of those things work just fine—but not all of them. You won't see me throw the RICE term around in this book. Each injury, to me, has specific treatment needs, and I'll delineate them in each section.

I disagree with total rest, first of all (you'll read about that in a moment). Ice? I love ice. Ice is Mother Nature's antiinflammatory. Compression and elevation work, too, but only on specific injuries (never compress a nerve compression injury, for example).

So when you don't see the term *RICE* in this book, don't automatically think that the treatments must be all wrong. Treatments aren't always as universal as an acronym.

niated disk. But the back muscles are also tied deeply into the kinetic chain, which means that back pain is interrelated with hamstring flexibility, hip flexor tightness, and core strength. The dreaded "back spasms" can be exacerbated by imbalances
in any or all of these areas. If you work to stay strong and flexible in your hammies and hips and you hit your core hard (I love planks for core stability), you'll greatly reduce the compressive forces around the back joints.

When you move upward to the shoulders, you're talking about a ball and socket and the least stable joint in the body. Your shoulder is very susceptible to muscular forces behind and in front of the joint. Ah, but the shoulder is also the joint most susceptible to strengthening. Weak muscles can create a lot of problems for swimmers, rowers, and anyone who plays an "overhead" sport in which your arms and shoulders work hard. Strong

muscles can stabilize the shoulder joint and reduce a host of problems.

Another useful thing to know about joints in the kinetic chain: They alternate for motion and stability.

ANKLE: Motion
KNEE: Stability
HIP: Motion
SPINE: Stability
SHOULDERS: Motion
ELBOWS: Stability
WRIST: Motion
KNUCKLES: Stability

Voilà, just like that you can see what will happen to a knee that is suddenly asked to be a "motion" joint. It just ain't gonna happen and you'll blow it out. Same with the spine—when the spine is straight, a football player can deadlift 500 pounds. But twist that spine the wrong way, ask it to be a motion joint, and you can throw out your back moving a basket of laundry. If you're mindful of how these joints are supposed to work with one another, you can prevent an injury.

Now, with all that in mind, how can you optimize your kinetic chain? You can alter your workout routines in many small but meaningful ways that will "train the chain." Here are some of my favorite techniques.

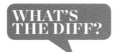

WHAT'S THE DIFF?

Separated shoulder and dislocated shoulder

Separated: A tear in the ligament connecting the collarbone to the shoulder blade. This generally happens when your shoulder takes a direct hit from the side.

Dislocated: The ball at the top of your arm bone pops out of the shoulder socket. This generally happens when you land on your outstretched arm.

10 Ways to Make Your Kinetic Chain Work Better, Achieve Total Body Fitness, and Prevent Injury

1 EXERCISE EVERY DAY.

I'm a big proponent of exercising every day. Not many people are willing to do this. Some say they don't have the time. More accurately, they won't make time. Some say they want to rest their bodies, let themselves recover from the previous day's workout. Well, human bodies are designed for everyday use. Our ancestors, from the caves to the farm fields, got their butts out the door early and sweated all day, every day. We can certainly find 30 minutes to an hour to break a sweat, no? The key is to avoid overuse. How do you do this?

Perform your central, sports-specific training however many times a week you need to in order to achieve your competitive goal. On the other days? Change it up. Think of them as workout vacation days, but instead of lying around, do something for fun. You'll see several terrific yet challenging options in this section. I'm a huge fan of yoga for strength and flexibility, and pilates for core strength. An "off day" is a great time for a class. Some other suggestions: Find a pool. Ride a bike. Play Ultimate Frisbee. Or maybe just get out for a brisk walk with your dog.

I look at daily exercise as a healthy addiction. We have such an obesity problem in this country, and so many obesity-related health issues are treated after they happen as opposed to being prevented in the first place. Hypertension and type 2 diabetes often are preventable with daily exercise. Exercise is medicine, preventive medicine, and it needs to be a daily ritual the same way brushing your teeth is.

My point is, a body that is used sensibly every day grows accustomed to being used and won't be as prone to injury.

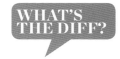

WHAT'S THE DIFF?

Common hernia and sports hernia

Common (inguinal): The lower abdominal wall around the inguinal canal becomes thin and weak enough to allow a bit of an internal organ, usually the large intestine, to poke through.

Sports (or sportsman's): A tearing of abdominal muscle, tendon, and/or fascia where it attaches to the pubic bone in the lower pelvis. It's caused by an abdominal/adductor muscle imbalance and is often mistaken for a chronic groin strain.

NOTE: I should mention actual exercise addiction. There are signals for it in both mind and body. In the mind: Does it dominate your life? Will you be seriously derailed for the day if you don't exercise? In the body: Chronic overuse injuries. These are signs that you're exercising in unhealthy ways and should talk to your doctor about it.

2 FORGET BICEPS AND ABS.

The "vanity muscles" are something of a fitness joke when it comes to athletic performance. Big biceps and defined abs don't do much for you, especially if you work them at the expense of the muscles around them. But if your biceps is trained in concert with your entire arm and shoulder? If your abs are part of a complete, well-conditioned core? Much better. That means forget the biceps curls and the crunches. It's far more important to do whole-body workouts, top to toe.

WHAT'S THE DIFF?

Muscle pull, muscle tear, and muscle cramp

Pull: Slang term for a muscle strain that can be overstretching or a muscle tear.

Tear: A muscle strain that involves a tear of the muscle and/or tendon (this usually occurs in more severe strains, such as grade 2 or 3).

Cramp: A sudden involuntary contraction of a muscle that can be incredibly painful. They're commonly caused by dehydration, a nutrition imbalance such as low sodium, and/or overuse.

Total-body conditioning takes into account your vanity muscles, but also all the supporting muscles that are even more important to having proper kinetic chain function and remaining injury free. The stronger the supporting muscles around each joint are, the less compressive force there is on the joint. Even if you have an arthritic knee, for example, if you strengthen around it, you'll reduce the symptoms.

Here are two fast ways to add total-body training to your regimen. First, whenever possible, add compound movements. Work as many muscles as possible in a single exercise. That means if you do a forward lunge, do it holding a medicine ball and add a core twist. And after that forward lunge? Do a reverse lunge and side lunges as well. Hit all directions.

Second, try individual single-leg exercises. I have people do single-leg squats, single-leg hops, single-leg lunges—things where they use their own body weight but also have to balance. That balancing act is huge. It gets all those small supporting muscles around the joints to fire. Very quickly you'll notice greater strength and stability around your ankles, knees, and hips.

3 DO PLYOMETRICS AND INTERVALS.

I touched on plyometric (explosive bodyweight) exercises previously, and I suggest adding in one or two total-body plyometric and interval (sprint) workouts each week. Neither one requires a gym or any equipment.

Why do this? Muscles have two types of fibers, fast twitch (used for sprinting and explosive movement) and slow twitch (used for longer distance and endurance exercise). Even if you run long distances exclusively or have a passion for endurance events, you still need to maintain a balance between fast- and slow-twitch fibers. This gives you more athletic ability, prevents overuse injuries, and keeps your body from becoming a one-trick pony.

Some examples of plyometric exercises are squat jumps, lunges, skater plyos (which mimic speed skating's side-to-side motion), and compound movements like burpees (from standing, squat, thrust your legs back into the pushup position, do a pushup, return to the squat position, then jump explosively; repeat until you can't walk!).

For intervals, choose a time interval appropriate to your fitness level (anything from 10 seconds on, 20 seconds off to 60 seconds on, 30 seconds off; listen to your body) and apply it to your normal activity, whether it's running, cycling, swimming, etc. For a taste of both, and if you're daring, try a plyometric Tabata workout (see #7, page xxvii).

4 TO STRETCH AND STRENGTHEN, DO YOGA AND PILATES.

Old-school static stretching—meaning that you don't move while you do it, like when you hold a hamstring stretch for 30 seconds—isn't nearly as effective for total-body flexibility as regular yoga and Pilates movements are. These techniques deliver dynamic, movement-based flexibility and can transform your body. Pilates also hammers your core. You'll feel more powerful, movement will be easier and more fluid, and most important, you'll reduce your injury risk.

5 TRY BAREFOOT TRAINING.

I told you how important your feet are when it comes to kinetic chain performance—they're your foundation. If you want to strengthen your feet, try barefoot training. Sound strange? Think about it: Humans haven't used shoes for very long—only a few hundred years.

If you try it, don't go too hard, too fast. Start with walking, and if you can, walk in sand. As your feet become stronger, graduate to running.

This kind of training naturally makes you shorten your stride,

WHAT'S THE DIFF?

Displaced fracture, nondisplaced fracture, and stress fracture

Displaced: The bone breaks into two or more pieces and is out of alignment. This generally requires surgery to repair.

Nondisplaced: The bone cracks part or all the way through but retains its proper alignment. Surgery usually is not necessary.

Stress fracture: The bone swells and cracks from the inside from repetitive use over time, not from a sudden event.

raise your footstrike cadence, and transfer your landing from your heel to your forefoot, all of which help prevent injury. The concept here is that the stronger your foot muscles are, the more you forefoot strike, and the less you heel strike, the less compressive force there is on your ankles, shins, knees, and back. Many injuries I see are caused by improper running form (see the next item). So foot strength and foot muscles have a direct bearing on how you land and how you adapt your natural stride.

The beach is perfect for barefoot training. If no beach is available, your lawn is just fine. Also, shoes now exist that are more like gloves for your feet, designed to give no support so you can build foot strength. These are great if you live in the city and need to work on concrete or asphalt. Another city option: Jog to the nearest park and take off your shoes in the grass. Talk about a nice change from a boring exercise routine!

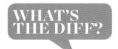

WHAT'S THE DIFF?

Adductor muscle and abductor muscle

Adductor: A muscle used to pull a body part toward the centerline of the body. Your adductor muscles in the inner sides of your thighs allow you to bring your legs together.

Abductor: A muscle used to move a body part away from the centerline of the body. Your abductor muscles in the outer sides of your hips allow you to move your legs away from each other.

6 TEST YOUR BODY FOR A RUNNING IMBALANCE.

Proper running form is important, as I've mentioned. How do you know if you have a muscle imbalance that might be affecting your form? I have runners in my office do a simple step-down test, once for each leg. They step down off a small box or stool and I look straight on at their pelvises. As they descend, the pelvic bones on either side—the bone points you can feel at the front of each hip—should be completely level, like a car's headlights. That means you have good pelvic stability.

Usually what I see when they step down is one hip sagging, the one that's on the weaker side. This result almost always comes from not training the whole body. Patients tell me they go to the gym and do leg extensions and hamstring curls, but those exercises target one muscle apiece and don't support that whole chain of motion. If you do that, you can end up with functional instability, which increases your injury risk. Total-body conditioning can help correct any muscle imbalance.

To do this test at home: Set up a box or stool or anything that lets you step down about 18 inches to 2 feet. Set this up in front of a mirror and slowly step down to the floor. Watch those pelvic bones as you do it, or have someone with a good eye watch them for you. Do the step-down test once for each foot. If one hip sags, add in some single-leg exercises on that side (squats, lunges, hops) to help reestablish balance. Retest yourself every week until you've fixed the imbalance.

7 TRY TABATA INTERVAL TRAINING.

This is a brutal method of interval training developed in Japan, and it's not for the faint of heart. It's pretty simple: Whatever your activity, sprint for 20 seconds, rest for 10, and repeat for eight sets. That's 4 minutes. I promise you, if you go full bore on each sprint, this will be one of the most difficult workouts you'll ever do. Try it after one of your regular workouts, or only after your body is warmed up and prepared for maximum effort. Do this once a week and you'll soon feel a difference in your performance, and your body will be in better condition and less susceptible to injury.

IMPORTANT: Whatever activity you do for Tabata training, *never sacrifice form*. The point is to work out safely and effectively. The second your form breaks down, you increase your chance of injury, so back off immediately. Build slowly. Be smart.

8 GET A COACH.

All of the suggestions I've presented so far will deliver better results if you have someone coach you. This could be a trainer, a sport-specific coach, a class instructor, anyone who has a legitimate base of knowledge about the area you want to improve in. A coach can not only help shape your activities, but also monitor your form, help you break bad habits, and motivate you. Anyone who's ever exercised knows how vital that can be.

9 SLEEP.

This is a huge blind spot for so many people, but sleep is the most important activity of your day, no joke, especially if you're training hard or exercising every day. Sleep is the only time your body has to regenerate itself, rebuilding muscle, strengthening bone, restocking red blood cells, and engaging in any number of other crucial processes that need time to take place. Not to mention REM sleep's importance in restoring your brain and helping you feel like a million bucks in the morning rather than a crumpled-up five-spot. Lack of sleep is tied to higher blood pressure, weight gain, elevated stress hormone levels, and other things that will detract from not just your athletic performance, but also your general health.

10 SMILE.

Some of you just did a double take on that one. Smile? Yeah, have a good time. Exercise, especially when you're training for a specific goal, can be such a dead-serious stretch of time. We forget that it's supposed to be fun. Get out there with some friends. Be intense if it ups your game, but at least enjoy the intensity. Exercise should be the most fun part of your day. Period.

What If You Still Get Hurt?

And you will. Even for the most diligent user, injury-prevention techniques aren't foolproof. Every active person has aches and pains and things worse than that. And I hate to say it, but simple bad luck stalks us all. When pain strikes, this book will help you figure out what's wrong, what you can do to alleviate your problem using home-based remedies, and when to see a doctor. But before we start talking about maladies and remedies, there's one more piece of advice I need to give you.

It's the most important advice in the book, in my opinion.

If you get hurt...***KEEP MOVING!***

What does that mean?

An injury does not grant you a vacation from fitness or exercise. You must continue to work out even if you need to rest another body part so it can heal. There are specific reasons for this, reasons that I've learned firsthand in my experience as a doctor and an athlete. There are also smart ways you can keep exercising without aggravating the body part that's hurt.

But first, the why:

There are several good reasons, but the first is based in science. More and more, doctors are moving away from the rest recommendation and encouraging injured patients to engage in physical activity. I'm one of them. Take osteoarthritis, for example, the most common form of arthritis that affects almost everyone over the age of 60. Usually when a patient had a flare-up, the prescription was rest and medication. Now studies have shown that weight loss combined with exercises that build up muscle to help support and improve joint function boosts patients' quality of life better than medication alone. Increased strength around an injured joint gives support to that joint. Regular activity helps replenish lubrication in the joint. As I said before: You can control pain with strength.

There's more.

Remember how I blew out my knee in med school? It kept me sidelined for a long time. And I'd never been sidelined before. I believe that the feel-good neurotransmitters secreted during exercise, like serotonin and dopamine, are very much like drugs, and exercise is one of our healthiest drugs. So when it's taken away, it can be clinically depressing for people. That's exactly how I felt when I hurt my knee and couldn't exercise.

That's why I believe, as a doctor and an athlete, that when you're hurt, total rest and "staying off it" are not just unwise, they're medically unhealthy.

Think about it: What happens when you can't do any physical activity?

• YOU'RE BORED. Your mind drifts into negativity. The research showing a positive mind-body connection through exercise is undeniable, so much so that exercise is often referred to as a natural antidepressant. I've noticed myself that young athletes in school have poorer academic performance when they're injured. More time on your hands isn't always a good thing.

• YOU NO LONGER GET YOUR REGULAR DOSE OF THE FEEL-GOOD NEUROTRANSMITTERS. Besides the pain of the injury, you simply don't feel as good as you normally do.

• YOUR BODY ATROPHIES. And not just your kinetic chain. The heart is a muscle, and like any other muscle, if you take 4 weeks off to rest, that muscle atrophies and your cardiovascular condition deteriorates. You'll have a lot of work to do to get back to where you were (hence the old maxim "It's easier to stay in shape than to get in shape").

• DEPRESSION SETS IN. I've felt it. I had surgery to fix the ACL, and aside from it being a painful experience that I hope is never repeated, the more than 6 months of rehab and only gradually being able to get back to the sports I loved was mental torture.

It was also enlightening.

You need to keep moving to fight all those negatives I just described. If you do, you'll keep some of your conditioning. You'll get your dose of neurotransmitters. You'll feel better. You'll be more positive. And you'll learn that no injury is the end of the world.

So, How Do You Exercise While Injured?

You do what I call dynamic rest. That means two things.

One, rest and rehab. Lay off the injured body part and do what you need to do to get it back to health. That could mean using specific remedies in this book or following something prescribed by a doctor you've seen, like targeted physical therapy or exercises.

And two, be dynamic, stay in motion as all this rest and rehab goes on. That's the trick. Here's how:

• FIND AN ACTIVITY THAT DOESN'T INTERACT WITH THE INJURY YOU HAVE. If you sprain your ankle, for example, do something that doesn't load your ankle. Hit the pool. Hit the upper-body weight training hard. Bad knee? Same concept. Whatever your injury, find its opposite counterpart and work it. Bad shoulder or elbow?

Run and do lower-body plyometrics. And here's a big one: Bad back? Simply move. Walk. Shuffle if you have to. Resting a bad back only deconditions the muscles and makes your back weaker. No matter what body part hurts, find something that doesn't aggravate it, and do not do "complete rest."

• GO HARD. Whatever your alternate activity is, up the intensity. This will get your heart pounding and your lungs heaving and keep your cardiovascular system in shape. Heck, it might even improve it. It'll also release those giddy neurotransmitters and you'll be the happiest hurt person on earth.

As you can see, injuries can hurt you, but they don't have to halt you. Knowledge is your best friend. And when it comes to treating injuries, there's a lot of half-baked information out there. The rest of the book is designed to deliver the good stuff, the accurate, medically sound, time-proven ways to help you heal and get you back to doing what you love most.

Exercise is one of the most important things we have for pursuing lifelong health and happiness. It's real preventive medicine. It doesn't just make you feel good. It keeps you from feeling bad. Don't let anyone or anything take that away from you.

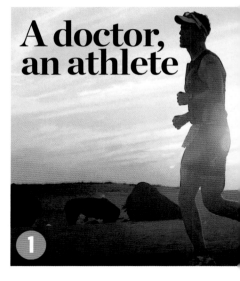

A doctor, an athlete

CLOCKWISE: 1 Mile 18 of the Hawaiian Ironman, feeling alive and on the brink at the same time. **2** Biking the Hawaiian lava fields at 130 degrees Fahrenheit. **3** If I'm ever having a tough day, I look at this pic. **4** With my brother Jamie after finishing the Hawaiian Ironman. **5** Strength-training class in Times Square!

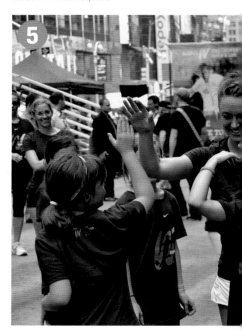

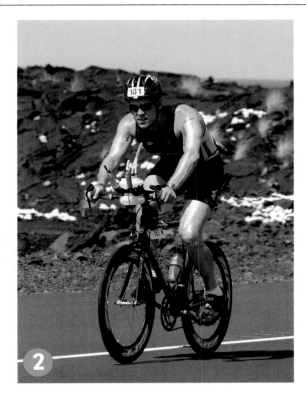

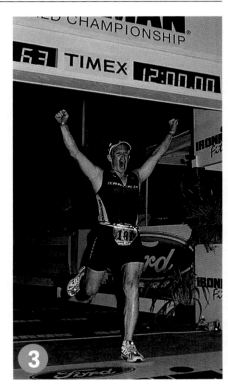

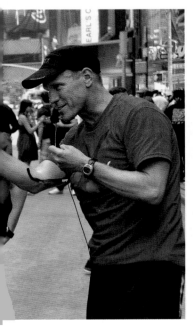

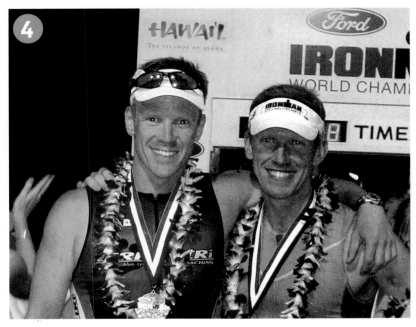

PART ONE
TELL ME WHERE IT HURTS

Here's your go-to guide to sports injuries. Each entry in this section is packed with information: key symptoms, a breakdown of how and why the injury occurs, as well as who has the highest risk. I'll also give you detailed instructions on how to treat the injury on your own and, just as important, how to prevent it in the first place. Understand, however, that no matter how good you think you are at self-diagnosis and self-care, there are definitely times when you need to see a professional for your problem. I cover that, too. The "When to Call a Doctor" section in each injury entry will give you the facts on making that all-important appointment and what to expect. Good luck, athletes, and get well soon!

FEET
ANKLES &
LOWER
LEGS

They're the foundation of virtually all athletic movement. Which is why it's so easy to hurt them—they're made up of lots of bones, muscles, and connective tissues, all of them concentrated in a small area and asked to withstand many times your weight in explosive force. And when one of them is hurt, it can literally take you off your feet. Let's not play that game. Let's get you back out there.

An anatomy lesson:
FEET, ANKLES & LOWER LEGS

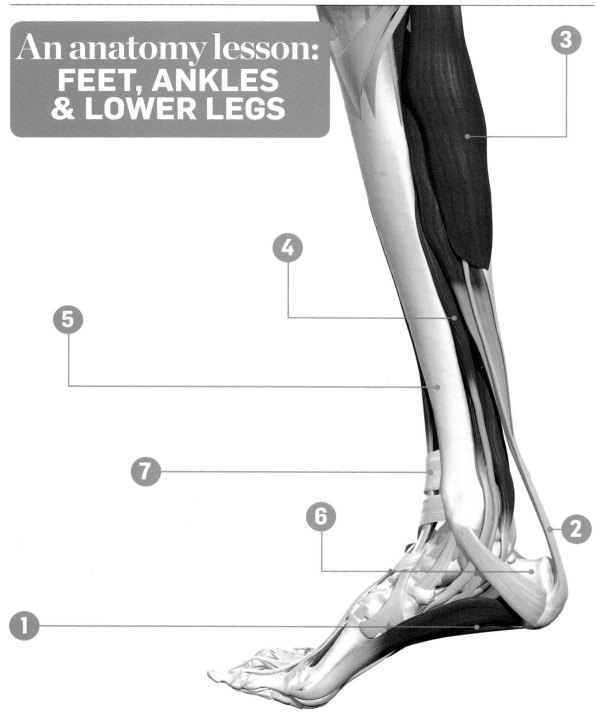

PLANTAR FASCIA

A tough, fibrous band of tissue running along the bottom of the foot from the calcaneus (6) to the toes. Fascia can be found around and in muscles and nerves throughout the body, and when it becomes tight or inflexible, it can cause pain and injuries.

ACHILLES TENDON

A.k.a., the calcaneal tendon. A long, thick tendon running down the back of the lower leg that attaches the gastrocnemius and soleus to the calcaneal. It's named after the Greek hero Achilles, whose only vulnerable point was the back of his heel.

GASTROCNEMIUS

The larger of two calf muscles (with the soleus), and the one closest to the surface of the skin. This muscle attaches to the femur above the knee, and to the calcaneus via the Achilles tendon. The primary duty of both calf muscles is to extend your ankle, though the gastrocnemius takes on a greater workload when the knee is straight.

SOLEUS

The smaller of two calf muscles (with the gastrocnemius). This muscle attaches below the knee and to the calcaneus via the Achilles tendon. The primary duty of both calf muscles is to extend your ankle, though the soleus takes on a greater workload when the knee is bent.

TIBIA

The larger of the two lower leg bones (with the fibula), commonly referred to as the shin bone. It connects the knee to the ankle. This bone is affected in a vast majority of shin splint cases, either through a stress injury that irritates the bone, or a stress fracture.

CALCANEUS

The heel bone. The Achilles tendon attaches to the upper side of this bone. The calcaneal tuberosity, near the posterior of the heel, is where the plantar fascia connects to the rear of the foot.

SYNDESMOTIC LIGAMENT

A large ligament that connects the tibia and fibula just above the ankle. This ligament is most commonly injured in a "high ankle sprain," usually when the foot is inverted and twisted.

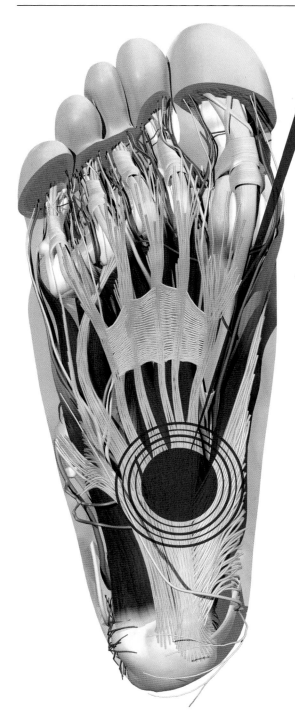

THE MALADY:
Plantar Fasciitis

THE SYMPTOMS

Nasty pain in the bottom of the foot, especially when running or even taking your first steps out of bed in the morning.

WHAT'S GOING ON IN THERE?

Plantar fasciitis is inflammation of the plantar fascia (plantar means the bottom of the foot, and its fascia is the band of connective tissue running from your heel bone to the front of your foot). This tissue helps support your foot's arch and give it shape, and it aids in stability when your foot strikes the ground and then pushes off.

The injury to the fascia usually begins where the fascia connects to the bony bump on the bottom of the heel called the calcaneal tuberosity, one of the most fun anatomical terms. The inflammation and pain come from excessive tension. The muscles above and the shape of the foot below contribute to its development. The calf muscles (specifically, the gastrocnemius and soleus) connect to the heel bone via the Achilles tendon. When those muscles are tight, the tendon pulls on the bone from above, stretching the fascia and causing strain. People with high arches are especially prone to plantar fasciitis because the arch itself also contributes tension to the fascia.

A mild case can turn major very quickly. Inflammation makes the fascia more prone to microtears, which can lead to debilitating pain. In other words, you can't walk, let alone exercise.

Bad cases can last months. My youngest brother was once sidelined for 10 months by plantar fasciitis, and I see many patients with similar stories.

FIX IT

- **Employ dynamic rest.** Take a break from the offending activity. The earlier you address plantar fasciitis, the better. How long you need to rest depends on the severity of the case, but expect to be sidelined for at least a couple of weeks. Stick with intense upper-body activity that doesn't load your foot. Does that stink? Sure. But it beats crippling yourself!

- **Stretch.** Use the stretches described in "Prevent It." Be gentle. Go slow. You're trying to relieve the tightness in the area, not prepare for a game or race. As the injury heals, adopt the stretching habit permanently.

- **Try an NSAID.** An antiinflammatory like ibuprofen or naproxen can help reduce pain and inflammation.

- **Consider night splints.** Foot splints are available (usually from $20 to $60) and can help if worn at night. It's best to have a doctor recommend the best one for your case, as there are several varieties. See "When to Call a Doctor."

- **Ease yourself back into the game.** Don't restart strenuous lower-body activity until you're pain free. If you mess around with this, you'll simply aggravate the injury and be out even longer.

PREVENT IT

- **Stay flexible.** The best way to stretch this area is to put your toes and the ball of your foot against the top of the vertical edge of a step with your heel on the floor and slowly lean forward, keeping your leg straight, until you feel the stretch at the top of your calf. Repeat the stretch with your knee bent, feeling the stretch farther down the leg near the Achilles tendon. Hold each stretch for 15 to 20 seconds and repeat several times in each position. Ideally, you'll do this daily, before and after exercise.

- **Roll it.** This is a simple preventive measure you can do anywhere, even sitting at your desk at work. Roll a tennis ball back and forth under each foot for a few minutes a day. The ball massages and loosens the fascia.

- **Try orthotics.** Over-the-counter (OTC) hard arch supports can be helpful, especially for you high-arched folks. Prescription orthotics are another option because they're custom-made for your foot, but I suggest trying the (much cheaper) OTC orthotics first because in my practice, about 90 percent of patients have good results with them. If they don't work, then see a podiatrist for a custom set.

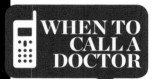

WHEN TO CALL A DOCTOR

If symptoms don't improve in about 2 weeks, make an appointment.

The doctor will probably have you do the home remedies listed here, as well as more aggressive treatments depending on the severity of the condition. These include a foot splint worn at night, a pair of sandals with big arches kept next to the bed for those first steps in the morning (which can reaggravate the injury before it heals completely), physical therapy, and corticosteroid injections to ease inflammation.

Another potential therapy involves platelet-rich plasma (PRP). It's new, but a lot of pro athletes have used it and gotten results. In areas of the body that don't have great blood supply, healing is slow. The doctor injects your own platelet-rich plasma into the injured area to promote faster healing. The upside is that it works for most people. The downside is that it's generally not covered by insurance. But if you can't get results from any other therapy, it doesn't hurt to investigate it.

DO YOU NEED SURGERY?

Not likely. Surgery is only required in extreme cases that don't respond to normal treatment.

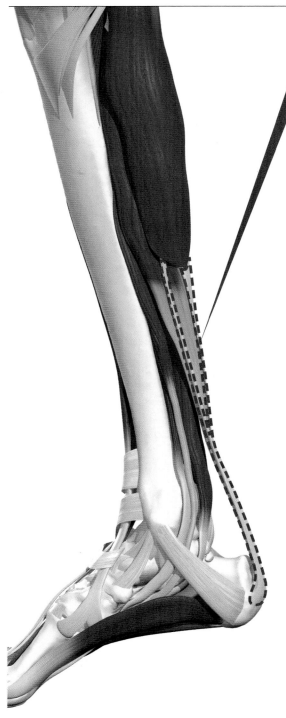

THE MALADY:
Achilles Tendinitis

THE SYMPTOMS
Pain in the back of the heel, the tendon just above it, or possibly up to where the calf muscles form a V on the back of the leg. The pain can be mild to debilitating.

WHAT'S GOING ON IN THERE?
The Achilles tendon, named for the legendary Greek warrior whose only vulnerability was his heel, is a thick, ropelike tendon about 4 inches long connecting the gastrocnemius and soleus muscles in the lower leg to their insertion points at the heel bone (calcaneus).

Achilles injuries can occur in several places. Occasionally they occur higher up in the muscle, in which case they're referred to as calf strains (see page 20). These injuries tend to heal quickly due to the abundant bloodflow to the muscle.

A more common injury location is the muscle-tendon junction, where the muscles converge into the tendon. This spot is about halfway down the back of the lower leg, where the muscles form a V. These injuries tend to heal spontaneously, but not as quickly as in the muscular area because the bloodflow isn't as generous.

The most serious Achilles injury is to the tendon itself. Inflammation of the tendon, called tendinitis, and chronic inflammation with fluid buildup, called tendinosis, are the most common of this type.

FIX IT

- **Employ dynamic rest.** With Achilles injuries, in general, swimming is fine and biking can work, but only if it's pain free. Running is a huge no-no and will make the injury worse.

- **Ice it.** Applying ice to the area for 15 minutes 4 to 6 times a day can help reduce inflammation and swelling.

- **Stretch it.** I don't advocate stretching if it brings pain. Once you can do so without pain, do the classic runner's stretch with your hands against a wall (see below).

- **Strengthen it.** A tendon like the Achilles starts to hurt because of the load on it. If you want to reduce the loading force, build up the muscles affecting that load so they can take the brunt of it. Once you're pain free, recondition your lower body. Start with eccentric calf raises: Stand with your heels hanging off a step, take 10 seconds to lower them, then raise them back up at a normal rate. Also add in plenty of plyometric lower-body work like squats, multidirectional lunges, squat thrusts, and so on (see next page for more info).

STRAIGHT-LEG CALF STRETCH

Stand about 2 feet in front of a wall in a staggered stance, right foot in front of your left. Place your hands on the wall and lean against it. Shift your weight to your back foot until you feel a stretch in your calf. Hold this stretch for 30 seconds on each side, then repeat twice for a total of three sets. Perform this routine daily, and up to 3 times a day if you're really tight.

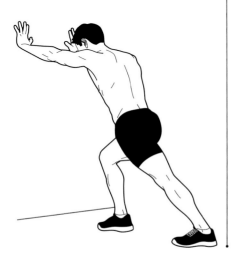

BENT-LEG CALF STRETCH

Perform this the same as the straight-leg calf stretch, only move your back foot forward so the toes of that foot are even with the heel of your front foot. Keeping your heels down, bend both knees until you feel a comfortable stretch just above the ankle of your back leg. Hold this stretch for 30 seconds on each side, then repeat twice for a total of three sets. Perform this routine daily, and up to 3 times a day if you're really tight.

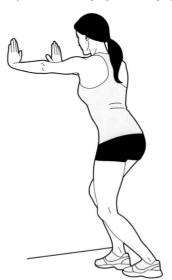

Cont'd on page 10

WHEN TO CALL A DOCTOR

A day or two of Achilles discomfort is fine, but pain that lasts for more than several days or, more important, results in limping or an altered gait needs to be checked out.

The prescription is generally suspension of the activity that caused the injury (running, usually). You may end up in a walking boot until you're pain free and can begin rehabilitation. In rehab, a therapist or athletic trainer will use ultrasounds, electrical-stimulation sessions, ice, and, eventually, a combination of stretching and strengthening to fix the problem.

DO YOU NEED SURGERY?

For general Achilles pain, no. But if persistent Achilles pain isn't given proper attention, tendinitis or tendinosis can lead to a degenerative tear in the tendon, often characterized as a lump on the side of the tendon. When this is present, there is risk of either chronic, career-threatening (your athletic career, that is) Achilles pain or Achilles tendon rupture. That's bad. Very, very bad. Don't let it get that far.

PREVENT IT

The best way to prevent Achilles tendinitis in the first place is by building limber lower legs. An underlying lack of flexibility, especially in your calf muscles, can be a primary cause of Achilles injuries. You can increase overall dynamic flexibility by using the Iron Strength workout section of this book (see page 256). But even if you don't use those specific workouts, the stretches and exercises here all target your lower leg and can be added to any workout.

SPLIT JUMP (WITH OR WITHOUT DUMBBELLS)

Stand in a staggered stance, your right foot in front of your left. Lower your body as far as you can. Quickly switch directions and jump with enough force to propel both feet off the floor. While in the air, scissor-kick your legs so you land with the opposite leg forward. Repeat, alternating back and forth with each repetition.

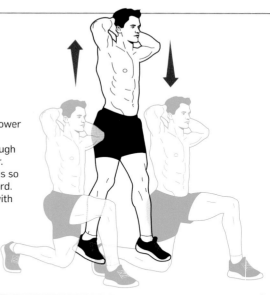

SINGLE-LEG STANDING DUMBBELL CALF RAISE

Grab a dumbbell in your right hand and stand on a step, block, or 25-pound weight plate. Cross your left foot behind your right ankle and balance yourself on the ball of your right foot, with your right heel on the floor or hanging off a step. Put your left hand on something stable—a wall or weight rack, for instance.

Lift your right heel as high as you can. Pause, then lower and repeat. Complete the prescribed number of reps with your right leg, then do the same number with your left (holding the dumbbell in your left hand).

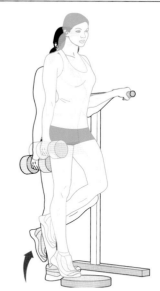

HOW YOUR CALF MUSCLES WORK

A pair of muscles, the soleus and gastrocnemius, make up your calf. Your soleus is more involved in extending your ankle when your knee is bent. Your gastrocnemius takes on a greater workload when your knee is straight. That means that bent-leg stretches and calf raises target your soleus, while standing calf raises and straight-leg stretches zero in on your gastrocnemius. To get the muscle growth and total flexibility you want, do both versions.

TWO ACHILLES-FRIENDLY TRAINING TIPS

Watch your foot mechanics.

Pronation (when the foot rolls inward as you walk or run) can contribute to Achilles injuries. Motion-control shoes and/or over-the-counter arch supports can help correct the problem.

Shorten your running stride.

Doing this while increasing your footstrike cadence may help you generate better stride mechanics because you'll be putting a lot less load on your feet, shins and knees. While running, count how many times your right foot strikes in 60 seconds. Shoot for 85 to 90 per minute.

THE EASY WAY TO STRONG LEGS

You don't need heavy weights to build powerful legs. Simple bodyweight exercises like squats, squat jumps, multidirectional lunges, mountain climbers, and skater plyos (which mimic the side-to-side motion of a speed skater) are all effective muscle builders.

SINGLE-LEG BENT-KNEE CALF RAISE

Using the same directions as the single-leg standing dumbbell calf raise, bend your knee and hold it that way as you perform the exercise.

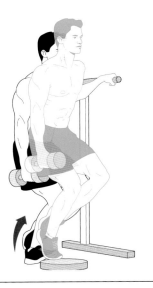

FARMER'S WALK ON TOES

Grab a pair of heavy dumbbells and hold them at your sides at arm's length. Raise your heels and walk forward (or in a circle) for 60 seconds. Be sure to stand as tall as you can and stick your chest out.

Choose the heaviest pair of dumbbells that allows you to perform the exercise without breaking form for 60 seconds.

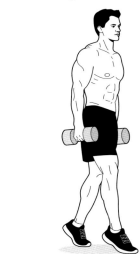

CALF ROLL

Place a foam roller under your right ankle, with your right leg straight. Cross your left leg over your right ankle. Put your hands flat on the floor for support and keep your back naturally arched.

Roll your body forward until the roller reaches the back of your right knee. Then roll back and forth. Repeat with the roller under your left calf. (If this is too hard, perform the movement with both legs on the roller.)

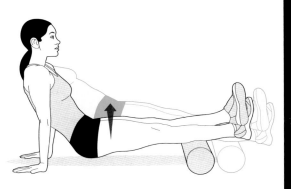

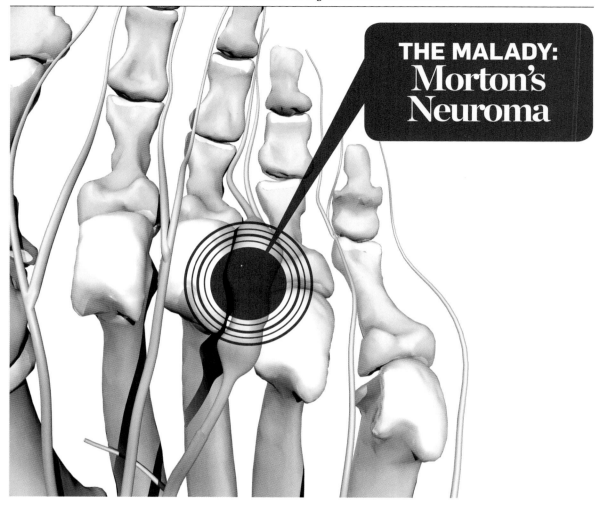

THE MALADY: Morton's Neuroma

THE SYMPTOMS

Burning pain in the forefoot that radiates into the toes and initially is worse during running, but eventually may occur when walking or at rest.

WHAT'S GOING ON IN THERE?

Morton's neuroma is a fibrous enlargement of the plantar nerve where it passes beneath the transverse metatarsal ligament. That's fancy doctor-speak saying that an important nerve in your forefoot is rubbing against a ligament and doesn't like it one bit.

Compression—usually from tight shoes—is the main cause of the problem because it comes from the nerve repeatedly being pressed against that ligament, which leads to inflammation. Running can worsen the condition once it starts.

Women are more susceptible to this problem because in addition to athletic shoes, high heels and other shoes that constrict the toes can exacerbate or accelerate a mild problem.

You can first try to ease or eliminate the symptoms with the home-based suggestions here, but understand that this will not fix the condition. It will only bring relief and delay further progression.

Morton's neuroma is not dangerous, but it can be extremely uncomfortable. Treatment can be delayed as long as the symptoms aren't too severe. However, some form of treatment will eventually be required to return to normal athletic performance.

FIX IT

- **Try an NSAID.** An antiinflammatory like ibuprofen or naproxen can help alleviate inflammation in the foot.

- **Change your shoes.** Switching both athletic and everyday shoes to pairs with larger toe boxes can help relieve pressure on the affected area.

- **If these suggestions don't help, see your doctor.** See "When to Call a Doctor."

PREVENT IT

- **Wear proper shoes.** A well-fitting shoe that doesn't compress the fore-foot and toes can help.

- **Women, wear high heels and toe-compressing shoes only when necessary.**

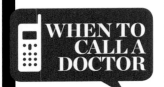

WHEN TO CALL A DOCTOR

If these home-based remedies don't help, see your doctor. If Morton's neuroma is diagnosed, the initial treatment is to identify the neuroma with an ultrasound and then inject cortisone directly into it to shrink it. If effective, this treatment relieves the pain and patients don't need surgery.

DO YOU NEED SURGERY?

Very doubtful. Surgery used to be more common for Morton's neuroma, but it's become rare because the therapies just discussed are so effective. If they're ineffective, however, surgery is the last resort. The surgical approach to the neuroma may be from the top of the foot or the bottom. Surgery can remove a neuroma but carries some risk of problems down the line because of subsequent forefoot instability.

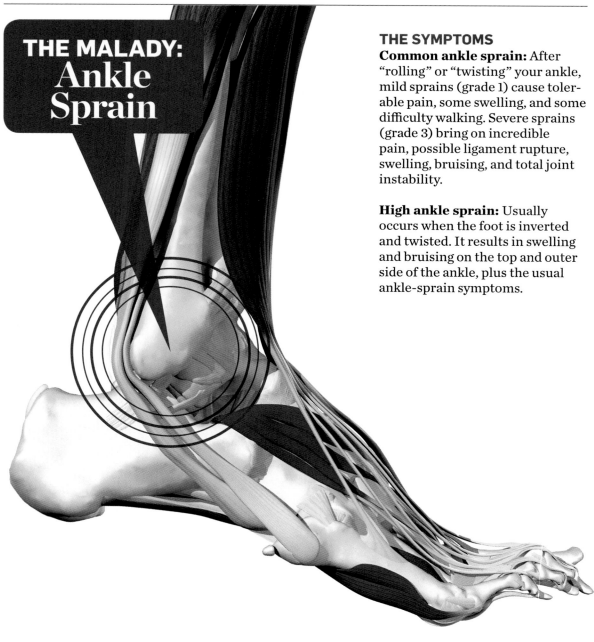

THE MALADY:
Ankle Sprain

THE SYMPTOMS

Common ankle sprain: After "rolling" or "twisting" your ankle, mild sprains (grade 1) cause tolerable pain, some swelling, and some difficulty walking. Severe sprains (grade 3) bring on incredible pain, possible ligament rupture, swelling, bruising, and total joint instability.

High ankle sprain: Usually occurs when the foot is inverted and twisted. It results in swelling and bruising on the top and outer side of the ankle, plus the usual ankle-sprain symptoms.

WHAT'S GOING ON IN THERE?

Everyone twists an ankle at some point. The question is, how badly. The most common variety is a lateral (or inversion) sprain, where the foot rolls outward, injuring the ligaments on the outer side of the ankle. The rarer medial ligament sprain is the opposite, with the foot rolling inward and injuring ligaments on the inner side of the ankle.

With your basic lateral sprain, the most commonly injured ligament is the talofibular, which connects the anklebone (talus) to the smaller calf bone (fibula). More severe sprains might also involve the calcaneofibular ligament, which connects the fibula to the heel (calcaneus).

As with all sprains, there are three grades. Grades 1 and 2 involve varying degrees of over-stretching or partial tearing of one or more ligaments. A grade 3 sprain is a complete tear (rupture) of one or more ligaments.

A high ankle sprain is different from a common ankle sprain. It usually occurs when the foot inverts (points downward) and twists, causing a stretch of the syndesmotic ligaments, which connect the tibia and fibula in the lower leg to the top of your foot. It's called a high sprain because it happens above the ankle, in the lower leg.

WHEN TO CALL A DOCTOR

If pain and swelling are severe, see a doctor to gauge how bad the damage is. Many things can go along with an ankle sprain—there are a lot of moving parts in the foot—including damage to the tendons, cartilage, and bones of the foot. Fractures are common, including avulsion fractures, which occur where ligaments or tendons attach to bone.

Severe ankle injuries can include full tears (ruptures) of the talofibular and other ligaments, as well as dislocation of the ankle.

DO YOU NEED SURGERY?

For typical ankle sprains, no. But if it's a bad sprain, only a doctor can answer that question. A pro needs to assess how bad your case is and what will be required to fix it (surgery, rehab, etc.).

FIX IT

- **Apply first aid.** For any sprain, ice and elevation for the swelling will help (don't ice an ankle for more than 15 minutes at a time). For anything above a grade 1 sprain, crutches are a good idea. As the sprain heals, compression with, for example, an elastic bandage can help with internal bleeding and swelling.

- **Employ dynamic rest.** Stay fit with upper-body work. Depending on the severity of your sprain, you could try swimming or running in a pool.

- **Try an NSAID.** An antiinflammatory like ibuprofen or naproxen can help with pain and inflammation.

- **Move it.** For simple sprains, as the pain becomes tolerable, perform basic range-of-motion exercises. During the first week, do only the following: Pull the foot upward, then point it away. Any side-to-side or rotating movement could aggravate the injured ligaments. After a week, add in rotation. With your ankle elevated, do ankle circles in one direction, then the other. Go slow at first if the injury is still painful, but up the speed and reps as the injury heals. This will help you get back the full range of motion.

- **Stay flexible.** Do some simple calf stretches, because these muscles tend to tighten up to inhibit ankle movement after an injury. You don't want to strain your calf as you get back to your normal activities.

Cont'd on page 16

PREVENT IT

No one can totally prevent an ankle sprain, but you can do certain stretches and exercises to improve ankle stability and your overall balance—which lowers your injury chances. This is especially important if you've sprained your ankle before. One of the best ways to do this is to improve strength and flexibility in your calves, as tight soleus and gastrocnemius muscles limit ankle motion. You can increase overall dynamic flexibility by using the Iron Strength workout section of this book (see page 256). But even if you don't use those specific workouts, the stretches and exercises here all target your lower leg and can be added to any workout.

CALF ROLL

Place a foam roller under your right ankle, with your right leg straight. Cross your left leg over your right ankle. Put your hands flat on the floor for support and keep your back naturally arched.

Roll your body forward until the roller reaches the back of your right knee. Then roll back and forth. Repeat with the roller under your left calf. (If this is too hard, perform the movement with both legs on the roller.)

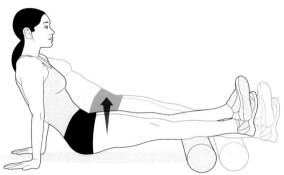

STRAIGHT-LEG CALF STRETCH

Stand about 2 feet in front of a wall in a staggered stance, right foot in front of your left. Place your hands on the wall and lean against it. Shift your weight to your back foot until you feel a stretch in your calf. Hold this stretch for 30 seconds on each side, then repeat twice for a total of three sets. Perform this routine daily, and up to 3 times a day if you're really tight.

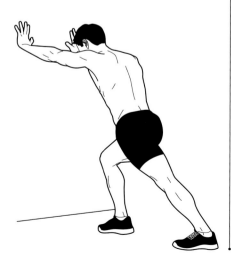

BENT-LEG CALF STRETCH

Perform this the same as the straight-leg calf stretch, only move your back foot forward so the toes of that foot are even with the heel of your front foot. Keeping your heels down, bend both knees until you feel a comfortable stretch just above the ankle of your back leg. Hold this stretch for 30 seconds on each side, then repeat twice for a total of three sets. Perform this routine daily, and up to 3 times a day if you're really tight.

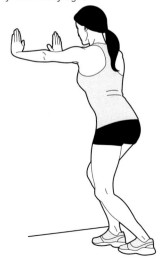

IMPROVE ANKLE STABILITY? EASY!

Simply balance on one foot. Add in complicating factors such as arm movement, twisting, and bending the knee. Also try it with your eyes closed. This is the most basic way to functionally work your ankle. (Be sure to work both sides equally to prevent imbalance.)

ISO-EXPLOSIVE BODYWEIGHT JUMP SQUATS

Place your fingers on the back of your head and pull your elbows back so that they're in line with your body. Perform a bodyweight squat until your thighs are parallel to the floor, then explosively jump as high as you can (imagine you're pushing the floor away from you as you leap). When you land, immediately squat and jump again. Hold dumbbells at your side to make it more challenging.

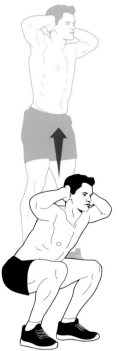

LUNGE (BODYWEIGHT OR WITH DUMBBELLS)

Stand tall with your feet hip-width apart. Brace your core and hold it that way for the entire exercise. Step forward with your right leg and slowly lower your body until your front knee is bent at least 90 degrees and your rear knee nearly touches the floor. Pause, then push yourself to the starting position as quickly as you can. Complete the prescribed number of repetitions, then do the same number with your left leg.

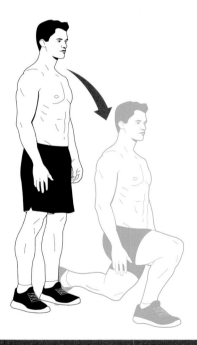

THE ZIGZAG SECRET

For better ankle mobility and stability, change direction. Add interval training with direction changes. Run figure-8 drills, use cones for obstacle runs, or even draw obstacles on a driveway with chalk. The point is to challenge your lower legs and ankles in ways you normally don't to add strength and flexibility.

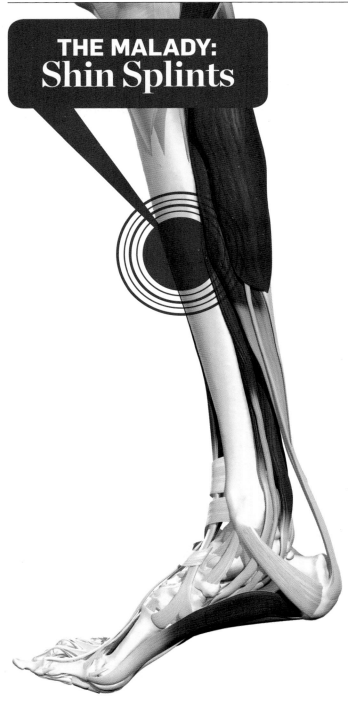

THE MALADY:
Shin Splints

THE SYMPTOMS

More common (roughly 90 percent of cases): Pain in the bony part of the shin, along the tibia, during and after exercise and when you press on the area.

Less common (about 10 percent of cases): A tightening pain in the soft, outside, muscular part of the shin. The pain is usually bad enough that running becomes impossible, and then it subsides when you stop running.

WHAT'S GOING ON IN THERE?

Shin splints have derailed many an athlete's hard-won training gains. They're among the most frustrating injuries because they make a basic act—running—impossible. But the term *shin splints* actually denotes more than one lower-leg ailment.

Bone-related shin pain, called medial tibial stress syndrome, can cover a broad spectrum of ailments, ranging from a stress injury—irritation of the bone—to a stress fracture, an actual crack in the bone. The area hurts during and especially after exercise, and the tibia hurts when touched or tapped.

Bone-related shin pain is more common than muscular shin pain (by about nine to one); the bone actually swells and, if irritated for long enough, a stress fracture can occur. It's generally the result of three variables: body mechanics, amount of activity, and bone density. Body mechanics include foot type, footstrike, and how your body is built. Activity can cause it if you up your training workload too soon. Bone density can be a bigger factor for women (see "When to Call a Doctor"). All three of these variables can be altered or compensated for to help alleviate the problem.

The less common muscular symptoms just mentioned usually signal exertional compartment syndrome (ECS). ECS can occur in any part of the lower leg and is characterized by a tightening in the shin that worsens during exercise. Patients often report that their legs feel so tight that they might explode. Eighty percent of ECS cases happen in the front part of the shin. The leg is pain free except during activity.

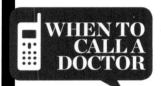

WHEN TO CALL A DOCTOR

For bone-related pain, it's best to get a doctor's diagnosis because then you'll know the severity of the injury. You'll need an MRI to determine if a stress fracture is present, because stress fractures don't show up on x-rays unless they're very severe or healing. Your doctor may also do a bone-density scan (using DEXA, dual-energy x-ray absorptiometry).

FIX IT

BONE RELATED:

- **See a doctor for a proper diagnosis.** Stress injuries can become stress fractures, which can sideline you for a long time.

- **Employ dynamic rest.** Find another activity that doesn't load your legs. Swimming and stationary biking are good choices.

MUSCULAR:

- **Foam roll it.** Part of the problem with ECS is tight fascia, the tough material that wraps most of our muscles. Run your shins and calves over a foam roller for several minutes several times a day to help loosen the fascia. Manual massage can help as well.

- **Try arch supports and motion-control shoes.** These can help correct biomechanical problems in the feet and take the stress off the affected muscles.

- **If these measures don't help, see a doctor.**

DO YOU NEED SURGERY?

Almost never. Conservative measures almost always cure bone-related shin splints. In rare cases where the bone is cracked, a rod could be installed. Also, for muscular pain, if foam rolling, massage, and footwear adjustments don't help, your doctor can test for exertional compartment syndrome by using a needle to measure the pressure inside the leg before and after exercise. When the pressure difference is high and other treatments don't work, a surgical procedure called a fasciotomy can be performed to open the fascia and give it room to expand. This procedure is rarely performed and requires 1 to 2 months of recovery.

PREVENT IT

BONE RELATED:

- **Change your shoes.** Try switching to a shoe that limits pronation. Arch supports can help as well.

- **Up your calcium and vitamin D intakes.** Try 1,300 milligrams of calcium and 400 micrograms of D per day. Easy food sources are milk and yogurt.

- **Follow the 10 percent rule.** Runners, never up your weekly mileage by more than 10 percent.

- **Train your hips and core.** Strengthening these areas will make you a stronger runner, which improves footstrike and body mechanics.

- **Shorten your running stride.** Doing this while increasing your footstrike cadence may help you generate better stride mechanics because you'll be putting a lot less load on your feet, shins, knees, and on up the kinetic chain. Count your footstrikes on one side for 1 minute. A good number is 85 to 90 strikes of one foot per minute.

MUSCULAR:

- **Foam roll and massage.** See above.

- **Try arch supports and motion-control shoes.** See above.

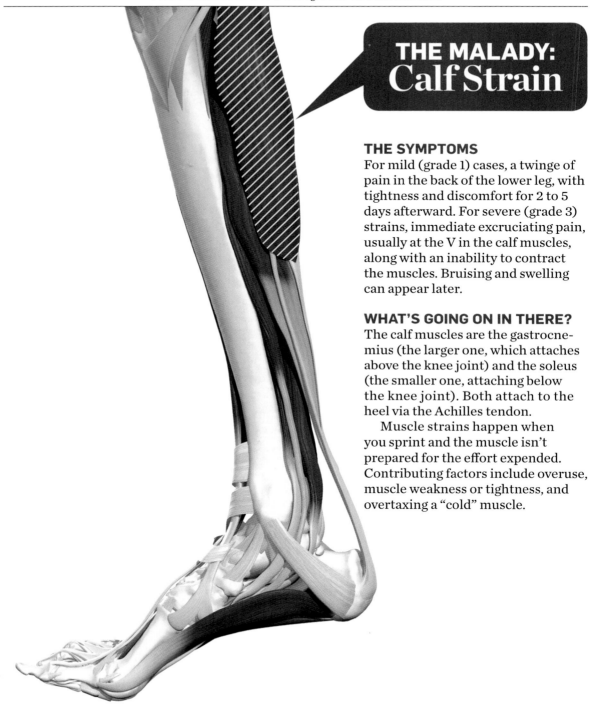

THE MALADY:
Calf Strain

THE SYMPTOMS

For mild (grade 1) cases, a twinge of pain in the back of the lower leg, with tightness and discomfort for 2 to 5 days afterward. For severe (grade 3) strains, immediate excruciating pain, usually at the V in the calf muscles, along with an inability to contract the muscles. Bruising and swelling can appear later.

WHAT'S GOING ON IN THERE?

The calf muscles are the gastrocnemius (the larger one, which attaches above the knee joint) and the soleus (the smaller one, attaching below the knee joint). Both attach to the heel via the Achilles tendon.

Muscle strains happen when you sprint and the muscle isn't prepared for the effort expended. Contributing factors include overuse, muscle weakness or tightness, and overtaxing a "cold" muscle.

All muscle strains are graded on a scale of 1 to 3. Grade 1, the mildest, usually involves only a small tear of roughly 10 percent of the fibers. Grade 2 involves up to 90 percent of the fibers, and grade 3 involves more than 90 percent. A full rupture, when the muscle tears in two, usually happens in the V of the calf muscle and also involves the Achilles tendon. This, obviously, isn't good.

Treating a muscle strain as soon after the injury as possible is crucial. If you neglect it or continue to exercise it, you'll only make it worse and put yourself out of the game for a longer stretch.

FIX IT

- **Dyanamic rest.** Avoid lower-leg work as much as possible. Do core and upper-body work to maintain your fitness.

- **Ice it.** Ice the muscles for 15- to 20-minute stretches during the first 24 hours to help reduce pain, inflammation, and muscle spasm.

- **Try a compression bandage.** Compression can help keep swelling down during the first 24 to 48 hours after the injury. Compression sleeves are easiest, and elastic bandages work, too, but be sure not to wrap it too tightly. If your foot turns color or gets cold, it's not getting enough blood.

- **Elevate it.** This can help draw fluid away from the injury. Try to keep your lower leg higher than your hip as much as possible during the first 48 hours after the injury.

- **Shorten the muscle.** For the first couple days after the injury, heel pads can raise the heel, shortening the muscle to reduce the strain on it.

- **Try an NSAID.** An antiinflammatory like ibuprofen or naproxen can help.

- **Rehab it.** Once you're able, follow the "Prevent It" measures to strengthen and stretch your calves (see next page).

- **Strengthen your calves.** Add single-leg calf raises to your exercise routine. If you're rehabbing from a strain, once you're pain free, try seated calf raises. Also use a Superband, Sport-Cord, or even a towel or belt to add resistance as you point your foot away from your body. Do two sets of 10 for all of these.

- **Work on flexibility.** Stretch the gastrocnemius by sitting on the floor with your leg straight out in front of you. Pull your toes and foot back, hold for several seconds, and relax. Repeat 10 times. To stretch the soleus, sit on the floor with your knees bent. Support yourself with your hands behind you as you lean back, lift your leg, and point your toes toward the ceiling, holding for several seconds. Repeat 10 times. Another good option? Regular yoga practice.

WHEN TO CALL A DOCTOR

For a severe strain, or if your symptoms don't improve, see a doctor. He or she can determine the grade of your strain, diagnose any underlying problems, and prescribe physical therapy if necessary.

DO YOU NEED SURGERY?

Almost never. If the strain is severe enough or you have a full rupture (when the muscle detaches from the bone), you could need surgery. A grade 3 strain is a serious injury, but surgical patients usually have a full recovery.

Cont'd on page 22

PREVENT IT

The best way to prevent a calf strain in the first place is building limber lower legs. An underlying lack of flexibility in your calf muscles and Achilles tendon is usually the primary cause of lower-leg problems. You can increase overall dynamic flexibility by using the Iron Strength workout section of this book (see page 258). But even if you don't use those specific workouts, the stretches and exercises here all target your lower leg and can be added to any workout.

STRAIGHT-LEG CALF STRETCH

Stand about 2 feet in front of a wall in a staggered stance, right foot in front of your left. Place your hands on the wall and lean against it. Shift your weight to your back foot until you feel a stretch in your calf. Hold this stretch for 30 seconds on each side, then repeat twice for a total of three sets. Perform this routine daily, and up to 3 times a day if you're really tight.

BENT-LEG CALF STRETCH

Perform this the same as the straight-leg calf stretch, only move your back foot forward so the toes of that foot are even with the heel of your front foot. Keeping your heels down, bend both knees until you feel a comfortable stretch just above the ankle of your back leg. Hold this stretch for 30 seconds on each side, then repeat twice for a total of three sets. Perform this routine daily, and up to 3 times a day if you're really tight.

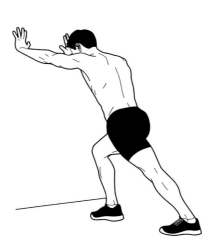

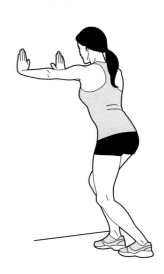

HOW YOUR CALF MUSCLES WORK

A pair of muscles, the soleus and gastrocnemius, make up your calf. Your soleus is more involved in extending your ankle when your knee is bent. Your gastrocnemius takes on a greater workload when your knee is straight. That means that bent-leg stretches and calf raises target your soleus, while standing calf raises and straight-leg stretches zero in on your gastrocnemius. To get the muscle growth and total flexibility you want, do both versions.

CALF ROLL

Place a foam roller under your right ankle, with your right leg straight. Cross your left leg over your right ankle. Put your hands flat on the floor for support and keep your back naturally arched.

Roll your body forward until the roller reaches the back of your right knee. Then roll back and forth. Repeat with the roller under your left calf. (If this is too hard, perform the movement with both legs on the roller.)

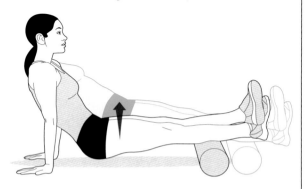

SINGLE-LEG BENT-KNEE CALF RAISE

Using the same directions as the single-leg standing dumbbell calf raise, bend your knee and hold it that way as you perform the exercise.

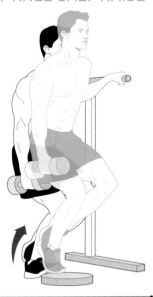

SINGLE-LEG STANDING DUMBBELL CALF RAISE

Grab a dumbbell in your right hand and stand on a step, block, or 25-pound weight plate. Cross your left foot behind your right ankle and balance yourself on the ball of your right foot, with your right heel on the floor or hanging off a step. Put your left hand on something stable—a wall or weight rack, for instance.

Lift your right heel as high as you can. Pause, then lower and repeat. Complete the prescribed number of reps with your right leg, then do the same number with your left (holding the dumbbell in your left hand).

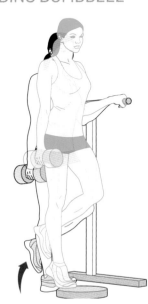

FARMER'S WALK ON TOES

Grab a pair of heavy dumbbells and hold them at your sides at arm's length. Raise your heels and walk forward (or in a circle) for 60 seconds. Be sure to stand as tall as you can and stick your chest out.

This exercise not only works your calves but also improves your cardiovascular fitness. Choose the heaviest pair of dumbbells that allows you to perform the exercise without breaking form for 60 seconds. If you feel that you could have gone longer, grab heavier weights on your next set.

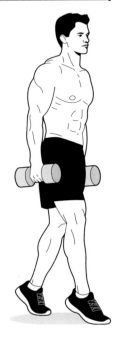

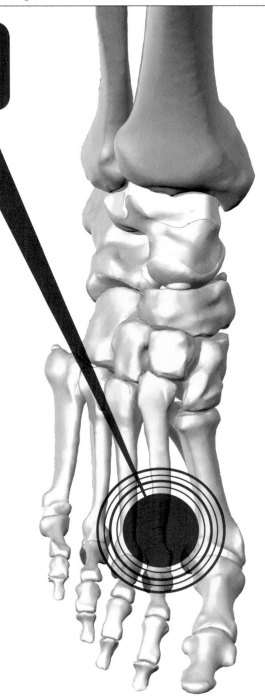

THE MALADY: Stress Fracture

THE SYMPTOMS
Pain that worsens over time, limits the sufferer's ability to load the bone, and is generally concentrated in one specific area.

WHAT'S GOING ON IN THERE?
This is the classic overuse injury. Unlike a bone break, which is the result of a trauma such as a twist or fall, a stress fracture develops over time due to repetitive loading. The demand on the bone simply exceeds the bone's ability to withstand force.

There are three risk factors for a lower-leg stress fracture:

• **Activity level.** Ramping up your athletic activity too fast can cause a stress fracture, such as when a runner training for a marathon adds too much mileage to his or her weekly rate.

• **Mechanics.** Pronation—the foot rolling inward as it strikes—while running has been correlated with a greater risk of stress fracture. Also, weak core and hip muscles can promote poor running mechanics.

• **Bone density.** This is common sense: The more brittle your bones, the easier it is to crack them. Low bone density (osteopenia) or very low bone density (osteoporosis) has several possible causes: genetics, as it tends to run in families; inadequate dietary calcium intake (1,300 milligrams a day is the recommended minimum); and, for women, a history of menstrual disorders, e.g., not getting a period for more than 6 months in a row, which can cause a low level of circulating estrogen.

We all acquire 90 percent of our bone density for life by age 18, and women reach their maximum bone density by age 32. After that, it's about maintenance.

FIX IT

• **Employ dynamic rest.** Cease the offending activity. For how long varies depending on the severity of your injury, but expect at least a month. Runners can cross-train with swimming and biking as long as they don't load the injury.

• **Support your arches.** Orthotics (arch supports) can help fix pronation and improve your running mechanics. Over-the-counter products usually work just fine, but if not, consider custom orthotics.

• **Supplement.** Eat more calcium- and vitamin D–rich foods or take supplements.

PREVENT IT

• **Change your shoes.** Try switching to a shoe that limits pronation. Arch supports can help as well.

• **Up your calcium and vitamin D intakes.** Try 1,300 milligrams of calcium and 400 micrograms of D per day. Easy food sources are milk and yogurt.

• **Follow the 10 percent rule.** Runners, never up your weekly mileage by more than 10 percent.

• **Shorten your stride.** A shorter running stride and faster foot cadence can reduce stress in your lower legs. Count your footstrikes for 1 minute on your right foot—shoot for 85 to 90 per minute.

• **Train your hips and core.** Strengthening these areas will make you a stronger runner, which improves footstrike and body mechanics.

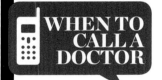

WHEN TO CALL A DOCTOR

With stress fractures, the earlier, the better. Your doctor can confirm the diagnosis with x-rays and MRIs. However, stress fractures typically don't show up on x-rays unless they're very serious or already in the healing stage. The key is to treat both the symptoms and the causes, which you can do with the home-based tips found here. Your doctor will guide your care.

Depending on your individual case and family history, your doctor may also do a bone-density scan (using DEXA, dual-energy x-ray absorptiometry). If you have low bone density, the doctor can treat you for osteopenia or osteoporosis.

Don't wait to see a doctor if you suspect you're developing a stress fracture. It only gets worse the more demand you put on it, and eventually it'll be so severe and painful that you won't be able to walk.

DO YOU NEED SURGERY?

Almost never, and only if a crack in the bone compromises bone stability and needs to be reinforced, for example, with a rod.

THE MALADY:
Ingrown Toenail

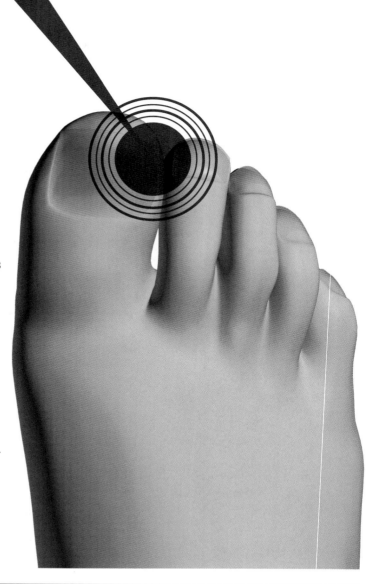

THE SYMPTOMS

Pain, sometimes worse than just annoying, where the toenail has grown into the skin around it. The entire area is usually red and tender to the touch.

WHAT'S GOING ON IN THERE?

Ingrown nails typically start when a nail, usually the one on the big toe, grows or is pushed into the soft, tender tissue alongside it. People whose toes are somewhat convex are more susceptible, but anyone can get one. Athletes who spend a lot of time in tight shoes or who put a lot of pressure on their toes with explosive movements are prime candidates for ingrown nails.

While they arise mostly as the result of improper cutting, ingrown nails can also be caused by any number of accidents or heavy use, such as in long-distance running. Stubbing your toe can also cause them, as can dropping a heavy object on your toe.

It's important to address ingrown nails quickly. Trying to ignore them will only lead to more pain while running, changing direction, or jumping—basically, all the things an athlete needs his or her feet for. If the area becomes infected, you'll have a serious problem. But most ingrown nails can be taken care of with the home-based remedies listed here.

FIX IT

- **Try an over-the-counter product.** Many products will help soften the skin and the nail, and many of them have a soothing antiinflammatory agent like tea tree oil or menthol. Dr. Scholl's Ingrown Toenail Pain Reliever and Outgro Pain Relieving Liquid are examples. Read and follow the directions to the letter and don't use these types of products if you have diabetes, impaired circulation, or any kind of infection.

- **Use cotton.** The ultimate solution is to have the toenail eventually grow out over the skin folds at its side. Start by soaking your foot in warm water for 5 to 10 minutes to soften the nail (add 1 teaspoon of salt for every pint of water). Dry it, then gently insert a wisp (not a wad) of sterile cotton beneath the burrowing edge of the nail. The cotton will lift the nail slightly so it will grow past the sore skin. Apply an antiseptic over the cotton as well to guard against infection. Change the cotton daily until the nail grows out.

PREVENT IT

- **Cut nails with precision.** Never cut your nails too short. Cut straight across with a sharp, substantial straight-edged clipper. Never cut a nail in an oval shape that causes the leading edge to curve down into the skin at the sides.

- **Buy the right shoes.** Tight shoes, especially around the toes, can help cause ingrown nails. When shopping for shoes, remember the following tips: Shop in the afternoon or evening, when your feet are at their largest, and wear athletic socks to get a proper fit. If ingrown nails are a chronic problem for you, wear wide-toed or open-toed shoes when you can.

- **Forget the V.** Don't fall for the old wives' tale about cutting a V-shaped wedge in the middle of the nail's top edge. The thinking is that the sides will grow toward the open center and away from the ingrown edge. Not true. All nails grow outward from the base.

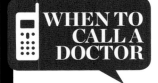

WHEN TO CALL A DOCTOR

If your toe becomes infected, you need to see a doctor. Signs to look for include swelling, redness, pain, and warmth when touched. Pus-filled blisters may also form. The doctor will most likely treat your infection with soaks, removal of infected skin, and antibiotics.

Allowing an ingrown toenail to get out of control spells serious trouble. If you have poor circulation, a nail infection can ultimately lead to gangrene.

DO YOU NEED SURGERY?

Ingrown toenails can lead to something you could technically call surgery. Sometimes a bloody growth, called proud flesh, builds up along the side of the nail. This inflamed soft tissue can become quite sensitive when it extends into the nail groove. Doctors may cut away a small portion of the ingrown nail during a minor operation and prescribe antibiotics to fight infection.

KNEES

Achilles had his heel, but the rest of us have our knees. Athletes hurt their knees more than virtually any other body part. Think of a sport and chances are it pounds on the knees. Endurance: marathons, triathlons. Explosive: tennis, gymnastics. Full contact: rugby, wrestling. And our most popular sports, football (American and soccer), basketball, and baseball. How many times have a pro team's playoff dreams been crushed when a quarterback, ace southpaw, or scoring machine goes down with a bum knee? When your knees hurt, it's scary. Bad knees can also compromise your overall health, for when you're off your feet, you're susceptible to weight gain and deconditioning. Here's all the info you need to know to figure out what's wrong and how to get yourself back in the game.

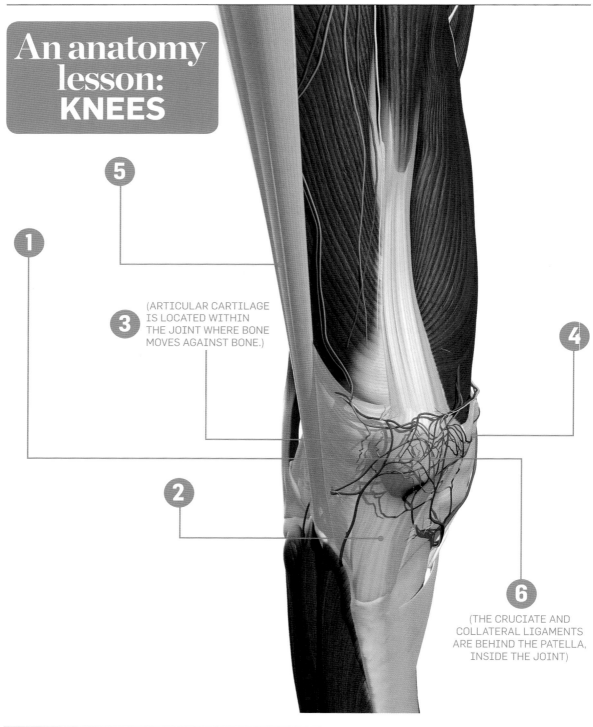

An anatomy lesson: KNEES

5

1

3 (ARTICULAR CARTILAGE IS LOCATED WITHIN THE JOINT WHERE BONE MOVES AGAINST BONE.)

4

2

6 (THE CRUCIATE AND COLLATERAL LIGAMENTS ARE BEHIND THE PATELLA, INSIDE THE JOINT)

2 PATELLAR TENDON

This tendon, located below the kneecap, attaches that bone to the tibia. It helps you extend your lower leg for kicking and jumping and is particularly vulnerable to overuse injuries like patellar tendonitis ("jumper's knee").

1 PATELLA

The kneecap. This bone protects the front of the knee joint. The patella is the largest sesamoid bone in the body (sesamoid, meaning it sits completely within tendons – in this case, the quadriceps tendon and the patellar tendon.

3 ARTICULAR CARTILAGE (KNEE)

Smooth, protective material found on bone in the joints to keep them moving smoothly ("articular" refers to movement). The patella helps protect the articular cartilage in the knee. This cartilage has no blood supply, so any injury to it is very slow to heal.

4 MENISCUS

A C-shaped piece of cartilage that cushions the knee between the femur and tibia. Each knee has a pair of menisci. Sudden stops and hard twisting can tear the menisci, however, it is possible to have a torn meniscus and have no pain or symptoms whatsoever.

5 ILIOTIBIAL BAND

A thick tendon that runs from the outer side of the hip down to the outer side of the tibia, crossing two joints (hip and knee). It helps support and stabilize the knee, as well as control the angle of the lower leg while running. It's also called the "iliotibial tract" or the "IT Band."

6 THE CRUCIATE AND COLLATERAL LIGAMENTS

Four ligaments that attach the femur to the tibia in the knee. The cruciate ligaments (anterior, ACL, and posterior, PCL) cross each other inside the knee. The collateral ligaments (medial, MCL, and lateral, LCL) run on either side of the knee.

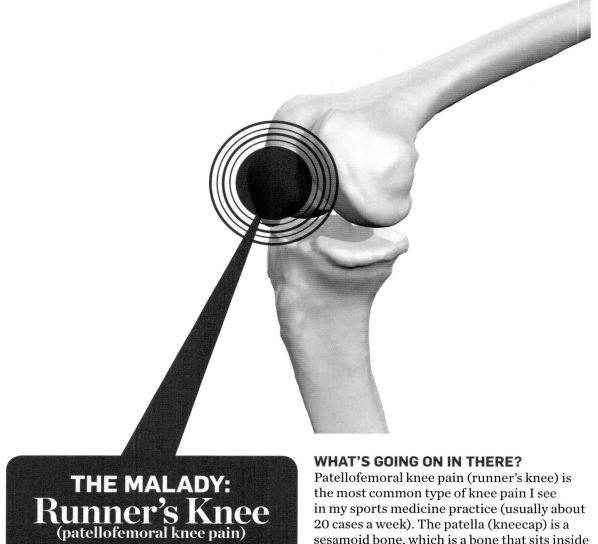

THE MALADY:
Runner's Knee
(patellofemoral knee pain)

THE SYMPTOMS

Pain beneath the kneecap that's worst after you finish an activity. It's especially sore going up or down stairs, tends not to swell, and typically becomes most aggravated after about an hour of running, when your quads start to tire.

WHAT'S GOING ON IN THERE?

Patellofemoral knee pain (runner's knee) is the most common type of knee pain I see in my sports medicine practice (usually about 20 cases a week). The patella (kneecap) is a sesamoid bone, which is a bone that sits inside a muscle-tendon unit. In the case of the knee, the patella is located inside the patellar tendon and connects to the quadriceps muscle group, the most powerful group in the body.

The patella has to withstand tremendous amounts of force, and the direction in which the patella moves is directly related to the forces that come from the quads. For example, if an athlete has a strong lateral

KNEES

(or outer) quad, the patella can be pulled to the outer side. The back of the patella is lined with a thin layer of cartilage known as articular cartilage. This layer helps the patella track up and down along the front of the femur.

Pain can come from several causes. One is an injury to the cartilage under the patella. Poor running or biking mechanics resulting from weak or tight muscles can contribute. Poorly conditioned glutes, core muscles, hips, and quads can lead to pelvic instability, which can affect the knees. Here's how: Ideally, your pelvis remains in a steady, level state as you run. But if your muscles are underconditioned, your pelvis will wobble as you run, just as a car will wobble on badly aligned tires. This stresses the knees and can cause runner's knee.

I see this condition in more women than men because of what is called the Q angle or the knock-kneed angle, which is caused by their wider hips and can result in overpronation (when the foot falls inward).

Obviously, these multiple causes of pain need to be addressed systematically to pinpoint what, exactly, the cause is. The multi-pronged attack listed here (in "Fix It") can help. Once the reasons for the pain are determined, treatment is usually successful.

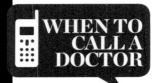

WHEN TO CALL A DOCTOR

Patellofemoral knee pain is very treatable and preventable, so if pain persists after 2 months of disciplined home-based treatment or if swelling appears, you could have a different problem and a doctor should evaluate you.

Another factor: Patients older than 50 should see a doctor for knee pain. X-rays can help diagnose patellofemoral arthritis, a wearing down of the cartilage beneath the kneecap.

An MRI might be done to evaluate the cartilage in the knee joint and is often recommended if the pain hasn't subsided after 2 months of treatment or if a cartilage injury is suspected.

DO YOU NEED SURGERY?

Almost never. The only way you run into further problems is if you don't address the pain in the first place, which could lead to cartilage and arthritis issues. But you're smart. You won't ignore your knee pain.

FIX IT

- **Employ dynamic rest.** As you work to rehab the injury, stay fit with vigorous upper-body work, plus pool running and/or biking if you can do so without knee pain. Meanwhile...

- **Strengthen your knees, quads, and hips.** All three areas can contribute to this type of knee pain. Weak or inflexible quads are a particular source of knee pain, but upping your strength and flexibility throughout your hips, quads, and knees will help both ease the pain and improve your form once you return to your normal training. Plyometric lower-body exercises can help with strength and flexibility, so add multidirectional lunges, planks, skater plyos, squats, and squat jumps to your workout (see next page for more ideas).

- **Work on body mechanics.** Poor running form can bring on this condition. A good way to see what your form looks like is to have a friend record you running toward a video camera or camera phone. You may see things you never realized you were doing. Do your knees fall inward? Do your feet roll inward or outward? You want your stride and footstrike to be smooth, straight, forward, and neutral to put the least amount of stress on the knee. Increasing your strength and flexibility can help your mechanics, but you may have to concentrate on proper form or seek out a coach to help you retrain yourself.

- **Try orthotics.** Arch supports and motion-control shoes can help with overpronation.

Cont'd on page 34

PREVENT IT

Patellofemoral knee pain (runner's knee) is only sometimes caused by a literal knee problem. More likely, muscle imbalances, tightness, or bad conditioning in the quads and hips is the issue. Building up your quads makes your knees more stable and less susceptible to injury. You can increase overall dynamic flexibility by using the Iron Strength workout section of this book (see page 258). But even if you don't use those specific workouts, the stretches and exercises here all target your quads and hips and can be added to any workout.

QUADRICEPS-AND-HIP-FLEXORS ROLL

Lie facedown on the floor with a foam roller positioned above your left knee. Cross your right leg over your left ankle and place your elbows on the floor for support.

Roll your body backward until the roller reaches the top of your left thigh. Then roll back and forth. Repeat with the roller under your right thigh. (If that's too hard, perform the movement with both thighs on the roller, as shown.)

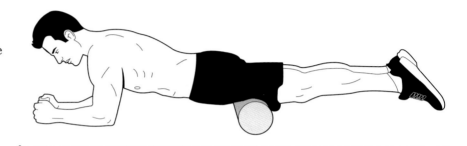

PRISONER SQUAT

Stand as tall as you can with your feet spread shoulder-width apart. Place your fingers on the back of your head (as if you have just been arrested). Pull your elbows and shoulders back, and stick out your chest. Lower your body as far as you can by pushing your hips back and bending your knees. Pause, then slowly push yourself back to the starting position.

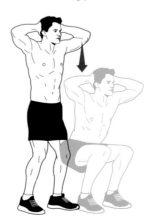

BODYWEIGHT BULGARIAN SPLIT SQUAT

Stand in a staggered stance, your left foot in front of your right 2 to 3 feet apart. Place just the instep of your back foot on a bench or chair. Pull your shoulders back and brace your core. Lower your body as deeply as you can, keeping your back foot on the bench. Keep your shoulders back and chest up through the movement. Pause, then return to starting position. Perform equal reps for each leg.

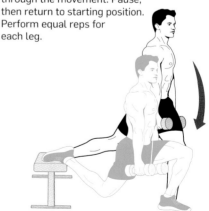

MOUNTAIN CLIMBERS

Get in pushup position with your arms straight (you can use the ground or a bench as your base). This is the starting position.

Lift your right foot and raise your knee as close to your chest as you can. Touch the ground with your right foot and then return to the starting position and repeat with your left leg. Go as fast as possible.

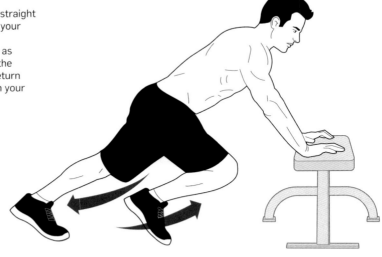

WALKING LUNGE (DUMBBELLS OPTIONAL)

Perform a lunge, but instead of pushing your body backward to the starting position, raise up and bring your back foot forward so that you move forward (as though you're walking) a step with every rep. Alternate the leg you step forward with each time.

When you complete the prescribed number of repetitions, perform back-ward walking lunges to return to your starting point.

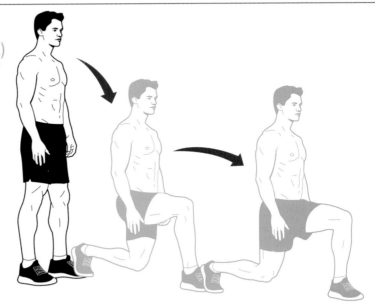

SHORTEN YOUR STRIDE

If you shorten your stride and raise your footstrike rate, you'll take a lot of stress off your knees. Count the number of foot-strikes of either the left or right foot over 1 minute as you run. A good number is 85 to 90 footstrikes per minute on one foot.

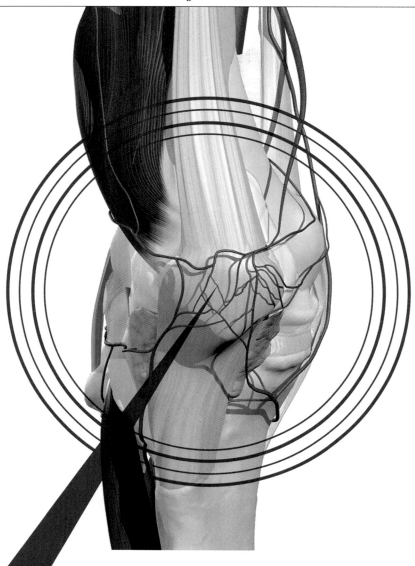

THE MALADY:
Knee Effusion
(swelling, or "water on the knee")

THE SYMPTOMS

Swelling of the knee that may also include pain, stiffness, and the inability to fully extend the leg.

WHAT'S GOING ON IN THERE?

Effusion is a fancy word for swelling. And swelling in a joint is never normal. The question is, *why is the knee swollen?* Answer that by starting with another question: *When did it first swell up?*

Within an hour or two of activity: Swelling that occurs soon after an activity is much more serious than swelling that shows up, say, the next day. Example: You twist your knee skiing and it swells up. This is a sign of bleeding within the knee, or hemarthrosis. Basically, something has been torn or broken. About 80 percent of hemarthrosis cases are caused by a torn anterior cruciate ligament (ACL). Sudden-onset effusion is a sign that something serious is going on.

Hours later or the day after activity: Swelling that arrives later is generally caused by excess synovial fluid (the lubricant in joints) in the knee, much like too much oil in a car (and why it's called water on the knee). Overuse and an underlying medical condition are the most common causes. Something in there is irritated or rubbing during activity and the body responds by overlubricating the knee to compensate. Osteoarthritis is one of the most common causes, but far less common maladies can also be the culprits, such as rheumatoid arthritis, infection, gout, bursitis, cysts, bleeding disorders, tumors, and Lyme disease. Advancing age and participation in sports that require sudden changes in speed and direction raise your risk.

FIX IT

- **See a doctor.** Anytime you have a swollen joint, you should see a doctor (check out "When to Call a Doctor" for more). This is especially true with sudden-onset effusion.

- **Employ dynamic rest.** Even if the swelling comes without pain, avoid loading the knee until the swelling subsides. Trade knee-loading exercises for intense upper-body and core work.

- **Ice it.** Apply ice for 15 minutes 4 to 6 times a day for the first 2 days of swelling. Elevating the knee as you ice it can also help reduce the swelling.

- **Try an NSAID.** Even if you have no pain, ibuprofen or naproxen could help with swelling due to inflammation.

PREVENT IT

- **Strengthen your legs.** Strong legs protect your knees. Be sure your workout regimen includes regular lower-body strength training in addition to any aerobic exercise of the legs (running, biking, etc.) that you do.

You may not be able to prevent knee effusion caused by health issues, but properly trained legs will help your knees recover in the long run no matter what the issue turns out to be.

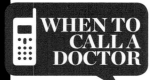

WHEN TO CALL A DOCTOR

My philosophy is that anytime you have joint swelling, you should see a doctor because you need to figure out what the problem is. Try to pinpoint when the effusion began in relation to your athletic activities, especially if your knee has swelled up with no discernible cause such as an overt injury and you have no other symptoms that suggest a related illness.

Also, if the knee is swollen but has some bonus symptoms like redness or warmth of the skin and/or you have a fever, it could signal an infection. Get to an ER pronto.

WILL YOU NEED SURGERY?

There's no way to tell until you see a doctor. The biggest issue with common knee swelling is figuring out the cause. A physician can help shed light on the mystery, whether by physical exam, analysis of fluid drawn from the knee, or review of images such as MRIs or x-rays.

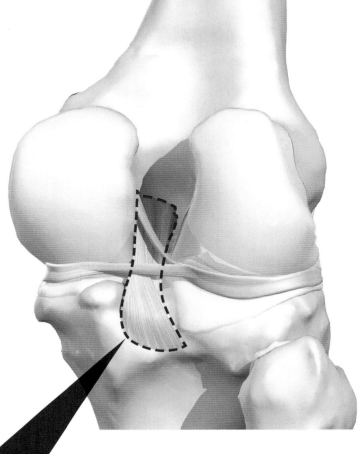

THE MALADY:
Knee Ligament Sprain

THE SYMPTOMS
Pain at the time of the injury (usually caused by an impact) and varying levels of pain afterward depending on the severity of the sprain. The location of the pain also depends on which knee ligament is damaged. Some swelling is common, as is joint instability, which makes you feel as if your knee might give out. Like strains, sprains are graded in severity from 1 to 3 (a grade 3 sprain is a complete rupture of a knee ligament; see page 42).

WHAT'S GOING ON IN THERE?
There are four main ligaments in the knee that keep the femur attached to the fibula and tibia in the lower leg. One or more of these ligaments

can be sprained at the same time. However, each ligament is vulnerable to certain impacts to the knee.

Medial collateral ligament (MCL): Medial means on the inner side, so this ligament is on the inner side of the knee. This is the most commonly sprained ligament because it's vulnerable to trauma to the outer side of the knee, which can easily be hit. Think of it this way: The outer side of the knee is hit, the knee bends inward, and the ligament on the inner side of the knee stretches. Pain will be localized on the inner portion of the knee.

Lateral collateral ligament: Lateral means on the outer portion, so this ligament is on the outer side of the knee. This is the counterpart of the MCL. The injury process is the opposite of that for the MCL: The inner part of the knee is hit, the knee bends outward, the ligament on the outer side of the knee stretches. Pain will be localized on the outer side of the knee.

Anterior cruciate ligament: One of two crossing (the meaning of cruciate) ligaments inside the knee joint that attach the femur to the tibia. The anterior is the one closest to the front of the knee. It's most commonly hurt when the knee twists and the foot remains planted.

Posterior cruciate ligament (PCL): The other crossing ligament inside the knee, this one running behind the ACL and thus being posterior. The PCL is thicker and stronger than the ACL, so it isn't injured as often. An impact on the front of the tibia while the knee is bent is the most common cause of a sprain.

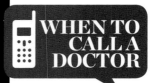

WHEN TO CALL A DOCTOR

A mild sprain (grade 1) probably won't feel bad enough to drive you to see a doctor—and you'll probably be okay—but really, any sprain symptoms should be checked out by a sports doctor. Be smart. The knee is simply too important to your future athletic performance for you to just "suck it up" and take the pain.

Severe sprains (grade 2 or 3) won't give you a choice. You won't be able to walk, or the knee will feel as though it's about to give out. Make the appointment.

The doctor will do a physical exam and any imaging (MRI, etc.) that's necessary to assess the damage. The fact is, even if you suspect a sprain, you could have other damage that needs attention. These decisions and diagnoses should be made by your doctor, not you.

WILL YOU NEED SURGERY?
Undetermined. Believe it or not, three of the four ligaments generally heal themselves—only the ACL needs help. Obviously, this all depends on how badly you're hurt. And again, that's why it's so important to see a doctor after any knee injury.

FIX IT

- **See a doctor.** Don't mess around. Any knee injury needs a diagnosis. Check out "When to Call a Doctor."

- **Employ dynamic rest.** Avoid loading the knee and continue with intense upper-body and core work to maintain fitness.

- **Ice it.** Apply ice for 15 minutes every 4 to 6 hours for the first 2 days to alleviate swelling. Elevating the knee above your heart can also help with swelling.

- **Try an NSAID.** An antiinflammatory like ibuprofen or naproxen can help with pain and inflammation.

- **Rehab and strengthen.** When pain subsides and activity can resume, perform mobility and balance exercises to improve joint stability and leg strength. A good start for basic strengthening: Uphill walking, cycling, or pool running. When you're pain free, build up all of your leg muscles with multidirectional lunges and squats. If you experience any pain, back off.

Cont'd on page 40

PREVENT IT

You may not be able to prevent an impact to your knee. But the strength and flexibility of your legs will help determine how quickly you'll recover if the problem isn't surgical. Your quads are of particular help here. Building them up also helps make your knees more stable and less susceptible to injury. You can increase overall dynamic flexibility by using the Iron Strength workout section of this book (see page 256). But even if you don't use those specific workouts, the stretches and exercises here all help build powerful legs and can be added to any workout.

QUADRICEPS-AND-HIP-FLEXORS ROLL

Lie facedown on the floor with a foam roller positioned above your left knee. Cross your right leg over your left ankle and place your elbows on the floor for support.

Roll your body backward until the roller reaches the top of your left thigh. Then roll back and forth. Repeat with the roller under your right thigh. (If that's too hard, perform the movement with both thighs on the roller, as shown.)

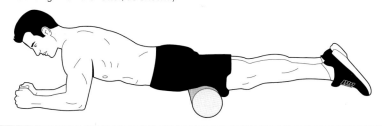

SQUAT THRUSTS

Stand with your feet shoulder-width apart and your arms at your sides (hexagonal dumbbells optional). Push your hips back, bend your knees, and lower your body as deep as you can into a squat.

As you squat down, place your hands on the floor in front of you, shifting your weight onto them. Kick your legs backward, so that you're now in a pushup position.

Quickly bring your legs back to the squat position. Stand up quickly and repeat the movement.

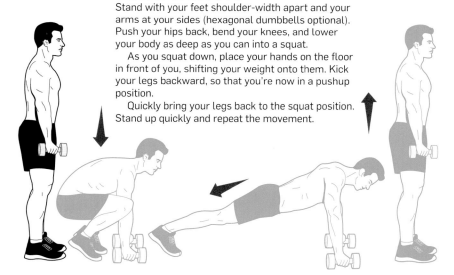

AVOID THE LEG EXTENSION MACHINE

Two good reasons: First, you're using only one group of muscles (quads) in a set range of motion that doesn't mimic any real-world movement. And second, researchers at the Mayo Clinic found that leg extensions stress your knees more than free-weight squats do. The machine puts the resistance near your ankles, which leads to high amounts of torque applied to your knee joint every time you lower the weight.

A BIG BONUS

You're not just keeping your knees safe. Research has shown that doing intense lower-body work, especially plyometric exercises, for 3 weeks can boost your vertical leap by as much as 9 percent.

LOW SIDE-TO-SIDE LUNGE

Stand with your feet set about twice shoulder-length apart, your feet facing straight ahead. Clasp your hands in front of your chest (dumbbells optional).

Shift your weight over to your right leg as you push your hips backward and lower your body by dropping your hips and bending your knees. Your lower right leg should remain nearly perpendicular to the floor. Your left foot should remain flat on the floor.

Without raising yourself back up to a standing position, reverse the movement to the left. Alternate back and forth.

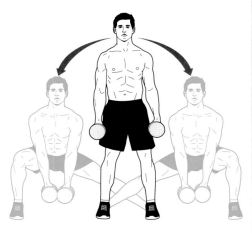

- Uphill walking
- Uphill sprinting
- Sprints with directional change, such as figure 8, shuttle runs (suicides), or cone drills
- Stairs
- Pool running or aerobics
- Cycling
- Indoor/outdoor rock climbing

BODYWEIGHT JUMP SQUATS

Place your fingers on the back of your head and pull your elbows back so that they're in line with your body. Perform a bodyweight squat until your thighs are parallel to the floor, then explosively jump as high as you can (imagine you're pushing the floor away from you as you leap). When you land, immediately squat and jump again. Hold dumbbells at your side to make it more challenging.

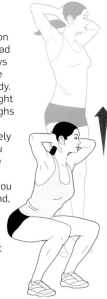

PISTOL SQUAT (WITH OPTIONAL PLYO)

Stand holding your arms straight out in front of your body at shoulder level. Raise your right leg off the floor and hold it there. Keeping your right leg straight, push your hips back and lower your body as far as you can without breaking form. As you do this, raise your right leg so that it doesn't touch the floor, and keep your torso as upright as possible. Pause, then push your body back to the starting position. Perform reps for each leg.

For a bigger challenge, as you rise out of the squat, add in a jump off your plant leg.

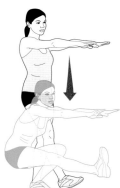

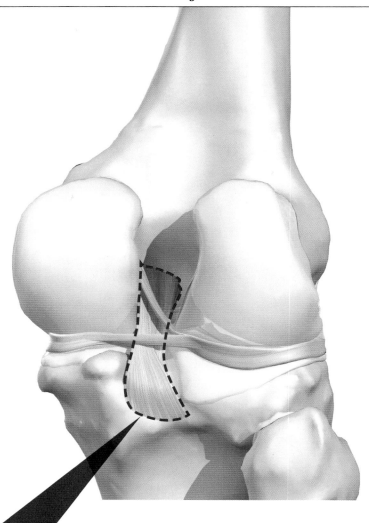

THE MALADY:
Knee Ligament Rupture (Tear)

THE SYMPTOMS
A snap or pop upon impact with the knee, followed by pain, swelling, and a feeling of weakness or looseness in the joint due to instability. The pain and instability can be severe enough to prohibit walking.

WHAT'S GOING ON IN THERE?
A rupture (a.k.a. a grade 3 sprain) is a complete tear of one or more of the four ligaments attaching the femur to the lower leg—the medial and lateral collateral ligaments and the

anterior and posterior cruciate ligaments (see "Knee Ligament Sprain" for complete descriptions).

Several types of knee trauma can cause a ligament to rupture:

- An impact on the front or side of the knee
- Twisting the knee while the foot is planted
- Bending the knee backward

A note on ACL tears: This injury is typically most painful immediately after the injury. Also, women are more prone to ACL tears than men are, possibly because of muscle imbalances and wider hips; the angles between a woman's hip, knee, and foot aren't the same as a man's.

FIX IT

- **See a doctor.** Your knee will tell you to go—and it won't be subtle about it.

- **Employ dynamic rest.** Avoid loading the knee. Continue intense upper-body and core workouts to maintain fitness.

- **Ice it.** Apply ice for 15 minutes 4 to 6 times a day for the first 2 days, then as needed to control swelling. Elevating the knee and compression wraps can also help with the swelling.

- **Rehab it.** Whether or not you require surgery, your doctor will recommend strengthening exercises to gradually return you to full activity. Take this process seriously. Generally, recovery from reconstructive knee surgery takes 6 to 12 months, and how you will perform for the rest of your life depends on how disciplined you are during the rehab process. I'm living proof—having competed in nine Ironman triathlons and more than two dozen marathons—that you can have normal or even better athletic performance after knee surgery if you do the work necessary.

PREVENT IT

- **Strengthen your legs.** You may not be able to prevent an impact to your knee. But the strength of your legs will help determine how badly you're hurt and how quickly you'll recover. A strong leg can mean the difference between a ligament rupture and a simpler sprain. Add a regular strength-training component to your workout regimen on top of any aerobic training that involves your legs (running, biking, etc.). Even if your knees are never injured, this training will help fend off wear and tear as you age.

WHEN TO CALL A DOCTOR

KNEES

As soon as you can after you feel that pop. The most serious symptom you can have isn't pain, but instability. If your knee feels as if it's going to give out, that usually signals a serious injury.

DO YOU NEED SURGERY?

Maybe; not every ligament tear needs to be fixed. This is a serious conversation to have with your doctor.

If needed, surgery generally includes reconstructing fully ruptured ligaments with replacements taken from parts of your hamstring or patellar tendon.

As far as determining who's a candidate for, say, ACL surgery goes, it depends. If the joint is unstable, I ask if the person wants to get back to twisting sports. What's his or her level of function? Is it a complete tear? All of these are considerations, but most younger athletes who want to return to their sports opt for surgery. The rehab time is 6 to 12 months, though. It's a big deal.

Some folks, especially those who have hit that age-40 threshold, opt out of surgery and still have normal, active lives. They can wear knee braces and perform general athletic activities (running, biking, even skiing).

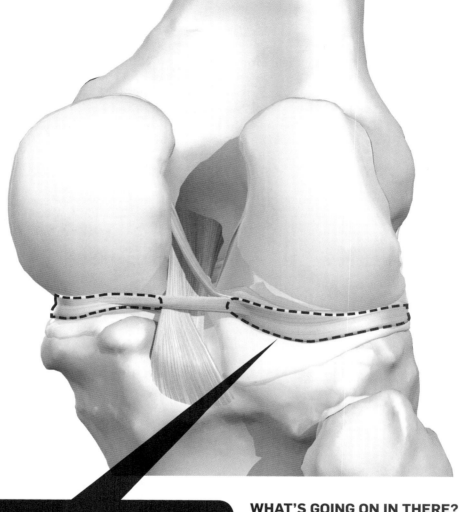

THE MALADY:
Torn Meniscus

THE SYMPTOMS
Pain (especially when twisting or rotating the knee), swelling, a popping or clicking sensation, and/or stiffness in the knee. You may not be able to fully extend it. You could also have knee instability, a feeling that it will give out.

WHAT'S GOING ON IN THERE?
Each knee has a pair of menisci, C-shaped pieces of cartilage that cushion your knee between the femur and the tibia.

Any forceful activity can lead to a torn meniscus. The most common causes: Hard twisting or pivoting, sudden stops and turns, or deep squatting while lifting something heavy. Basically, any athlete is at risk for a torn meniscus, but especially those playing football, basketball, and tennis. Your risk increases with age, and some older adults have meniscus tears from the degeneration that occurs with age.

Oddly enough, you could have a torn meniscus and have no pain or symptoms whatsoever. Some studies peg the incidence of meniscus tears in pain-free knees at between 30 and 40 percent. (Similar studies of volunteers with no back pain showed that 40 to 50 percent had herniated disks.) I have two meniscus tears myself and have no problems.

The fact is, a torn meniscus isn't necessarily a catastrophic knee injury, though it can be painful and require surgery. It's very individualized, but many tears that produce symptoms can be treated without surgery and be fine (see "Fix It").

FIX IT

- **Employ dynamic rest.** Avoid loading your knee until the pain and swelling subside. Concentrate on intense upper-body and core workouts to maintain fitness.

- **Ice it.** Apply ice to your knee for 15 minutes every 4 to 6 hours for the first 2 days after the injury to help with swelling. Ice it as needed afterward.

- **Try an NSAID.** An antiinflammatory like ibuprofen or naproxen can help with pain and swelling.

- **Get back in game condition.** When you're pain free, add in lower-body exercises to strengthen the leg muscles (squats and lunges are some of the simplest and most effective exercises). The goal is to be stronger than you were when you originally got hurt.

PREVENT IT

- **Strengthen your legs—and more.** The stronger your legs, the safer your knees. Revise your training plan to include a comprehensive lower-body and core program. Leg, knee, and hip strength are obvious goals, but a strong core will also affect how you move during your activity. The greater your strength and agility—and your core is a big part of both—the better prepared your body will be to handle the starts and stops that could cause a meniscus tear.

- **Wear your gear.** If your game requires knee protection, don't leave it in your gym bag.

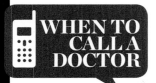

WHEN TO CALL A DOCTOR

If you have symptoms, see a doctor for a proper diagnosis. Generally, a torn meniscus can be diagnosed with physical examination of the knee. An MRI will confirm the diagnosis.

DO YOU NEED SURGERY?

Here's where it can get complicated. I have had patients come in complaining of knee pain after already having had an MRI show a meniscus tear, and they wanted to know if they needed surgery. After examining them, I found that the knee pain was the far more common patellofemoral knee pain (pain under the kneecap). The meniscus tear was asymptomatic.

Here's my advice: See your doctor and verify that your problems are indeed caused by a meniscus tear and not some other issue. Understand that a tear that requires surgery usually causes pain in the back inside part of the knee, swelling, and clicking in the knee. An MRI should be accompanied by a thorough physical examination. Physical therapy and home remedies can usually be tried before opting for surgery. However, if surgery is necessary, the results are generally good.

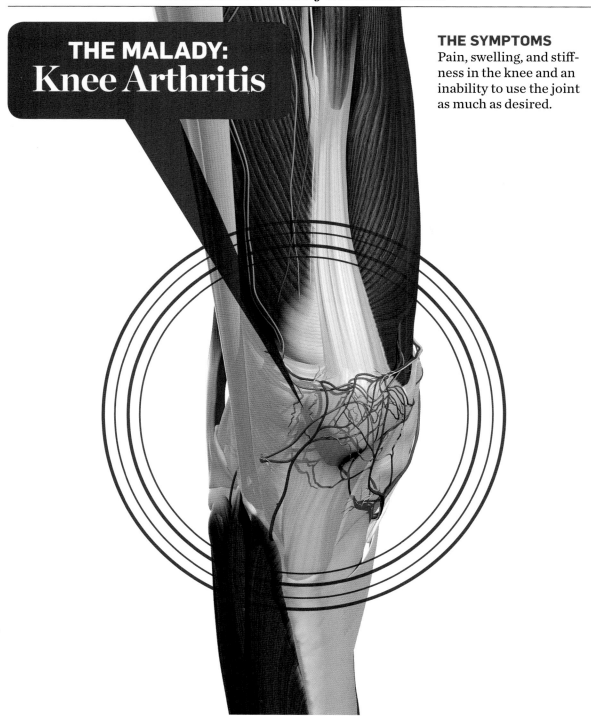

THE MALADY:
Knee Arthritis

THE SYMPTOMS
Pain, swelling, and stiffness in the knee and an inability to use the joint as much as desired.

WHAT'S GOING ON IN THERE?

There are more than 100 types of arthritis, including postinfectious arthritis, which is related to infections such as Lyme disease; arthritis related to a chronic disease such as inflammatory bowel disease; and arthritis related to an autoimmune disease, with the best-known example being rheumatoid arthritis, in which the immune system attacks the organs and joints. All types of arthritis can develop in any joint, but the knees, ankles, wrists, and shoulders are the typical locations.

The most common form of arthritis, osteoarthritis, affects 30 million Americans, and that number will increase over the next 20 years as the population ages.

It is, simply, the wearing out of a joint's lining, leaving bone to grind on bone. It's caused by a combination of factors, including old injuries (folks with ACL tears, for example, are 50 percent more likely to develop arthritis than folks without them), genetic predisposition, overuse, and sometimes just bad luck.

Arthritis gets worse over time, of course. But it's also possible to continue at your current level of fitness. The strategy I recommend is to find ways to train and maintain fitness while reducing the wear and tear on your knees. Squats, stairs, and high-mileage running are problems for folks with arthritic knees. But there are many other options.

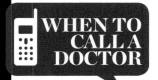

WHEN TO CALL A DOCTOR

If you suspect you have arthritis in your knee, it's a good idea to see a sports doctor, who can verify it easily with an x-ray (which is a better diagnostic tool for arthritic joints than an MRI). A full-on assessment of biomechanical factors such as strength, flexibility, and foot mechanics, as well as of external factors such as shoe type, running surface, bike fit, and training regimen, can be a huge help.

A doctor can also administer more aggressive treatments if warranted. For example, prescription antiinflammatories and injectable forms of hyaluronic acid (a substance that occurs naturally in cartilage and helps cushion joints) can help alleviate symptoms.

Last, since arthritis is a degenerative condition, it's a good idea to see a doctor early in its course to establish a baseline for your condition. Your doctor can use it to assess later changes as he or she continues your care.

DO YOU NEED SURGERY?

Generally, no. As you get older, however, knee replacement surgery may be an option if your condition no longer responds to regular therapies.

FIX IT

• **Build super legs.** Resting through arthritis, unless you're in the middle of a significant flare-up, is a bad move. More and more research shows that activity and building strength are better options. It's simple: The stronger your legs, the better you can support your knee without irritating the joint. If you rest or scale back on your activity level, you lose muscle and the condition worsens. I suggest biking and swimming to build leg strength. Quad-, hip-, and glute-strengthening exercises are musts. Multidirectional lunges as well as squats, squat jumps, and squat thrusts once you're able to do them are all good muscle builders.

• **Fix foot mechanics.** Pronation (when the foot turns inward as it strikes) puts extra pressure on the knee joint. Arch supports and motion-control shoes can help relieve excess knee pounding. Also, when you're running, try to shorten your stride and raise your footstrikes to 90 per minute.

• **Try supplements.** Glucosamine and chondroitin can help people with arthritis pain. You may hear mixed things about this supplement. The scientific data don't prove there's a definitive benefit, but many of my patients report that they have no doubt that it helps.

• **Try an NSAID.** An antiinflammatory like ibuprofen or naproxen can help with pain and swelling.

• **Change the conditions.** If possible, switch to a softer running surface. Blacktop is softer than concrete, dirt and grass are softer than blacktop, and the all-weather track at your local high school or college is best of all. Your knees will thank you.

Cont'd on page 48

PREVENT IT

I say it often: Strength controls pain. The stronger, more flexible, and better conditioned your kinetic chain, the more support your knees will get from muscles, ligaments, and tendons. The lining of the knee will receive less stress and irritation, and you'll have less knee pain. Your quads are of particular help here. Building them up helps make your knees more stable and less susceptible to pain. You can increase overall dynamic flexibility by using the Iron Strength workout section of this book (see page 256). But even if you don't use those specific workouts, the stretches and exercises here all help build powerful legs with minimal impact on the knees and can be added to any workout.

QUADRICEPS-AND-HIP-FLEXORS ROLL

Lie facedown on the floor with a foam roller positioned above your left knee. Cross your right leg over your left ankle and place your elbows on the floor for support.

Roll your body backward until the roller reaches the top of your left thigh. Then roll back and forth. Repeat with the roller under your right thigh. (If that's too hard, perform the movement with both thighs on the roller.)

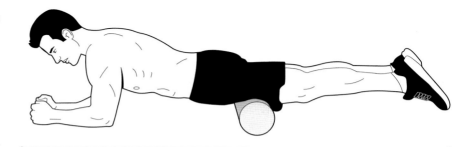

OVERHEAD DUMB-BELL SQUAT

Stand with your feet slightly wider than hip-width apart. Hold a pair of dumbbells straight over your shoulders, your arms completely straight. Brace your core and lower your body as far as you can by pushing your hips back and bending your knees. Pause, then slowly push yourself back to the starting position. Note: Keep your torso as upright as possible and don't let the dumbbells fall forward as you squat.

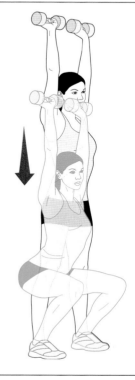

PRISONER SQUAT

Stand as tall as you can with your feet spread shoulder-width apart. Place your fingers on the back of your head (as if you have just been arrested). Pull your elbows back, and shoulders back, and stick out your chest. Lower your body as far as you can by pushing your hips back and bending your knees. Pause, then slowly push yourself back to the starting position.

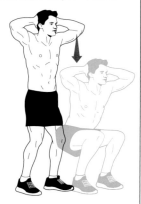

DUMBBELL LUNGE

Grab a pair of dumbbells and hold them at arm's length next to your sides, your palms facing each other. Brace your core and step forward with your right leg and slowly lower your body until your front knee is bent at least 90 degrees. Pause, then push yourself to the starting position as quickly as you can. Complete the prescribed number of repetitions with your right leg, then do the same number with your left leg.

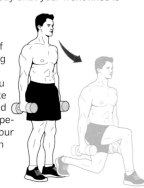

DON'T IGNORE THESE LOW-IMPACT LEG BUILDERS...

- Cycling
- Swimming
- Rowing
- Pool running or aerobics
- Indoor rock climbing
- Elliptical machines
- Versaclimber machines

KNEES

LOW SIDE-TO-SIDE LUNGE

Stand with your feet set about twice shoulder-length apart, your feet facing straight ahead. Clasp your hands in front of your chest (or use dumbbells as illustrated).

Shift your weight over to your right leg as you push your hips backward and lower your body by dropping your hips and bending your knees. Your lower right leg should remain nearly perpendicular to the floor. Your left foot should remain flat on the floor.

Without raising yourself back up to a standing position, reverse the movement to the left. Alternate back and forth.

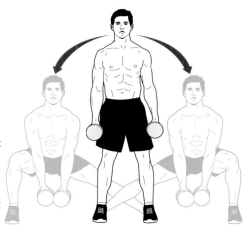

LEAN BODY, HAPPY KNEES

Many athletes depend on extra weight for their performance (think football and wrestling). People also tend to put on weight as they age. But if you're at risk for knee arthritis, such as from a previous knee injury, or if you have arthritis already, drop whatever weight you don't need for athletic performance, especially as you get older. The math is simple: The less weight you have to carry around, the less your knees have to bear. A lean physique also makes any strength gains in your legs that much more effective at supporting your knees.

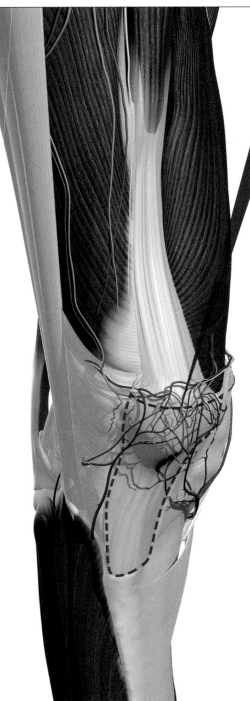

THE MALADY:
Patellar Tendinitis
("jumper's knee")

THE SYMPTOMS

Pain just below the kneecap and at the top of the tibia (the shinbone). The pain sharpens during leg exertion, but if the tendinitis progresses enough, any knee movement will hurt, especially doing stairs.

WHAT'S GOING ON IN THERE?

The patellar tendon connects your kneecap to your tibia. It's one of the main reasons you're able to extend your lower leg, whether it's to kick a soccer ball or jump to block a launched basketball.

Patellar tendinitis is a classic overuse injury—usually caused by violating the "too" rule: too much, too fast. Repeated stress on the tendon causes irritation that the body can't repair fast enough, and pain results.

Anyone can get jumper's knee, but obviously it's more common in people who play jumping sports like basketball and volleyball. You can also irritate the patellar tendon if you increase your training load too quickly or suddenly fire up the intensity.

Ignoring the pain is a bad idea. Overusing an already overused and irritated tendon can cause tendinosis, a buildup of fluid in the tendon. Eventually, it could tear. Start treatment as soon as you feel the pain and you'll shorten both your suffering and your recovery time.

FIX IT

- **Employ dynamic rest.** Lay off hard exertion of the knee, especially jumping. Swimming is possible if you can do it pain free. Otherwise, do intense upper-body and core workouts to maintain fitness.

- **Ice it.** Apply ice for 15 minutes several times a day to help relieve pain.

- **Try a strap.** A patellar tendon strap that goes around your leg just under the knee can support the tendon and relieve pain.

- **Massage it.** Rubbing the area may help lessen the pain and promote healing.

- **Rehab with the strategies suggested in "Prevent It."**

PREVENT IT

- **Stretch your quads and hammies.** Inflexible quadriceps and hamstrings can put extra stress on the patellar tendon. Basic, disciplined stretches of both muscles can help prevent tendinitis and help heal it.

- **Try eccentric training.** Do leg extensions—however, lower the weight slowly after lifting it at normal speed. If you're rehabbing the tendon, you can first do this old school by having a partner apply resistance to your lower leg and then move to a leg extension machine as

your rehab progresses. Lowering the weight slowly challenges the tendon and the muscles around it, making them all stronger. This helps prevent future cases.

NOTE: Normally I'm not a fan of leg extensions as a regular training exercise— they don't mimic any real-world movement and put excessive torque on the knee—but in cases of rehabbing patellar tendinitis, used as described, they can be effective.

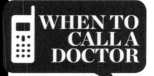

WHEN TO CALL A DOCTOR

Basic conservative measures and time are usually enough to cure patellar tendinitis, depending on the severity. However, if these treatments don't help, see your doctor. He or she will examine and diagnose you and, if warranted, prescribe anti-inflammatories and physical therapy.

The use of platelet-rich plasma (PRP) is one potential new treatment. The patient's own platelets are injected into the area to speed healing. This is effective in parts of the body that have poor bloodflow and therefore heal slowly. It can be expensive and is not always covered by insurance. But for some cases, it's worth investigating, especially if tendonosis has developed.

DO YOU NEED SURGERY?

Almost never. In rare cases, surgery may be an option if your condition hasn't improved after 12 months. This is obviously a last resort, and it isn't generally needed. But if it is, the surgeon can go in and repair tears in the tendon or excise damaged tissue. Recovery takes 6 to 18 months, but this usually fixes the problem.

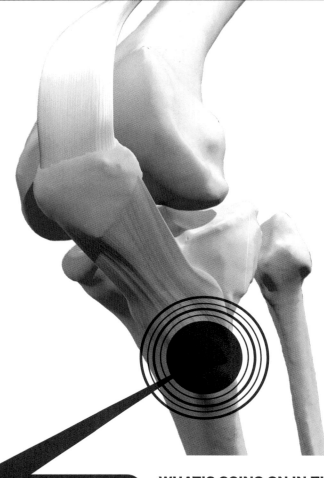

THE MALADY:
Osgood-Schlatter Disease

THE SYMPTOMS

Pain in the tibia an inch or two below the knee-cap (in one knee or both) in young adolescents. The bone can protrude as a lump. The intensity of the pain varies from child to child, but it gets worse with activity and improves with rest.

WHAT'S GOING ON IN THERE?

As a child grows, "growth plates" form at the ends of the long bones in the arms and legs. These plates are made of cartilage. Bone's tougher than cartilage, obviously, so irritation or stressing of the growth plate by the bone can cause pain.

Osgood-Schlatter is most common in kids who participate in sports involving running and explosive changes in direction. Why? During these movements, the quadriceps muscles put stress on the patellar tendon, which connects the kneecap to the tibia. This can pull the tendon away from the bone, causing pain. The body compensates by growing new bone in that space, resulting in a bony lump below the kneecap.

About one in five kids participating in sports develops Osgood-Schlatter. It's more common in boys and usually hits between the ages of 12 and 15. The discomfort can last for weeks or months depending on how the child's tibia grows. However, when they're done growing, the situation resolves itself.

FIX IT

There is no "fix," technically, but the following can help alleviate the pain.

- **Moderate activity.** Competitive sports will aggravate the condition. It's up to you and your child to determine how much it hurts and how much he or she can do. If the pain interferes with everyday activities, back him or her off sports and tone down the running and jumping. Biking and swimming are good low-impact options to keep the kid moving.

- **Try a strap.** A patellar tendon strap that goes around the leg just under the knee can offer support and relieve pain.

- **Use a pain reliever.** Acetaminophen or ibuprofen can help with the pain.

PREVENT IT

- **Keep the quads and hammies loose.** Introduce your child to basic quadriceps and hamstring stretches. Keeping these muscles loose can help take stress off the patellar tendon and possibly prevent it from pulling away from the bone.

- **Put the kid on a bike.** Strengthening the quads is also a good way to stabilize the knee. Kids this age aren't ready for weight training, so biking is a good way for them to build up their quads.

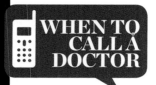

WHEN TO CALL A DOCTOR

If the pain is debilitating or prevents the child from doing everyday activities, see a doctor for an x-ray. Also, if the knee is red or swollen or feels warm to the touch and/or the child has a fever, this could signal an infection.

Generally, the doctor will perform range-of-motion tests in the knee and hip. Treatment is usually conservative—using the remedies given here and physical therapy to stretch muscles—because the pain will eventually resolve after the bone growth takes place. However, the doctor can also verify that nothing else is wrong in the joint.

DO YOU NEED SURGERY?
No.

KNEES

THE MALADY: Iliotibial Band Impingement Syndrome

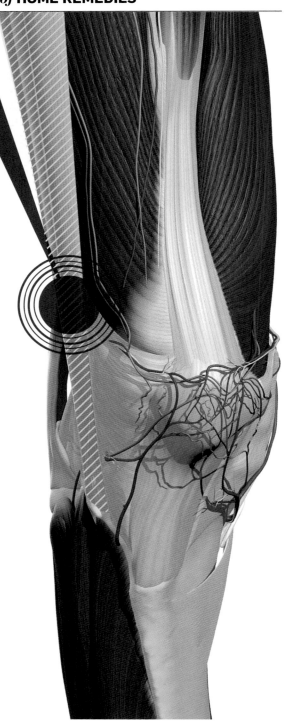

THE SYMPTOMS

Hip or knee pain, or both. Specifically, pain on the outer side of the knee where the bone bumps out above the joint, or on the outer side of the hip. The pain usually starts after 10 minutes of running. Walking usually causes no pain.

WHAT'S GOING ON IN THERE?

The iliotibial band (ITB) is a thick tendon that runs the length of and connects the tensor fascia lata muscle—which starts on the outer side of the hip—to the outer side of the tibia, the major bone in the lower leg. So you're talking about a tendon that stretches from your hip to your knee; that's one long, important piece of tissue. It also crosses two joints, the hip and the knee, and helps control the angle of the lower leg while running. The ITB can also cause a pinching pain on the outside of the hip joint with trochanteric bursitis. In the knee, a tight ITB causes similar pinching.

Here's how the pain happens: A small, fluid-filled sac called a bursa sits between the tendon and the outside of the femur near the knee. You also have a bursa at the hip joint. When the ITB is tight, it increases the tension on the outer sides of the hip and knee. The ITB then pinches these two sites and the bursa (one or both) swells. Over time, the bursa becomes enlarged—big enough to cause pain every time you begin to run (which is why pain usually starts within 10 minutes of activity).

FIX IT

• **Stretch it.** A tight ITB needs some love. There are many stretches for the ITB, though none of them are terrific. It's a tough area to stretch because it covers so much distance. Try both of these tosee which one brings you the best results.

FIGURE-4 STRETCH: This targets the upper, more muscular half of the ITB. Lie on your back and cross one ankle over the other knee so your legs resemble the numeral 4. Pull the bent leg up toward the chest. You'll feel the stretch in the outside of the hip. Hold for a few seconds and release. Repeat 5 times for both legs.

ROLL IT (SEE ILLUSTRATION BELOW): A 6- by 36-inch foam roller is the best tool for stretching the ITB. Lie on your side with the roller under your leg and roll it from your hip to your knee, using your body weight to knead the area. The pressure will help loosen the tendon and the fascia, almost like a self-massage. Do this at least once a day for several minutes, and make it a permanent part of your exercise activity.

IMPORTANT: Rolling the ITB will probably hurt like crazy for the first couple of weeks. This is normal. Don't stop. The pain is simply a signal that the ITB is tight and you need the treatment. As your ITB loosens, the pain gradually gets better. That's a terrific sign of progress.

• **Beef up your glutes and hips.** Weak butt and hip muscles contribute to ITB impingement syndrome. Make sure your lower-body work includes squats, especially single-leg squats, as well as multidirectional lunges (for more ideas, see next page).

• **Try orthotics.** As is the case with many lower-body injuries, foot mechanics often play a role. A motion-control shoe along with over-the-counter arch supports can help tremendously.

• **Cyclists, having a properly fitted bike can help you and triathletes who suffer from ITB impingement while riding.**

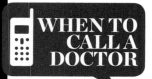

WHEN TO CALL A DOCTOR

If home-based care doesn't help, see a doctor. If your doctor diagnoses ITB impingement syndrome and physical therapy to strengthen and loosen tissue doesn't help, injection of a corticosteroid—a steroid that reduces swelling—into the bursa often helps. We also use this treatment when a patient has a race or athletic event coming up and a fast fix is needed.

Also, and this is important, remember that ITB pain generally occurs only while you're running. If your knee or hip pain comes while walking or doing other basic daily activities, see a doctor because you may not have ITB impingement syndrome. For example, arthritis in the hip or knee can cause pain while running and walking. Also, pain from a tear in the lateral meniscus, part of the cartilage inside the knee that sits just beneath the ITB, can mimic ITB pain. Again, this pain will come with both running and walking. Either way, you need to see your doctor for a proper diagnosis and treatment.

DO YOU NEED SURGERY?
Almost never.

Cont'd on page 56

PREVENT IT

Always remember: A strong butt is the key to a happy life. Weak glutes and hip muscles contribute to ITB impingement syndrome. A computer-driven lifestyle makes it easy for that area of your body to become deconditioned; the more you sit and stare at a screen, the weaker your glutes become, contributing to hip imbalances and instability. Build up your glutes and you reinforce the body's largest and potentially most powerful muscle group. You can increase overall dynamic flexibility by using the Iron Strength workout section of this book (see page 256). But even if you don't use those specific workouts, the stretches and exercises here all help build up your glutes and hip flexors and can be added to any workout.

LYING GLUTE STRETCH

Lie faceup on the floor with your knees and hips bent. Cross your left leg over your right so that your left ankle sits across your right thigh. Grab your left knee with both hands and pull it toward the middle of your chest until you feel a comfortable stretch in your glutes. Hold for 30 seconds, then repeat on the opposite side. Repeat twice for a total of three sets—and several times a day if you're really tight.

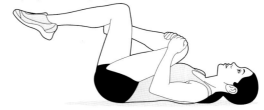

REVERSE HIP RAISE

Lie chest-down on the edge of a bench or Roman chair so that your torso is on the bench but your hips aren't. Keeping your legs nearly straight, lift them until your thighs are in line with your torso. Squeeze your glutes as you lift your hips. Pause, then lower to the starting position. **NOTE:** You can also do this exercise while lying on a Swiss ball with your hands flat on the floor.

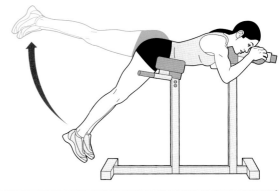

HIP RAISE

Lie faceup on the floor with your knees bent and your feet flat on the floor. Place your arms out to your sides at 45-degree angles, your palms facing up. Raise your hips so your body forms a straight line from your shoulders to your knees. Squeeze your glutes as you raise your hips. Make sure you're pushing with your heels. To make it easier, you can position your feet so that your toes rise off the floor. Pause for 5 seconds in the up position, then lower your body back to the starting position.

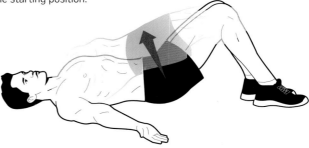

A BIG (BUTT) BONUS

Strong glutes don't just help prevent ITB impingement syndrome. As the largest muscle group, they're one of your body's biggest calorie burners. Plus, strong glutes and hip flexors keep your hips in alignment, reducing the chance of back pain and improving your posture.

LOW SIDE-TO-SIDE LUNGE

Stand with your feet set about twice shoulder-length apart, your feet facing straight ahead. Clasp your hands in front of your chest (or hold dumbbells at your sides).

Shift your weight over to your right leg as you push your hips backward and lower your body by dropping your hips and bending your knees. Your lower right leg should remain nearly perpendicular to the floor. Your left foot should remain flat on the floor.

Without raising yourself back up to a standing position, reverse the movement to the left. Alternate back and forth.

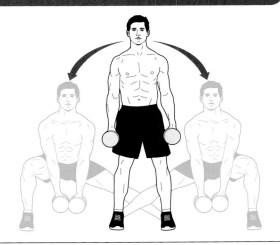

STANDING RESISTANCE-BAND HIP ABDUCTION

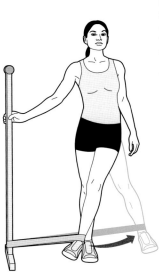

Secure a miniband to a sturdy object, then loop it around your left ankle. Start with your legs as close to each other as you can while keeping resistance on your working leg. Place your hand on a sturdy object for support. Raise your left leg straight out to the side, as far as you can. Pause, then return to the starting position. Perform the prescribed number of repetitions, then turn around and do the same number with your right leg. **NOTE:** This exercise can also be done with an ankle strap on the low pulley of a cable station.

LATERAL BAND WALKS

Place both legs between a miniband and position the band just above your knees. Take small steps to your right for 20 feet. Then sidestep back to your left for 20 feet. That's one set.

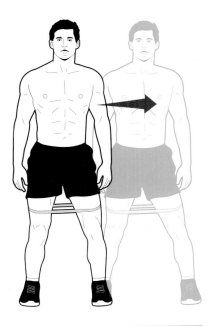

HAMSTRINGS
HIPS
GLUTES
& GROIN

This is one of the most complex and interrelated sections of the kinetic chain. When you really start talking about muscles and connective tissues working together, complementing one another, much of it happens in the space between your knees and belly button. As you read, you'll see that what you feel as groin pain may have nothing to do with your groin, and that sometimes the butt's not involved in a classic "pain in the butt." These are injuries you want to address quickly because ignoring them can have such massive impacts on all the other parts working around it. Let's see how it all works.

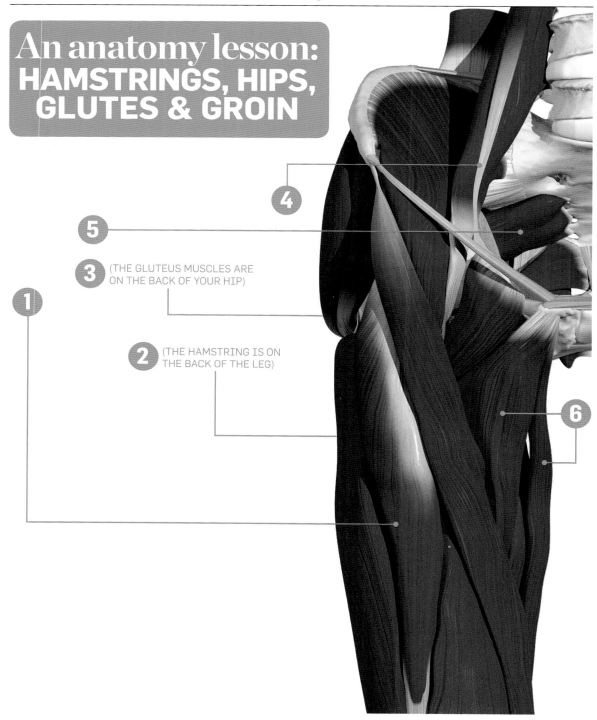

An anatomy lesson:
HAMSTRINGS, HIPS, GLUTES & GROIN

4

5

3 (THE GLUTEUS MUSCLES ARE ON THE BACK OF YOUR HIP)

1

2 (THE HAMSTRING IS ON THE BACK OF THE LEG)

6

2 HAMSTRING

A set of three muscles running behind your upper leg—the biceps femoris, semitendinosus, and semimembranosus. They help bend your knee and also work with your glutes to extend your hip. They also help rotate your thigh inward and outward.

1 QUADRICEP

A group of four muscles in the upper leg, the vastus lateralis, vastus medialis, vastus intermedius, and rectus femoris. The latter runs from the hip to the knee, crossing both joints. The quads help you extend your leg at the knee, and they also act as knee stabilizers.

3 GLUTEUS MUSCLES

Three muscles make up the gluteus group: the gluteus maximus (the biggest muscle in the body), gluteus medius, and gluteus minimus. They are your "butt" muscles, which help stabilize your pelvis and help with virtually any athletic lower-body movement (running, jumping, etc).

5 PIRIFORMIS

This muscle lies deep within the pelvis, running behind the hip joint over the sciatic nerve. It helps with external hip rotation. Too much sitting can make the muscle tighten, irritating the sciatic nerve.

4 ILIOPSOAS, A.K.A. HIP FLEXORS

(pronounced ILL-ee-o-so-AS) are two large bands of muscle, one on either side of your spine, that attach to the vertebrae in your lower back and run through the pelvis to hook up with the inner sides of each femur. The band is comprised of the psoas and iliacus, which helps draw your knees up to your chest.

6 ADDUCTOR

A collection of muscles running from the groin down along the inside of the femur. Commonly referred to as your "groin" muscle—i.e., a strained groin—the adductors are working anytime you bring your knees and thighs together.

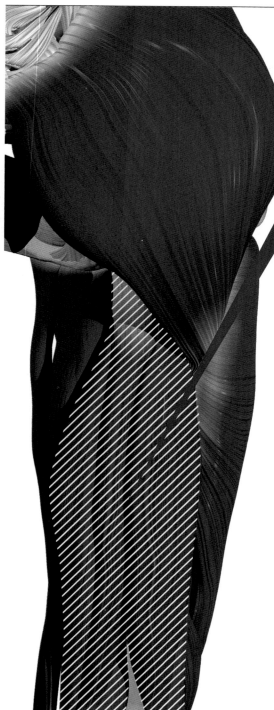

THE MALADY:
Strained (Pulled) Hamstring

THE SYMPTOMS

Tightness or pain, sometimes severe, when you apply pressure to the hamstring or load the muscle group.

WHAT'S GOING ON IN THERE?

The hamstring is a combination of three muscles that originate at the ischial tuberosity (the part of the pelvis you feel when you sit down) and run along the back of the leg until they connect with bone just below the knee. Since the muscle group spans both the hip and the knee, the hamstring responds to two sets of forces from top to bottom, serving as both a hip extensor and a knee flexor.

Unfortunately, the hamstrings aren't ideally constructed for sports. The proximal hamstring, the section at the top near the hip, and the distal hamstring, the lower section near the knee, have poor blood supplies. This means slow healing rates. The middle, meaty portion of the hamstring has an excellent blood supply and heals much more quickly.

When the hamstring is injured, the key to fixing it is to first recognize the injury. A hamstring strain is typically the result of pushing too hard and, most important, not paying enough attention to pain cues.

For information on the more specific "pain in the butt" hamstring strain, see "Proximal Hamstring Strain" on page 66.

FIX IT

- **Stop.** When you feel hamstring pain, stop what you're doing. Trying to push through it will only make it worse.

- **Employ dynamic rest.** Avoid hamstring-loading activities and do intense upper-body and core workouts to maintain fitness.

- **Ice it.** As soon as you can after the injury, start applying ice to the muscle for 15 minutes at a time 4 to 6 times a day for the first 2 days.

- **Stretch it—gently.** After a few days, perform gentle hamstring stretches several times a day (see below). Depending on the severity of the strain, expect a healing time of anywhere from 2 to 8 weeks.

- **Work it—gradually.** As the pain recedes, ease yourself back into activity, particularly speed and hill work. If you feel pain, don't push it. Also, use the "Prevent It" exercises on the following pages to rehab the muscle.

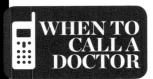

WHEN TO CALL A DOCTOR

Severe hamstring strains generally heal after 8 weeks. If you still have pain after that, see a doctor. MRIs and ultrasounds can show the details of what's going on in the muscle and how much damage you have, along with any other issues you may not know about.

A sports doc can also prescribe professional physical therapy and other remedies. Newer treatments such as platelet-rich plasma (PRP) may offer some hope to those suffering from lingering hamstring injuries. In this treatment, the patient's own plasma is injected into the injury site to speed healing because areas with poor bloodflow (like the proximal and distal hamstring) heal slowly. Many sports docs are involved in clinical trials to assess the efficacy of PRP, and so far the results have been encouraging.

DO YOU NEED SURGERY?

Hamstring surgery is rare but not unheard of, and it is used only to repair significant tears or ruptures. If that's your problem, trust me, you'll know it.

STANDING HAMSTRING STRETCH

Place your right foot on a bench or secure chair. Your right leg should be completely straight. Your left leg should be slightly bent. Stand tall with your back naturally arched. Place your hands on your hips. Without rounding your lower back, bend at the hips and lower your torso until you feel a comfortable stretch. Hold the stretch for 30 seconds on each side, then repeat 2 times. Do the routine up to 3 times a day if you're really tight.
NOTE: Bending your plant knee more increases the stretch near your hip; keeping it straight increases the stretch at your knee. Rotating the toes of your stretching leg outward emphasizes the inner portion of your hamstring; rotating your toes inward emphasizes the outer portion.

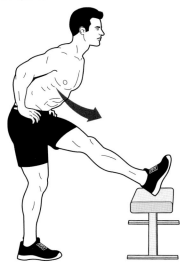

LYING GLUTE STRETCH

Lie faceup on the floor with your knees and hips bent. Cross your left leg over your right so that your left ankle sits across your right thigh. Grab your left knee with both hands and pull it toward the middle of your chest until you feel a comfortable stretch in your glutes. Hold for 30 seconds, then repeat on the opposite side. Repeat twice for a total of three sets—and several times a day if you're really tight.

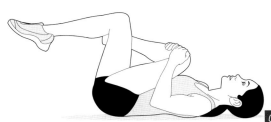

Cont'd on page 64

PREVENT IT

The point can't be made enough: A strong butt is the key to a happy life. You need to work your glutes, hip flexors, quads, and core as well as your hamstrings if you want to prevent a pulled hammie. All these muscles work together and need to be strong, flexible, and balanced. Isolated hamstring curls can work the hamstrings alone, but for better results stick with multimuscle exercises. You can increase overall dynamic flexibility by using the Iron Strength workout section of this book (see page 256). But even if you don't use those specific workouts, the stretches and exercises here can be added to any workout.

HIP RAISE

Lie faceup on the floor with your knees bent and your feet flat on the floor. Place your arms out to your sides at 45-degree angles, your palms facing up. Raise your hips so your body forms a straight line from your shoulders to your knees. Squeeze your glutes as you raise your hips. Make sure you're pushing with your heels. To make it easier, you can position your feet so that your toes rise off the floor. Pause for 5 seconds in the up position, then lower your body back to the starting position.

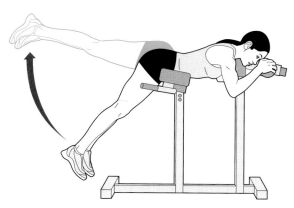

REVERSE HIP RAISE

Lie chest-down on the edge of a bench or Roman chair so that your torso is on the bench but your hips aren't. Keeping your legs nearly straight, lift them until your thighs are in line with your torso. Squeeze your glutes as you lift your hips. Pause, then lower to the starting position.
NOTE: You can also do this exercise while lying on a Swiss ball with your hands flat on the floor for stability.

A BIG BONUS

Strong hamstrings and glutes don't just prevent injury. Your anterior cruciate ligaments (ACLs) rely on your hamstrings to help them stabilize your knees. And your glutes, the biggest muscle group in your body, help you burn more calories as well as provide pelvic stability, which improves posture. Hammies and glutes can also play a big part in lower-back pain—keeping them strong and flexible is a key to eliminating backaches.

DON'T FORGET THESE IMPORTANT HAMSTRING BUILDERS...

- Sprints/intervals
- Sprints with directional change, such as figure 8, shuttle runs (suicides), or cone drills
- Hill sprints
- Stairs
- Indoor/outdoor rock climbing

AVOID A QUAD/HAMSTRING IMBALANCE

An *American Journal of Sports Medicine* study found that 7 out of 10 athletes with recurring hamstring injuries had muscle imbalances between their quadriceps and hamstrings. After correcting the imbalance by strengthening the hamstrings, every person in the study went injury free for the entire 12-month follow-up.

BACK EXTENSION

Position yourself in the back extension station and hook your feet under the leg anchors. Keeping your back naturally arched, place your fingers on the back your head and lower your upper body as far as you comfortably can. Squeeze your glutes and raise your torso until it's in line with your lower body. Pause, then slowly lower your torso back to the starting position.

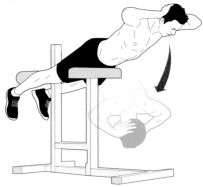

DUMBBELL STEPUP

Hold a pair of dumbbells at arm's length at your sides. Stand in front of a bench or step and place your right foot firmly on the step. The step should be high enough that your knee is bent 90 degrees. Press your right heel into the step and push your body up until your right leg is straight and you're standing on one leg, keeping your left foot elevated. Lower your body back down until your left foot touches the floor. That's one rep. Complete the prescribed number of reps with your right leg, then do the same number with your left leg.

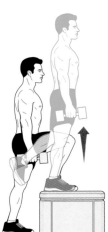

WALKING LUNGE (DUMBBELLS OPTIONAL)

Perform a lunge, but instead of pushing your body backward to the starting position, raise up and bring your back foot forward so that you move forward (as though you're walking) a step with every rep. Alternate the leg you step forward with each time.

When you complete the prescribed number of repetitions, perform backward walking lunges to return to your starting point.

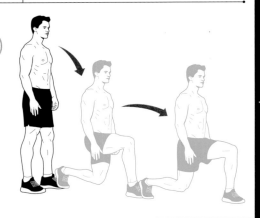

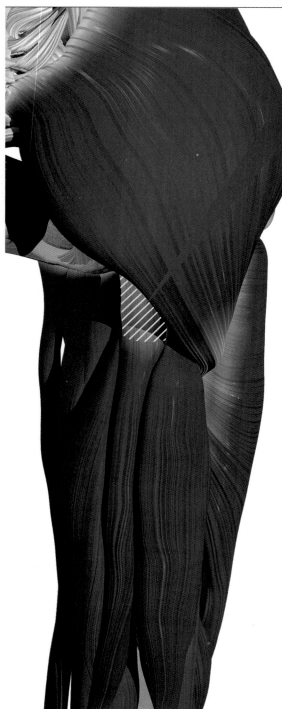

THE MALADY:
Proximal Hamstring Strain
(aka pain in the butt)

THE SYMPTOMS

Discomfort in the gluteus muscle where the hamstring originates, especially during the push-off phase of running and other sports. The harder you push, the harder it grabs.

WHAT'S GOING ON IN THERE?

Gluteal pain can signal several injuries— a strained glute or piriformis muscle, or inflammation of the sciatic nerve—but when the pain is associated with the push-off phase of running, it's a hamstring strain.

The hamstring, a set of three muscles running from your ischial tuberosity (the pelvic bones you feel when you sit down) down the back of your leg to just below the knee, is divided into three sections: the distal hamstring (the section near the knee), the middle hamstring, and the proximal hamstring (the section near the hip). The "pain in the butt" hamstring strain is in the proximal hamstring, and it presents difficulties that are different from those posed by lower hamstring strains.

Strains come from overuse, pushing the muscle too hard, or weakness in the surrounding muscles. A mild strain begins as a dull ache in the buttock, and if not treated, it progresses to a sharp pain that prohibits you from using the leg with any power.

What's worse, the proximal hamstring has a lousy blood supply, which means it takes longer to heal than middle hamstring strains do.

FIX IT

- **Stop.** As soon as you feel gluteal pain, stop your athletic activity immediately. If you try to push through the pain, you'll make the injury worse.

- **Employ dynamic rest.** Avoid hamstring-loading activities and do intense upper-body and core workouts to maintain fitness.

- **Ice it.** As soon as you can after the injury, start applying ice to the muscle for 15 minutes at a time 4 to 6 times a day for the first 2 days.

- **Stretch it—gently.** After a few days, perform gentle hamstring stretches several times a day (see below). Depending on the severity of the strain, expect a healing time of anywhere from 2 to 8 weeks. More severe strains could take longer.

- **Work it—gradually.** As pain recedes, ease yourself back into activity, particularly speed and hill work. If you feel pain, don't push it. Also, use the "Prevent It" exercises on the following pages to rehab the muscle.

STANDING HAMSTRING STRETCH

Place your right foot on a bench or secure chair. Your right leg should be completely straight. Your left leg should be slightly bent. Stand tall with your back naturally arched. Place your hands on your hips. Without rounding your lower back, bend at the hips and lower your torso until you feel a comfortable stretch. Hold the stretch for 30 seconds on each side, then repeat 2 times. Do the routine up to 3 times a day if you're really tight.
NOTE: To target the proximal hamstring, bend your plant knee more to increase the stretch near your hip. Keeping the plant leg straight increases the stretch at your knee. Rotating the toes of your stretching leg outward emphasizes the inner portion of your hamstring; rotating your toes inward emphasizes the outer portion.

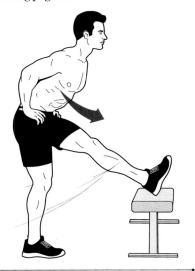

LYING GLUTE STRETCH

Lie faceup on the floor with your knees and hips bent. Cross your left leg over your right so that your left ankle sits across your right thigh. Grab your left knee with both hands and pull it toward the middle of your chest until you feel a comfortable stretch in your glutes. Hold for 30 seconds, then repeat on the opposite side. Repeat twice for a total of three sets—and several times a day if you're really tight.

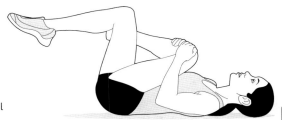

WHEN TO CALL A DOCTOR

If a tincture of time and gradual stretching and activity hasn't fixed the problem after 8 weeks, see a doctor. An ultrasound or MRI can identify a severe injury or tear. A sports doc can give you a more targeted prescription based on your individual case, including a physical therapy plan that can help you rehab as well as a progressive program of stretching and strengthening to get you back to normal activity.

Platelet-rich plasma (PRP) is new, but is increasingly being used with good results on proximal hamstring strains that don't heal within 6 months. The procedure entails the patient's own plasma being injected into the affected area to speed healing.

DO YOU NEED SURGERY?

Hamstring surgery is rare but not unheard of, and it is used only to repair significant tears or ruptures. If that's your problem, trust me, you'll know it.

Cont'd on page 68

PREVENT IT

I say it because it's true: A strong butt is the key to a happy life. Weak glutes create activation problems for the muscles that come off the pelvis and allow pelvic rotation and instability, which can cause injuries. Strong butt muscles keep your pelvis level. You can increase overall dynamic flexibility by using the Iron Strength workout section of this book (see page 256). But even if you don't use those specific workouts, the stretches and exercises here build powerful glutes, hamstrings, quads, and hips and can be added to any workout.

HAMSTRINGS ROLL

Place a foam roller under your right knee, with your leg straight. Cross your left leg over your right ankle. Put your hands flat on the floor for support. Keep your back naturally arched.

Roll your body forward until the roller reaches your glutes. Then roll back and forth. Repeat with the roller under your left knee.

NOTE: If rolling one leg is too difficult, perform the movement with both legs on the roller, as shown.

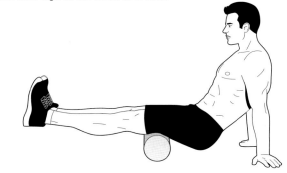

GLUTES ROLL

Sit on a foam roller with it positioned on the back of your right thigh, just below your glutes. Cross your right leg over the front of your left thigh. Put your hands flat on the floor for support.

Roll your body forward until the roller reaches your lower back. Then roll back and forth. Repeat with the roller under your left glute.

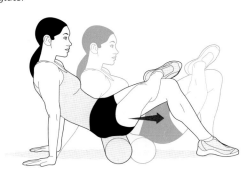

BODYWEIGHT JUMP SQUATS

Place your fingers on the back of your head and pull your elbows back so that they're in line with your body. Perform a bodyweight squat until your thighs are parallel to the floor, then explosively jump as high as you can (imagine you're pushing the floor away from you as you leap). When you land, immediately squat and jump again. Hold dumbbells at your side to make it more challenging.

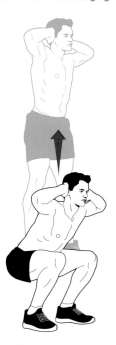

SHORTEN YOUR STRIDE

Distance runners, shortening your stride can reduce stress on the hamstring. To test the length of your stride, time yourself. Your right foot should strike the ground 85 to 90 times a minute.

DON'T FORGET THESE IMPORTANT HAMSTRING BUILDERS...

- Sprints/intervals
- Sprints with directional change, such as figure 8, shuttle runs (suicides), or cone drills
- Hill sprints
- Stairs
- Indoor/outdoor rock climbing

REFIT YOUR BIKE
Cyclists, checking the fit of your bike—specifically the height of your saddle—can help. A too-high saddle puts more stress on the hamstring.

SPLIT JUMP (WITH OR WITHOUT DUMBBELLS)

Stand in a staggered stance, your right foot in front of your left. Lower your body as far as you can. Quickly switch directions and jump with enough force to propel both feet off the floor. While in the air, scissor-kick your legs so you land with the opposite leg forward. Repeat, alternating back and forth with each repetition.

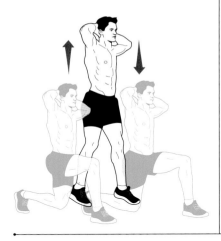

PISTOL SQUAT (WITH OPTIONAL PLYO)

Stand holding your arms straight out in front of your body. Raise your right leg off the floor. Keeping your right leg straight, push your hips back and lower your body as far as you can without breaking form. As you do this, raise your right leg so that it doesn't touch the floor, and keep your torso as upright as possible. Pause, then push your body back to the starting position. Do equal reps for each leg.

For a bigger challenge, as you rise out of the squat, add in a jump off your plant leg.

PLANK

Get into pushup position, but bend your elbows and rest your weight on your forearms. Your body should form a straight line from your shoulders to your ankles. Brace your core and hold. Let your fitness level determine how long you hold the plank, but 30 seconds to a minute is good, while I recommend 3 to 6 minutes total plank time.

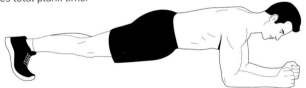

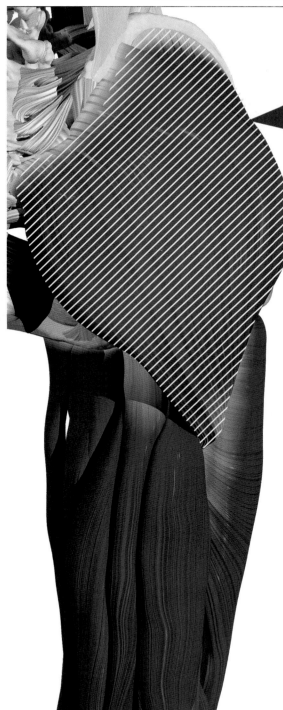

THE MALADY:
Postworkout Quad and/or Glute Soreness
(including delayed-onset muscle soreness)

THE SYMPTOMS

General muscle soreness, especially the day after an intense workout or starting a new activity. However, delayed-onset muscle soreness, a specific and serious condition, can be incredibly painful.

WHAT'S GOING ON IN THERE?

When muscle tissue is injured by exercise, the fibers tear. Ideally, in a day or two the fibers repair themselves and are stronger than before. This is the basis of building muscle, and normal muscle soreness after a workout—especially during the first few weeks of intensified activity—is to be expected.

If your muscle soreness is intense and doesn't begin until 24 to 48 hours after the muscle injury, however, you may have a serious condition called delayed-onset muscle soreness (DOMS). It can happen when you apply an excessive loading force to muscle cells. It's important to distinguish the symptoms of DOMS from the everyday aches and pains that come after hard exercise. This pain can be severe.

Why is DOMS serious? When muscle tissue is injured, a process called rhabdomyolysis causes it to release a protein called myoglobin. We all have a bit of myoglobin released after hard athletic events, and some of it is processed by the kidneys. Several studies that looked at healthy athletes after marathons found mild to moderate amounts of myoglobin in their urine, a condition called myoglobinuria. When the muscle injury is more serious, however, the amount of myoglobin can be quite large. The urine can be a dark color, and in some cases kidney damage and even kidney failure can result.

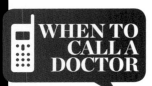

WHEN TO CALL A DOCTOR

If your muscle pain and soreness are severe and seemed to come on 24 to 48 hours after hard activity and your urine is dark, see your doctor immediately.

Your doctor will do a urinalysis to check your myoglobin level and, if necessary, perform blood tests to determine if there's been any kidney damage.

DOMS is much more common than most athletes realize. Why some athletes experience DOMS and others don't is not yet understood, but one of the most important factors is dehydration before, during, and after intense activity. However, regardless of their hydration status, some athletes just seem prone to developing DOMS and get it often, probably because of biological and genetic factors affecting their muscle tissue.

The good news: DOMS is usually preventable with education and smart pre-exercise behavior.

DO YOU NEED SURGERY?
No.

FIX IT

Normal postworkout soreness:

- **Hydrate, fuel up, sleep well.** Give your body the best opportunity to repair muscle damage and come back strong. Drink fluids until your urine is clear, eat smart, and get a great night's sleep. The best restoration and recovery happen while you sleep.

- **Try an NSAID.** An antiinflammatory like ibuprofen or naproxen can help alleviate soreness.

Delayed-onset muscle soreness:

- **Hydrate and see your doctor.** If you suspect you have DOMS, start drinking lots of fluids and call your doctor. A sports doctor is a better bet than a primary care physician because he or she will have more experience identifying DOMS.

PREVENT IT

- **Hydrate.** Proper hydration before engaging in any exercise or athletic event can help ease common postexercise muscle soreness and, more important, prevent DOMS. Factors to consider: temperature and humidity level (Vegas versus Seattle), the intensity of effort you plan on reaching (race versus easy run), and your overall health during the previous week (even a mild stomach bug or case of diarrhea can dehydrate you). Drink enough fluids to keep your urine running clear.

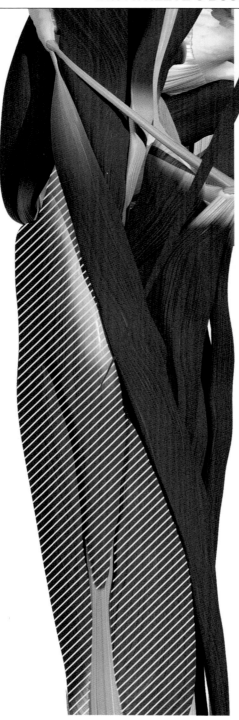

THE MALADY:
Strained Quad

THE SYMPTOMS

Anything from a twinge to a sharp pain in the thigh, depending on the severity of the strain. Trying to straighten the leg against resistance causes pain. Swelling and bruising are possible. For grade 2 or 3 strains, the pain affects walking.

WHAT'S GOING ON IN THERE?

The quadriceps group, at the front of the upper leg, is a set of four muscles (thus quads): the vastus lateralis, vastus medialis, vastus intermedius, and rectus femoris. The last muscle is the one most commonly strained because it runs from the hip to the knee and crosses both joints, thus facing the double jeopardy of hip and knee stress. However, the most common site of a strain is at the point where the muscle turns into tendon just above the knee.

Sprinting, jumping, or kicking is usually the cause, though any movement can cause a strain.

FIX IT

- **Employ dynamic rest.** Avoid loading the leg, especially in the acute stage (the first 48 to 72 hours after the injury, depending on the severity). Concentrate on intense upper-body and core work to maintain fitness.

- **Ice it.** Apply ice for 15 minutes 4 to 6 times a day for the first 2 days.

- **Compress and elevate.** Applying a compression bandage and elevating the leg can help with swelling and inflammation.

- **Stretch it—gently.** Several days after the strain, if it's comfortable, perform gentle quad stretches for 20 to 30 seconds several times a day. Also do hip flexor stretches: Kneel with the knee on the strained side on the floor and the other leg out front with the knee bent (sort of like a lunge, but with the back knee on the floor). Keeping your back straight, push your hips forward until you feel the stretch in the hip and thigh. Hold for 20 to 30 seconds. Do 3 reps several times a day (also try the stretch illustrated below).

- **Strengthen it—gradually.** Three quad exercises work well for rebuilding the injured muscle. Ease into them slowly and do only as many reps as comfort allows. As time goes on, you should be able to do them more easily and with more intensity. For the straight-leg raise, sit on the floor with your back straight and your legs straight out in front of you. Slowly raise the strained leg, keeping it straight. Hold for a moment, then lower it. The other two exercises are common lunges and squats. For single-leg exercises, be sure to do equal reps with both legs to avoid muscle imbalance (see the next page for more ideas).

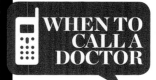

WHEN TO CALL A DOCTOR

For a severe strain (if walking is difficult), or if you don't get adequate relief for a milder strain with home-based treatment, see a doctor.

A sports doc uses an MRI to determine the extent and specifics of the injury. In addition to suggesting stretching and strengthening exercises, a doctor or physical therapist can prescribe ultrasound or electro-stimulation treatment, as well as sports massage.

DO YOU NEED SURGERY?

Only in the case of a full rupture, which is very rare.

KNEELING HIP FLEXOR STRETCH

Kneel down on your left knee, with your right foot on the floor and your right knee bent 90 degrees. Reach up with your right hand as high as you can. Contract your butt, brace your abs, and bend your torso to the right. Then rotate your torso to the right as you reach with your right hand as far behind you as you can. You should feel the stretch in your left hip and quad. Hold this position for 30 seconds. Then kneel on your right knee, switch arms, and repeat. Do two more sets for a total of three. Perform this stretch daily, or up to 3 times a day if you're really tight.

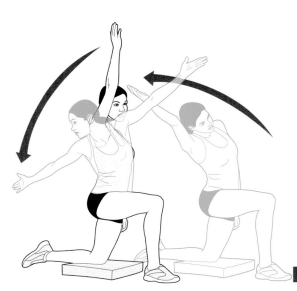

Cont'd on page 74

PREVENT IT

Strong, flexible, and balanced muscles throughout your lower body will help prevent quad strains (or any strains, for that matter). But your quads are of particular help when it comes to potentially more serious injuries. Building them up also helps make your knees more stable and less susceptible to breakdown. You can increase overall dynamic flexibility by using the Iron Strength workout section of this book (see page 256). But even if you don't use those specific workouts, the stretches and exercises here all help build powerful legs and can be added to any workout.

QUADRICEPS-AND-HIP-FLEXORS ROLL

Lie facedown on the floor with a foam roller positioned above your left knee. Cross your right leg over your left ankle and place your elbows on the floor for support.

Roll your body backward until the roller reaches the top of your left thigh. Then roll back and forth. Repeat with the roller under your right thigh. (If that's too hard, perform the movement with both thighs on the roller.)

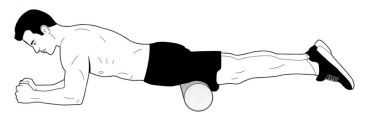

REVERSE LUNGE WITH REACH BACK

Stand tall with your arms hanging at your side. Brace your core and hold it that way. Lunge back with your right leg, lowering your body until your left knee is bent at least 90 degrees.

As you lunge, reach back over your shoulders and to the left. Reverse the movement back to the starting position.

Complete the prescribed number of reps with your right leg, then step back with your left leg and reach over your right shoulder for the same number of reps. Keep your torso upright for the entire movement.

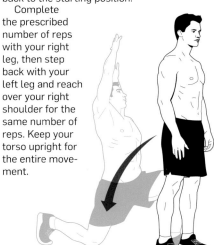

BODY-WEIGHT JUMP SQUATS

Place your fingers on the back of your head and pull your elbows back so that they're in line with your body. Perform a bodyweight squat until your thighs are parallel to the floor, then explosively jump as high as you can (imagine you're pushing the floor away from you as you leap). When you land, immediately squat and jump again. Hold dumbbells at your side to make it more challenging.

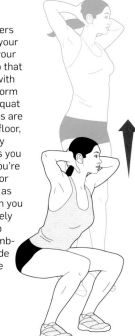

PISTOL SQUAT (WITH OPTIONAL PLYO)

Stand holding your arms straight out in front of your body at shoulder level, parallel to the floor. Raise your right leg off the floor and hold it there. Keeping your right leg straight, push your hips back and lower your body as far as you can without breaking form. As you do this, raise your right leg so that it doesn't touch the floor, and keep your torso as upright as possible. Pause, then push your body back to the starting position. Perform equal reps for each leg.

For a bigger challenge, as you rise out of the squat, add in a jump off your plant leg.

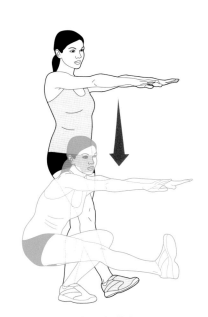

SPLIT JUMP (WITH OR WITHOUT DUMBBELLS)

Stand in a staggered stance, your right foot in front of your left. Lower your body as far as you can. Quickly switch directions and jump with enough force to propel both feet off the floor. While in the air, scissor-kick your legs so you land with the opposite leg forward. Repeat, alternating back and forth with each repetition.

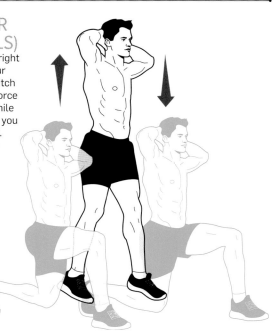

DON'T FORGET ABOUT THESE INCREDIBLE LEG BUILDERS...

- Uphill walking
- Uphill sprinting
- Sprints with directional change, such as figure 8, shuttle runs (suicides), or cone drills
- Stairs
- Pool running or aerobics
- Cycling
- Indoor/outdoor rock climbing

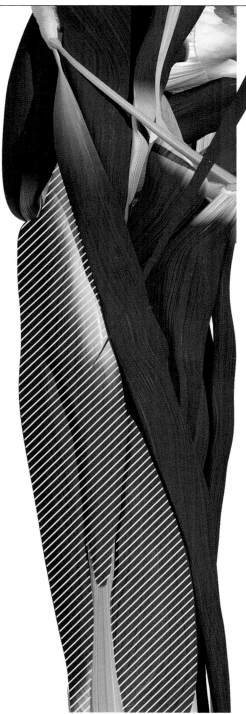

THE MALADY:
Quad Cramp

THE SYMPTOMS
An involuntary and painful contraction of a quad muscle that refuses to relax.

WHAT'S GOING ON IN THERE?
Several things can trigger a muscle cramp. The most common are nutritional: You're dehydrated or don't have enough sodium (salt) in your body. Fatigue and working a muscle when it's "short"—not fully extended—are less common causes. The triggering factor, whatever it is, makes the muscle edgy and it anticipates contraction, which can lead it to simply contract on its own. This is why muscle cramps are more common at the end of a race or game.

Of the four quad muscles, the rectus femoris is most prone to cramping because it attaches above the hip and below the knee, crossing both joints. The other three muscles—the vastus lateralis, vastus medialis, and vastus intermedius—connect only at the top of the femur and at the knee. This simply means that the rectus femoris has more opportunity to contract when it's short because two things can shorten it—knee extension and hip flexion (imagine yourself sitting with your leg out straight and lifting it while keeping it straight—that's how you shorten the rectus femoris). This muscle works harder than its quad buddies.

FIX IT

- **Break the cramp.** The fastest way to break a cramp is to stretch the contracted muscle, i.e., slowly extend it from its contracted state. In the quads' case, pull your foot back toward your butt to stretch out the muscle. Don't yank it. Gently and gradually stretch it.

- **Watch the hammie.** If one muscle cramps, another one might as well, and when you stretch the quad, you shorten the hamstring. To prevent a reciprocal hammie cramp, be mind-ful not to contract or fire the muscle as you stretch out the quad. This may sound difficult, but just concentrate on relaxing your leg as you stretch.

- **Hydrate and get salty.** Pound the fluids and up your salt intake—pretzels and pickle juice are fast sources. This strategy will also help prevent other cramps.

PREVENT IT

- **Get in better shape.** Train a muscle so it's stronger and less prone to fatigue and you'll prevent cramping. In the case of quads, explosive bodyweight exercises like squats and lunges are musts. If you're a cyclist prone to having cramps, increase your training to put more distance between the mileage you need to complete and your fatigue threshold.

- **Stretch.** Regular quad stretching can help keep the muscles loose and your legs limber.

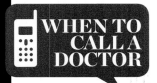

WHEN TO CALL A DOCTOR

Cramping isn't normally something that sends you to a doctor. However, if you get chronic cramps that no amount of training and home-based treatment seems to help, it's worth it to consult with a sports doctor.

The doctor will try to determine if your cramps are caused by a nutritional or functional trigger. If it's nutritional, the problem may be fixed by increased fluid and salt intake. If it's functional, you'll start working on stretching and strengthening.

DO YOU NEED SURGERY?
No.

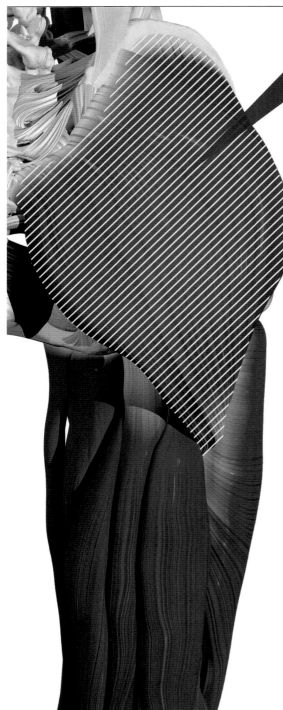

THE MALADY: Strained Glute Muscle

THE SYMPTOMS

A sharp pain or pulling sensation in the glutes, its intensity depending on the grade of the strain. In mild cases, the pain increases after activity but doesn't make you stop doing it. More severe strains could have you limping off the field immediately. Running, jumping, and lunging will cause pain, but you'll also feel pain walking up or down stairs, walking uphill, and possibly even sitting.

WHAT'S GOING ON IN THERE?

Three muscles make up the gluteal group: the gluteus maximus, gluteus medius, and gluteus minimus. They connect on the pelvis and the femur. They help stabilize the pelvis and are integral to running, jumping, squatting, and lunging.

Strains most commonly occur when the muscles contract while in the middle of a stretch. Examples include suddenly accelerating while running, doing weighted squats in a gym, and jumping. Naturally, athletes in football, basketball, track and field, and soccer are prime candidates for glute strains. They also can occur during weight training. The older you are and the less you warm up before an activity, the greater your strain risk.

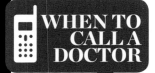

WHEN TO CALL A DOCTOR

FIX IT

- **Employ dynamic rest.** Avoid running, jumping, lunging, and stairs. Swimming could work if you can do it pain free. Do intense upper-body workouts to maintain fitness.

- **Ice it.** Apply ice for 15 minutes 4 to 6 times a day for the first 2 days.

- **Try an NSAID.** An antiinflammatory like ibuprofen or naproxen can help with swelling and inflammation.

- **Stretch and strengthen your glutes.** When you can perform these simple exercises without too much discomfort, start slowly and gradually increase your effort until you can do a set of 10 to 20 reps 3 times a day.

GLUTEAL STRETCH: Lie on your back. Raise your knee to your chest and use your hands to pull the knee toward your opposite shoulder.

Hold for several seconds. That's 1 rep. Do both sides even if only one side is injured.

GLUTEAL BRIDGE: Lie on your back with your knees raised and your feet flat on the floor. Brace yourself with your hands and arms and raise your hips until your knees, hips, and shoulders are in a straight line. You should feel your glutes flex. Hold for several seconds, then lower yourself. That's 1 rep.

CHAIR SQUATS: Stand in front of a chair and do a squat onto the chair, then stand. Work your way up to six sets of 15 reps. Then do one-legged chair squats, up to several sets of 15 reps on each leg. All of this will get you strong enough to do squats without the chair.

- **Also try . . .**

In the case of a grade 3 strain (rupture), you'll have no choice but to see a doc. But for less severe cases, 2 to 6 weeks is the general time frame for healing. If pain persists longer, see a sports doctor.

Physical therapy, including ultrasound and electrostimulation treatments, can help heal the muscle.

DO YOU NEED SURGERY?

For a rupture, surgery may be required. In that case, you generally will be out of action for 6 months or more.

LYING GLUTE STRETCH

Lie faceup on the floor with your knees and hips bent. Cross your left leg over your right so that your left ankle sits across your right thigh. Grab your left knee with both hands and pull it toward the middle of your chest until you feel a comfortable stretch in your glutes. Hold for 30 seconds, then repeat on the opposite side. Repeat twice for a total of three sets—and several times a day if you're really tight.

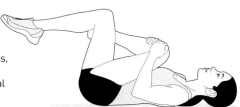

GLUTES ROLL

Sit on a foam roller with it positioned on the back of your right thigh, just below your glutes. Cross your right leg over the front of your left thigh. Put your hands flat on the floor for support.

Roll your body forward until the roller reaches your lower back. Then roll back and forth. Repeat with the roller under your left glute.

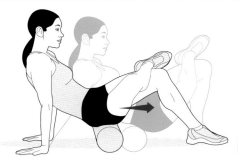

Cont'd on page 80

PREVENT IT

I keep saying it because it's true: A strong butt is the key to a happy life. Weak glutes create activation problems for the muscles that come off the pelvis and allow pelvic rotation and instability, which can cause injuries. Strong butt muscles keep your pelvis level. The secret? Pay attention to your core, hips, and hamstrings. Your glutes work closely with that entire system of muscles—they form a big part of the kinetic chain—and weakness or instability in one or more of those areas can affect how your glutes perform. You can increase overall dynamic flexibility by using the Iron Strength workout section of this book (see page 256). But even if you don't use those specific workouts, the stretches and exercises here build powerful glutes, hamstrings, quads, and hips and can be added to any workout.

HAMSTRINGS ROLL

Place a foam roller under your right knee, with your leg straight. Cross your left leg over your right ankle. Put your hands flat on the floor for support. Keep your back naturally arched.

Roll your body forward until the roller reaches your glutes. Then roll back and forth. Repeat with the roller under your left knee.

NOTE: If rolling one leg is too difficult, perform the movement with both legs on the roller, as shown.

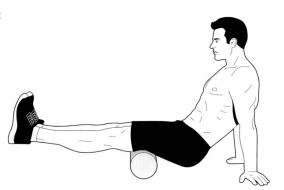

BODYWEIGHT JUMP SQUATS

Place your fingers on the back of your head and pull your elbows back so that they're in line with your body. Perform a bodyweight squat until your thighs are parallel to the floor, then explosively jump as high as you can (imagine you're pushing the floor away from you as you leap). When you land, immediately squat and jump again. Hold dumbbells at your side to make it more challenging.

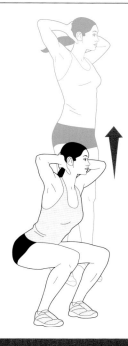

GIVE US THIS DAY, OUR DAILY PLANK
While giving a group of muscles time to recover after a workout is standard procedure for athletes, it's generally safe to work your core and glutes every day. But that's not an excuse to overwork them, either. Listen to your body.

BURPEES

Stand with your feet shoulder-width apart and arms at your sides (hexagonal dumbbells optional). Lower your body into as deep a squat as you can. Now kick your legs backward so that you're in pushup position. Do a pushup, then quickly bring your legs back into the squat position. Stand up quickly and jump. That's 1 rep.

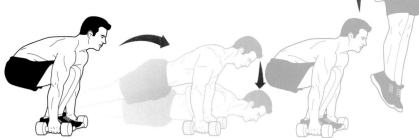

DON'T FORGET THESE IMPORTANT HAMSTRING AND GLUTE BUILDERS...

- Sprints/intervals
- Sprints with directional change, such as figure 8, shuttle runs (suicides), or cone drills
- Hill sprints
- Stairs
- Indoor/outdoor rock climbing

DUMBBELL SPLIT SQUAT

Hold a pair of dumbbells at arm's length next to your sides, your palms facing each other. Stand in a staggered stance, your right foot in front of your left, with your feet set 2 to 3 feet apart. Slowly lower your body as far as you can. Pause, then push yourself back up to starting position as quickly as you can. Keep your torso upright and brace your core for the entire movement. Halfway through the prescribed time, switch feet.

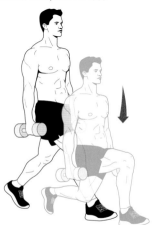

PLANK

Get into pushup position, but bend your elbows and rest your weight on your forearms. Your body should form a straight line from your shoulders to your ankles. Brace your core and hold. Let your fitness level determine how long you hold the plank, but 30 seconds to a minute is good, while I recommend 3 to 6 minutes total plank time.

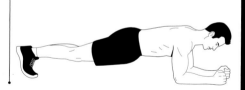

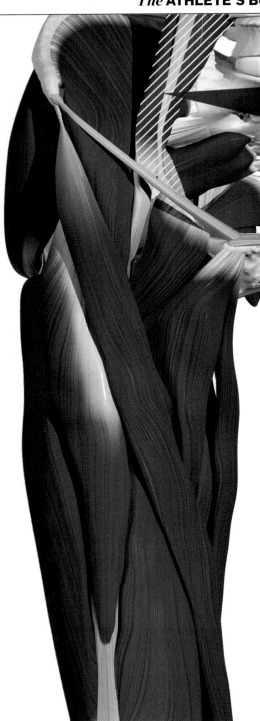

THE MALADY:
Iliopsoas (Hip Flexor) Strain and/or Tendinitis

THE SYMPTOMS

Pain in the front of the pelvis on either side, especially when the knees are raised toward the chest for an extended period (as when you pull your knee to your chest to tie your shoe, for example). Lower-back pain and patellar knee pain can also be symptomatic of iliopsoas problems.

WHAT'S GOING ON IN THERE?

The iliopsoas (pronounced ILL-ee-o-so-AS) is the combination of the psoas and iliacus muscles (a.k.a. the hip flexors), and they are seriously underrated muscles. They don't get nearly the press that hamstrings, glutes, and quads do, but they're equally as—if not more—important when it comes to everyday movement, as well as explosive athletic movement.

Why? First, consider the sheer size of the iliopsoas. They attach to the vertebrae in your lower back, one on either side, and run down through the pelvis to attach on the inner side of the femur. A well-developed iliopsoas can be several inches thick. These are big muscles.

Their role is twofold. First, they help support the spine. They help you bend forward at the waist (which is why a tight iliopsoas can cause lower-back pain). And second, they're your hip flexors, meaning that they help you draw your knee up to your chest. An injured iliopsoas is very bad news for an athlete.

Injuries usually happen due to one of two issues: an awkward or unexpected movement straining the muscle, or overuse caused by lots and lots of hip flexion or external rotation of the thigh, which can also lead to tendinitis. Name your sport and you're vulnerable: running (especially uphill), soccer, gymnastics, dance, rowing, and even resistance training.

To make matters worse, a tight iliopsoas can cause other injuries through the kinetic chain. Tight iliopsoas muscles can tilt the pelvis, which can bring on lower-back issues as well as affect your running stride, which in turn can lead to knee problems like patellar tendinitis.

Another iliopsoas issue is the so-called snapping hip syndrome, where a clicking or snapping sensation or sound occurs with hip flexion. If you have pain along with the snap, that could signal iliopsoas tendinitis or bursitis.

So you see, as I said in the introduction to this section, all of these muscles are interrelated and depend on one another for optimal performance.

FIX IT

- **Employ dynamic rest.** Avoid movement that stresses the iliopsoas (running, bending at the waist, any activity that forces you to raise your knee). Use intense upper-body workouts to maintain fitness.

- **Ice it.** Apply ice for 15 minutes 4 to 6 times a day for the first 2 days.

- **Try an NSAID.** An antiinflammatory like ibuprofen or naproxen can help with swelling and inflammation.

- **Stretch it.** As pain allows, gradually and gently begin basic hip flexor stretching: Kneel with one knee on the floor and the other leg out in front with your knee bent (sort of like a lunge, but with the back knee on the floor). Keeping your back straight, push your hips forward until you feel the stretch in the hip and thigh. Hold for 20 to 30 seconds. Do 3 reps several times a day. Don't hold your breath during the stretch.

You can also add a rectus femoris stretch to this move. Begin the hip flexor stretch as described, but instead of leaving the lower part of the rear leg on the floor, reach back and pull the foot up toward your butt. Again, push your hips forward and hold for 20 to 30 seconds for each of 3 reps performed several times a day.

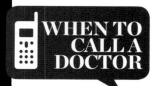

WHEN TO CALL A DOCTOR

If your pain doesn't improve, or if you have persistent issues with your lower back and/or knee, see a sports doctor. An MRI or ultrasound can help identify hip problems and also shed light on any other issues that may be contributing to your pain.

Another useful diagnostic test involves injecting a corticosteroid mixed with a local anesthetic like lidocaine into the iliopsoas. If your pain disappears, the source of your problem is clear. This requires a delicate injection because the tendon sheath of the iliopsoas is so small. Using ultrasound imaging to guide the injection has made this a much more effective therapy.

Chronic iliopsoas issues could respond to physical, chiropractic, or massage therapy to recondition and loosen the muscles. This is especially true in cases where the iliopsoas contributes to lower-back pain.

The good news: These home-based and medical therapies usually work wonders. Recovery, depending on the severity of the problem, generally takes 2 to 8 weeks.

DO YOU NEED SURGERY?

Never say never, but almost never. That's how rare it is.

Cont'd on page 84

PREVENT IT

Pay attention to your core, quads, glutes, and hamstrings. Your iliopsoas work closely with that entire system of muscles—they form a big part of the kinetic chain—and weakness or instability in one or more of those areas can affect all the others. You can increase overall dynamic flexibility by using the Iron Strength workout section of this book (see page 256). But even if you don't use those specific workouts, the stretches and exercises here build powerful glutes, hamstrings, quads, and hip flexors and can be added to any workout.

QUADRICEPS-AND-HIP-FLEXORS ROLL

Lie facedown on the floor with a foam roller positioned above your left knee. Cross your right leg over your left ankle and place your elbows on the floor for support.

Roll your body backward until the roller reaches the top of your left thigh. Then roll back and forth. Repeat with the roller under your right thigh. (If that's too hard, perform the movement with both thighs on the roller.)

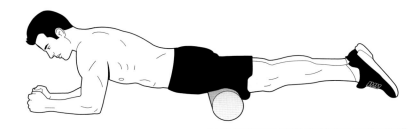

MOUNTAIN CLIMBERS

Get in pushup position with your arms straight. This is the starting position. Lift your right foot and raise your knee as close to your chest as you can. Touch the ground with your right foot and then return to the starting position and repeat with your left leg. Go as fast as possible.

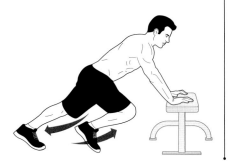

SWISS-BALL PIKE

Assume a pushup position with your arms completely straight. Position your hands slightly wider than and in line with your shoulders. Rest your shins on a Swiss ball. Your body should form a straight line from your head to your ankles. Without bending your knees, roll the Swiss ball toward your body by raising your hips as high as you can (push them toward the ceiling). Pause, then return the ball to the starting position by lowering your hips and rolling the ball backward.

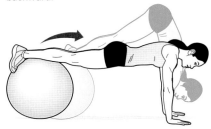

A BIG BONUS

Making good pelvic stability a priority doesn't just prevent hip flexor strains. Maintaining strength, flexibility, and balance in the glutes, hip flexors, hamstrings, and quads will prevent more serious injuries in your lower back and knees.

BODYWEIGHT JUMP SQUATS

Place your fingers on the back of your head and pull your elbows back so that they're in line with your body. Perform a bodyweight squat until your thighs are parallel to the floor, then explosively jump as high as you can (imagine you're pushing the floor away from you as you leap). When you land, immediately squat and jump again. Hold dumbbells at your side to make it more challenging.

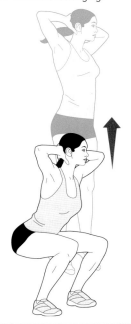

REVERSE LUNGE WITH REACH BACK

Stand tall with your arms hanging at your side. Brace your core and hold it that way. Lunge back with your right leg, lowering your body until your left knee is bent at least 90 degrees.

As you lunge, reach back over your shoulders and to the left. Reverse the movement back to the starting position.

Complete the prescribed number of reps with your right leg, then step back with your left leg and reach over your right shoulder for the same number of reps. Keep your torso upright for the entire movement.

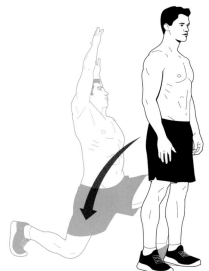

FUN AND HIP-FLEXOR-FRIENDLY ACTIVITIES...

- Sprints/ intervals (get those knees up!)
- Sprints with directional change, such as figure 8, shuttle runs (suicides), or cone drills
- Hill sprints
- Stairs
- Cycling
- Rowing
- Indoor/outdoor rock climbing

PLANK

Get into pushup position, but bend your elbows and rest your weight on your forearms. Your body should form a straight line from your shoulders to your ankles. Brace your core and hold. Let your fitness level determine how long you hold the plank, but 30 seconds to a minute is good, while I recommend 3 to 6 minutes total plank time.

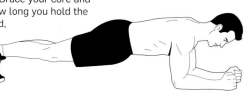

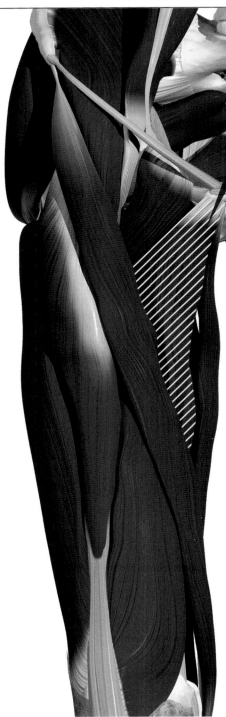

THE MALADY:
Strained Adductor
(groin strain)

THE SYMPTOMS

Pain in the inner thigh close to the groin. The pain can be sharp and severe with sudden injuries or a dull ache that gets worse over time with minor strains that become chronic because you "play through the pain." The amount of pain depends on the grade of the strain.

WHAT'S GOING ON IN THERE?

The adductor is a collection of muscles running from the groin down along the inside of the femur. They help you move from side to side as well as bring your knees together.

Injuries most often occur during an explosive change of direction or side-to-side movement, as well as sudden acceleration during a sprint. Kicking and twisting the leg can also be a factor. Which means that virtually all athletes are at risk.

Even bigger risk factors: Weakness and lack of flexibility in the adductor group. As with any muscle group, if it isn't trained for the job, it will fail when put to the test. See "Prevent It" for strengthening strategies.

A good way to determine if your injury is an adductor strain and not some other hip injury (a strained hip flexor, for example) is to try moving your knee inward toward the other knee against resistance. Pain in the inner thigh is your main clue. Depending on the grade of the strain, expect the healing time to range from a few days to more than a month, though grade 3 strains will require more time and a doctor's care (see "When to Call a Doctor").

FIX IT

- **Employ dynamic rest.** Avoid lower-body movement that will aggravate the adductor. Use intense upper-body workouts to maintain fitness. You can also work your core, but be careful to avoid movements that cause pain in the injured area—the hips and core work together in many movements.

- **Ice it.** Apply ice for 15 minutes 4 to 6 times a day for the first 2 days.

- **Try an NSAID.** An antiinflammatory like ibuprofen or naproxen can help with swelling and inflammation.

- **Stretch it.** When you can do so with little or no pain, begin basic stretching and strengthening exercises. Try these:

SITTING GROIN STRETCH: Sit on the floor with your knees bent to the sides and the bottoms of your feet pressed together. Press the tops of your knees down toward the floor with your elbows. Hold for 10 to 15 seconds, then release. Repeat 3 to 5 times.

STANDING GROIN STRETCH: Stand with your legs shoulder-width apart. Shift your weight to one side, bending your knee slightly. Stop when you feel a stretch in your adductor. Hold for 10 to 15 seconds, return to the starting position, and repeat 3 to 5 times.

- **Strengthen it.** When you can do so with little or no pain, do side and diagonal lunges, which are standard lunges except you do them to each side as well as diagonally to each side (forward and backward). Do a set of 5 in each direction, upping your reps and sets as you get stronger and become completely pain free.

PREVENT IT

- **Train your groin.** The best prevention for strains is to have a strong and supple set of adductors. Core work, multidirectional lunges, squats, and squat jumps should be staples of your lower-body work (yes, your core works with your adductors). Also add in skater plyos, which are explosive side lunges that mimic the motion of a speed skater: In a controlled manner, jump sideways from your right foot to land on your left foot while bringing your right foot behind the left leg and your right arm across your body to touch the floor outside your left foot. Lunging to both sides is 1 rep. Repeat 10 times.

- **Learn the slider:** If you have access to one, a lateral slide board, used with special sliding socks worn over your sneakers, gives your adductors a terrific workout.

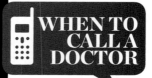

WHEN TO CALL A DOCTOR

Understand that the adductor muscles have a lousy blood supply and an abundant nerve supply, which means an injury will be painful and take longer to heal than other muscle strains. Home-based self-care as described here is usually effective, but expect complete healing in weeks rather than days. Platelet-rich plasma (PRP) injections have been used successfully and could be an option in cases that don't respond to conservative measures.

Severe strains, however, need medical attention. Any loss of function—if you have difficulty bringing one knee closer to the other—signals a severe tear or rupture. You'll need imaging (MRI and/or ultrasound) for your doctor to determine just how much damage there is and if it involves muscles, tendons, or both, as well as whether there's any nerve involvement.

DO YOU NEED SURGERY?

Surgery is a real possibility in the worst cases (though it's not guaranteed), and if it is needed, it will probably keep you out of action for 3 to 6 months. Patients usually have a full recovery.

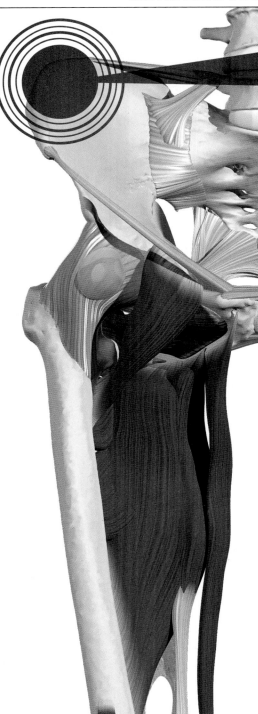

THE MALADY:
Hip Pointer

THE SYMPTOMS
Sudden pain—sometimes extreme—in the protruding point of the hip bone (the iliac crest) after being hit there.

WHAT'S GOING ON IN THERE?
A hip pointer is essentially a contusion of the tissue and/or bone around the iliac crest (the part of your pelvis on either side that feels literally like a bony point). Depending on how hard you're hit, the pain can be excruciating. The tissues in the area, including the bone and overlying muscle, are severely bruised.

Hip pointers most commonly happen in high-contact sports like football and hockey, though soccer players have their share as well. Basically, playing any sport where the hip bone can take a direct hit puts you at risk. Pre-teen and teen athletes are also at risk of damaging the growth plate in this area.

FIX IT

- **Employ dynamic rest.** Avoid any activity that causes pain, but what activities these are will vary with the severity of your injury. Maintain fitness with intense upper-body workouts, but engage the lower body as you're able to.

  IMPORTANT: While activities like swimming and stationary cycling may be possible, don't do them if you feel pain. This is especially true of running. If you try to "fight through it" and work with the pain, you could unconsciously alter your gait or other movements to compensate. That could cause another injury. If it hurts, back off immediately.

- **Ice it.** Apply ice for 15 minutes 4 to 6 times a day for the first 2 days. This is crucial for this kind of injury.

- **Try an NSAID.** An antiinflammatory like ibuprofen or naproxen can help with swelling and inflammation.

PREVENT IT

- **Use your pads.** If you play a full-contact sport like football or hockey, wear hip pads that completely cover the hip bone. You may not be able to prevent being hit, but there's no excuse for not being as protected as you can be while you play.

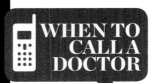

WHEN TO CALL A DOCTOR

A hip pointer generally doesn't require a doctor visit. However, if the pain hasn't improved after a week of home-based care, see a doctor to rule out a more serious injury. Hip pointers don't usually include a fracture, but it is possible.

DO YOU NEED SURGERY?
No.

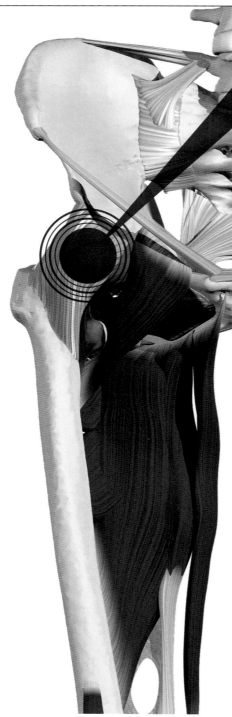

THE MALADY:
Hip Pain in Front of or in the Joint

THE SYMPTOMS

Pain emanating from the front or inside of the hip joint, not to be confused with groin pain and other nonhip injuries that can mimic a hip problem (see "What's Going On in There" to help yourself recognize the difference).

WHAT'S GOING ON IN THERE?

Hip injuries are common, and generalized hip and/or groin pain can mean a lot of different things. But the closer you look at the problem, the easier it probably will be to pinpoint exactly what you may be dealing with. If your hip joint and the region around it hurt and you don't know what the problem is, run through these quick self-diagnostic exercises for some of the most common conditions I see. This is no substitute for an actual sports doctor's exam, but these quick looks can point you in the right direction and help you determine if you should make the appointment.

• Does the pain hurt most at the footstrike when running or hopping on just that leg? Does it also hurt at night? It could be a stress fracture in the neck of the femur, where the bone leads into the ball-and-socket joint.
See "Hip Stress Fracture" on page 94.
• Does the pain come when you lift your knee, such as during the striding phase of running? It could be a strain or tendinitis of the iliopsoas muscle group. See "Iliopsoas (Hip Flexor) Strain and/or Tendinitis" on page 82.

• Does the pain come from the inside of the joint and without a specific source or trigger during general flexing of the hip? You could have arthritis. Osteoarthritis pain in the groin is achy and often hurts at night and first thing in the morning. If you also experience a "catching" sensation or locking of the joint, you could be dealing with a tear

in the labrum (the ring of cartilage around the rim of the socket that holds the ball of the femur in place). You could also have a tear of the articular cartilage inside the joint, which acts as a cushion. Read on for some home-based ways you can help yourself, but also check out "When to Call a Doctor" for more details about when to seek help.

FIX IT

The following remedies are effective for a cartilage tear and for relieving osteoarthritis symptoms.

• **Employ dynamic rest.** Rest the hip and especially avoid any jarring impacts on the joint. This will allow inflammation in the hip to calm down and relieve the pain. Concentrate on upper-body and core workouts to maintain fitness.

• **Try an NSAID.** An antiinflammatory like ibuprofen or naproxen can help with swelling and inflammation.

• **Strengthen the surrounding muscles.** The stronger the muscles around a joint, the more support the joint has during any activity. As your pain improves, gradually add and intensify core and low-impact lower-body exercises. Pilates, swimming, and cycling can all help strengthen the area. Don't start running or any other high-impact activity until you're pain free.

PREVENT IT

• **Intensify your conditioning.** You may not be able to prevent an acute hip injury that comes from a hit, bad twist, or fall. But overuse and degenerative conditions can be slowed or halted with proper conditioning. No matter what your sport is, prioritize

core and lower-body conditioning to protect your hips. Planks, multidirectional lunges, squats, squat jumps, burpees, and skater plyos are some of the simplest exercises to add to your regular program.

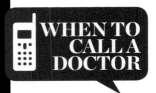

WHEN TO CALL A DOCTOR

See a doctor for hip pain that doesn't respond to home-based care within several weeks to a month. An exam with x-ray and MRI should give you a proper diagnosis, and you can move on from there with a more targeted approach.

If you have osteoarthritis, understand that since it's a degenerative condition, your symptoms will wax and wane as time goes on. The key for you is conditioning. Keep the muscles in the lower body strong.

DO YOU NEED SURGERY?
Not necessarily. A lot of people have labrum tears that show up on an MRI but aren't the source of their problem. If your doctor is leaning toward surgery, be sure to ask about the prevalence of false positives for labrum tears seen on MRIs. Also make sure you exhaust all conservative therapies and strengthening options before considering surgery.

If you do need it, expect a recovery time of 4 to 6 months. The vast majority of patients fully recover.

For arthristis sufferers, over time, the most severe cases can lead to hip replacement surgery, but that's usually in older patients.

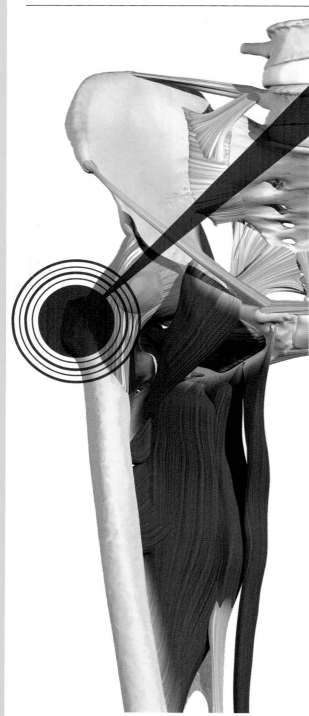

THE MALADY: Hip Pain on the Side, Away from the Joint

THE SYMPTOMS

Pain in the outer area of the hip, especially on the bump where the bone protrudes, during and after activities like running. The pain may intensify when you squat, get out of a chair, go up stairs, or push on that area. Lying on that side can also be painful.

WHAT'S GOING ON IN THERE?

The good news: Having pain in the outer part of the hip is much better than having pain in front of or inside the hip joint. Why? Pain in those other areas can signal cartilage tears, hip flexor strains or tendinitis, osteoarthritis, and other problems that can keep you out of action for a while (or become chronic and/or degenerative).

Side hip pain is most commonly caused by bursitis, inflammation of a fluid-filled sac called a bursa that helps cushion bones, tendons, and muscles where they come in contact with each other. In this case, the trochanteric bursa on the outside of the hip can be pinched by a tight muscle called the tensor fascia lata (TFL), which is the muscle that eventually becomes the iliotibial band (ITB), the muscle running down the side of your upper leg. In other words, a little sac of fluid is being bothered by a tight band of tissue. Pain results.

It's caused by various things: an impact on that area from a fall or being hit, overuse, or even possibly from lying on that side for too long.

FIX IT

- **Employ dynamic rest.** Avoid stressing the joint to allow the inflammation to subside. Do upper-body workouts to maintain fitness.

- **Ice it.** Apply ice for 15 minutes 4 to 6 times a day for the first 2 days.

- **Try an NSAID.** An antiinflammatory like ibuprofen or naproxen can help with swelling and inflammation.

- **Stretch it.** When the pain allows it, stretch the ITB and TFL by lying on your back, lifting the affected leg until it's vertical, then lowering it across your body until your knee is across your midline. Lower it as far as possible in that orientation and hold for 15 seconds, then raise the leg back up and return to the starting position. Do 3 to 5 reps.

- **Strengthen it.** The exercises recommended under "Prevent It" will strengthen your hips against injury.

PREVENT IT

- **Work the hips, TFL, and ITB.** Bursitis caused by an impact to the side of your hip may not be preventable, but the better shape that area is in, the better chance you have of avoiding or lessening the injury. First, be sure that core and lower-body training is a regular part of your program. The basics include planks, multidirectional lunges, squats, single-leg squats, squat jumps, and skater plyos. Second, use a foam roller regularly to help keep your ITB and TFL flexible, because it's very easy for them to tighten up. With the foam roller beneath you, lie on your side and roll up and down the length of your thigh from the hip bone to the knee. Repeat for several minutes on each side. Then do the same for your glutes. The perfect time to do this is while you're warming up for a workout. It may feel painful at first—that's okay. It just means the ITB and TFL are tight and you're working them. As you do this regularly over time, the pain will disappear.

WHEN TO CALL A DOCTOR

Trochanteric bursitis usually responds to home-based treatment and resolves by itself within a few days to a few weeks. If you still have pain after that period, see a sports doctor for a full exam.

Common treatments for tougher bursitis cases include physical therapy, electrostimulation, and corticosteroid injections. Doing one or all of these generally does the trick.

DO YOU NEED SURGERY?

It's rare. If surgery is needed, that usually means removal of the bursa.

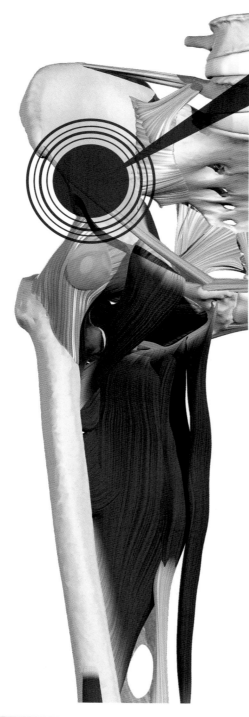

THE MALADY: Hip Stress Fracture

THE SYMPTOMS

Pain in the hip joint (sometimes perceived as groin pain) that worsens at the footstrike when running or hopping on just that leg. It can also hurt when lying down. With continued activity, the pain usually gets worse over time.

WHAT'S GOING ON IN THERE?

Hip injuries are common in all athletes, but this type of injury is especially common in runners and triathletes. A femoral neck stress fracture—a crack near the ball at the top of the femur—is the most serious. Stress fractures are almost always caused by overuse, usually by runners who try to "load" miles too fast in preparation for a big race. The bone simply cannot take the pounding.

If you have this type of pain, here are two questions to ask yourself: Have I upped my training workload too fast, too soon? And, How is my bone density? These aren't the only two factors involved, but they are the most common. (Then again, as the T-shirt says, sometimes stuff just happens.)

Low bone density (osteopenia) or very low bone density (osteoporosis) have several possible causes: genetics, as it tends to run in families; inadequate dietary calcium intake (1,300 milligrams a day is the recommended minimum); and for women, a history of menstrual disorders, e.g., not getting a period for more than 6 months can cause a low level of circulating estrogen.

The good news is that these variables can be altered or compensated for to help alleviate the problem.

FIX IT

- **Employ dynamic rest.** Stop any activity that impacts the hip joint. Use intense upper-body and core workouts to maintain fitness.

- **Supplement.** Eat more calcium- and vitamin D–rich foods or take supplements.

- **Slowly strengthen.** Your lower body will need some work once you're ready to resume activities. When you are pain free, gradually add lower-body strengthening exercises back into your workouts. Multidirectional lunges and squats will help, but avoid high-impact activity until your doctor gives you the all clear.

PREVENT IT

- **Up your calcium and vitamin D intakes.** Easy food sources are milk and yogurt, or take supplements. This is especially important if you have a family history of osteoporosis.

- **Follow the 10 percent rule.** Runners, never up your weekly mileage by more than 10 percent.

- **Train your hips and core.** The stronger the muscles in your core, glutes, hip, and leg are, the more support your hip joint will have against repetitive impacts. Make sure planks, multidirectional lunges, squats, squat jumps, and skater plyos are regular parts of your workouts.

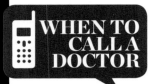

WHEN TO CALL A DOCTOR

With stress fractures, the earlier the better. Your doctor can confirm the diagnosis with x-rays and MRIs. However, stress fractures typically don't show up on x-rays unless they're very serious or already in the healing stage. The key is to treat both the symptoms and the causes, which you can do with the home-based tips found here. Your doctor will guide your care.

Depending on your individual case and family history, your doctor may also do a bone-density exam (using DEXA, or dual-energy x-ray absorptiometry). If you have low bone density, the doctor can treat you for osteopenia or osteoporosis.

Don't wait to see a doctor if you suspect you're developing a stress fracture. It will only get worse as you put more demand on it, and eventually it'll be so severe and painful that you won't be able to walk.

DO YOU NEED SURGERY?

Almost never, but in rare cases the hip stress fracture is large enough or in a worrisome location and requires surgery.

HAMSTRINGS, HIPS, GLUTES & GROIN

95

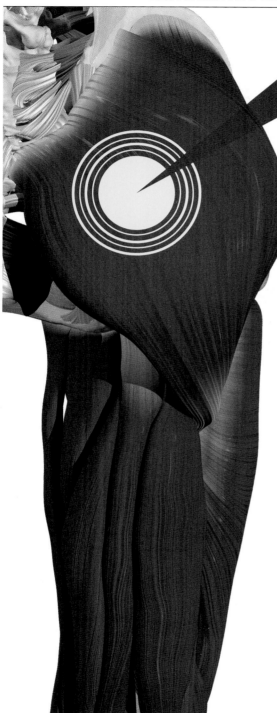

THE MALADY: Piriformis Syndrome

THE SYMPTOMS

Pain in the lower back and/or buttocks, sometimes feeling as if it's deep inside the buttock muscles. It may be too painful to sit on the affected buttock. The pain and/or tingling can radiate down the backs of the legs as well.

WHAT'S GOING ON IN THERE?

The piriformis muscle runs behind the hip joint and aids in external hip rotation, or turning your leg outward. The catch here is that the piriformis crosses over the sciatic nerve. The piriformis muscle can become tight from, for example, too much sitting (a problem many working people can relate to). The muscle can also be strained by spasm or overuse. In piriformis syndrome, this tightness or spasm causes the muscle to compress and irritate the sciatic nerve. This brings on lower-back and buttock pain, sometimes severe. The diagnosis is tricky because piriformis syndrome can very easily be confused with sciatica.

The difference between these diagnoses is that traditional sciatica is generally caused by some spinal issue, like a compressed lumbar disc. Piriformis syndrome becomes the go-to diagnosis when sciatica is present with no discernible spinal cause.

Runners, cyclists, and rowers are the athletes most at risk for piriformis syndrome. They engage in pure forward movement, which can weaken hip adductors and abductors, the muscles that allow us to open and close our legs. Throw in some weak glutes, and all those poorly conditioned muscles put extra strain on the piriformis. And you've got a painful problem.

Another risk for runners: Overpronating (when your foot turns inward) can cause the knee to rotate on impact. The piriformis fires to help prevent the knee from rotating too much, which can lead to overuse and tightening of the muscle.

FIX IT

- **Employ dynamic rest.** Stop the offending activity (if your pain is moderate to severe, you'll want to anyway). Use upper-body workouts to maintain fitness. Core work will probably be a problem, because your lower back and glutes will hurt. Let the pain be your guide and back off immediately if you do anything that hurts.

- **Try an NSAID.** An antiinflammatory like ibuprofen or naproxen can help with swelling and inflammation.

- **Stretch your hip rotators.** As pain allows, try to gradually open up your hips by stretching your hip flexors and rotators. These two stretches can help.

SEATED PIRIFORMIS STRETCH:
While sitting in a chair with your back straight, rest your ankle on your opposite knee. Then gently press down on your knee until you feel a stretch in your hip. Hold for 10 to 15 seconds. Repeat several times for each hip.

LYING PIRIFORMIS STRETCH:
Lie on your back with your knees raised and your feet flat on the floor. Put your right ankle on your left knee. Raise your left foot while pressing down on your right knee until you feel the stretch in your hip and buttock. Hold for 10 to 15 seconds. Repeat several times, then reverse the leg positions to stretch the left side and do a few reps.

You can find additional hip flexor stretches in the "Iliopsoas (Hip Flexor) Strain and/or Tendinitis" section on page 82.

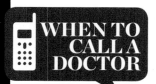

WHEN TO CALL A DOCTOR

If home-based care doesn't improve your symptoms in a week (or sooner if the pain is severe), see a doctor. A sports doctor may continue with conservative treatments like those mentioned here, but you'll also have a thorough examination to confirm the diagnosis, which, as I mentioned, can be tricky to determine given the similarity to sciatica. Also, a doctor may prescribe muscle relaxers that could be more effective than over-the-counter NSAIDs.

If conservative treatments fail, your doctor could opt for injections. A local anesthetic (lidocaine), corticosteroids, or even Botox—or a combination of them—can be used. Injections are tricky because of how deep the piriformis is in the hip, but injections guided by ultrasound for appropriate needle placement generally bring good results.

DO YOU NEED SURGERY?
Surgery is very rare.

Cont'd on page 98

PREVENT IT

Many of the interconnected muscles in this region—piriformis, glutes, hip flexors, hamstrings, quads—support one another, and weakness in one area can mess up the works. In short, if you want healthy piriformis muscles, you need to prioritize total-body fitness. You can increase overall dynamic flexibility by using the Iron Strength workout section of this book (see page 256). But even if you don't use those specific workouts, the stretches and exercises here build powerful glutes, hamstrings, quads, and hip flexors and can be added to any workout.

GLUTES ROLL

Sit on a foam roller with it positioned on the back of your right thigh, just below your glutes. Cross your right leg over the front of your left thigh. Put your hands flat on the floor for support.

Roll your body forward until the roller reaches your lower back. Then roll back and forth. Repeat with the roller under your left glute.

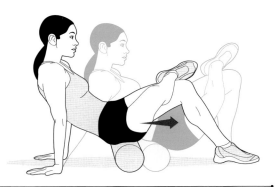

FIRE HYDRANT IN-OUT

Get down on your hands and knees with your palms flat on the floor and shoulder width apart. Relax your core so that your lower back and abdomen are in their natural positions. Without allowing your lower-back posture to change, raise your right knee as close as you can to your chest (your knee may not move forward much). Keeping your right knee bent, raise your thigh out to the side without moving your hips. Kick your raised right leg straight back until it's in line with your torso. That's 1 rep.

STANDING RESISTANCE-BAND HIP ABDUCTION

Secure a miniband to a sturdy object, then loop it around your left ankle. Start with your legs as close to each other as you can while keeping resistance on your working leg. Raise your left leg straight out to the side, as far as you can. Pause, then return to the starting position. Be sure to perform equal reps for each leg. **NOTE:** This exercise can also be done with an ankle strap on the low pulley of a cable station.

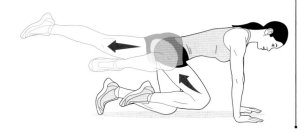

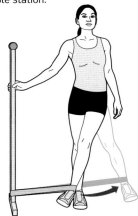

TRY ORTHOTICS
Motion-control shoes and over-the-counter arch supports can help with overpronation and reduce the chain reaction between the knee and the piriformis.

LATERAL BAND WALKS

Place both legs between a miniband and position the band just above your knees. Take small steps to your right for 20 feet. Then sidestep back to your left for 20 feet. That's one set.

BODYWEIGHT JUMP SQUATS

Place your fingers on the back of your head and pull your elbows back so that they're in line with your body. Perform a bodyweight squat until your thighs are parallel to the floor, then explosively jump as high as you can (imagine you're pushing the floor away from you as you leap). When you land, immediately squat and jump again. Hold dumbbells at your side to make it more challenging.

DON'T FORGET ABOUT THESE INCREDIBLE LEG BUILDERS...

- Uphill walking
- Uphill sprinting
- Sprints with directional change, such as figure 8, shuttle runs (suicides), or cone drills
- Stairs
- Pool running or aerobics
- Cycling
- Indoor/outdoor rock climbing

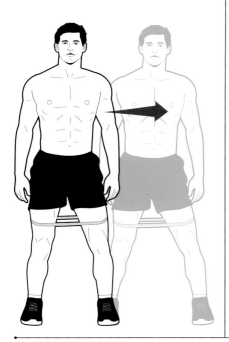

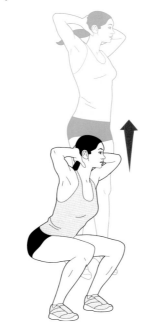

PLANK

Get into pushup position, but bend your elbows and rest your weight on your forearms. Your body should form a straight line from your shoulders to your ankles. Brace your core and hold. Let your fitness level determine how long you hold the plank, but 30 seconds to a minute is good, while I recommend 3 to 6 minutes total plank time.

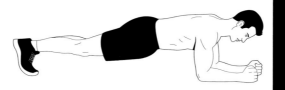

LOWER BACK

Lower-back pain is a very common complaint among my patients. Roughly four out of five people will have lower-back pain at some point. Why is it so prevalent? As wonderful a structure as the spine is—bending, twisting, holding us up—it's also vulnerable. It's a long string of nerves, muscles, and bones that all work in conjunction with the rest of the kinetic chain. When it's hurt, besides the pain (which can be excruciating), an injured back robs us of movement, strength, and flexibility. In short, we can't do a blessed thing. Another reason problems are so common: Issues with your core, hips, glutes, and hamstrings can all help set off the pain. Put simply, there are a lot of ways to hurt your back. Because it's so common, we now have several effective ways to treat it, especially home-based remedies. Read on and find out how to banish back pain for good.

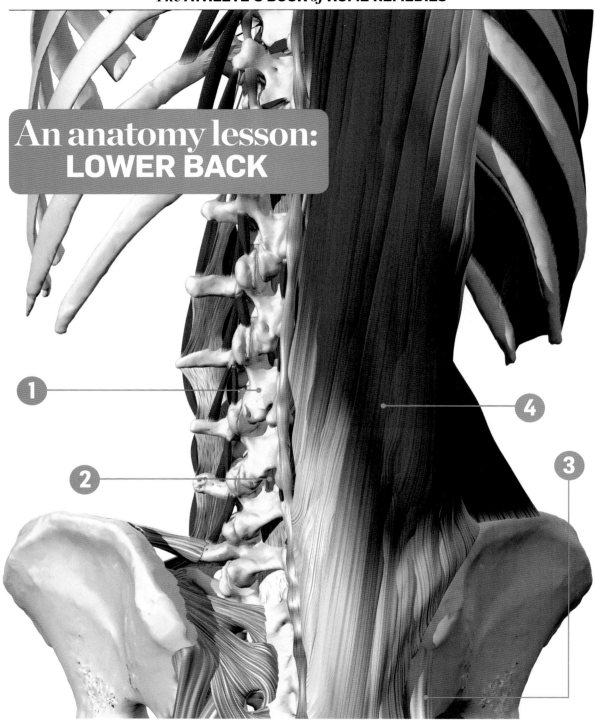

An anatomy lesson:
LOWER BACK

①

②

④

③

② INTERVERTEBRAL DISK

Shock absorbing tissue between vertebrae. A disk, made of cartilage, resembles a compressed marshmallow. They tend to degenerate with age and activity. If part of the disk lining tears, the interior material of the disk may bulge outward and affect nerves of the spinal cord.

① LUMBAR VERTEBRAE

The vertebrae in the lower section of the spine (the thoracic and cervical being the middle and upper sections, respectively). Each vertebra has its own designation from L1 to L5 and disco-genic lower back pain originates from one or more of these points.

③ SCIATIC NERVE

A thick, rope-like nerve that's com-prised of several nerve roots in the lumbar spine that merge into one. "Sciatica,' or irritation of this nerve, generally occurs in the area where the nerves have joined together.

④ PARASPINOUS MUSCLES. A.K.A. THE ERECTOR SPINAE MUSCLES

The muscles that help support, stabi-lize, and move the spine. They run next to the spine from the back of the hip up to the bottom of the skull. They're among the body's strongest muscles.

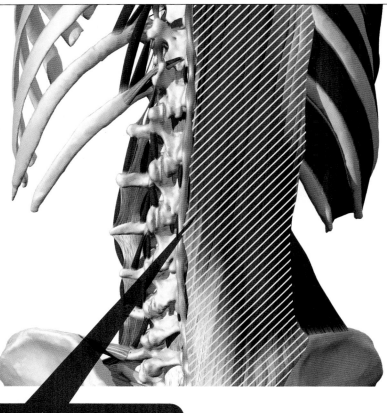

THE MALADY:
Lower-Back Spasms
(muscular back pain)

THE SYMPTOMS

Muscular back pain usually comes on instantly. Pain radiates from both sides of the spine and the muscles feel as though they're locked up. It can be severe and debilitating.

WHAT'S GOING ON IN THERE?

Muscular back pain is the most common type of back pain. It involves the paraspinal muscles, also known as the erector spinae muscle group, which are strong muscles on either side of the spine that enable you to move, twist, and bend the spine. These muscles run from the back of the hip, along the spine, and all the way up to the bottom of the skull. They're among the strongest muscles in the body.

So what brings on the pain? In general, the paraspinous muscles are too tight, too weak, or both. A sudden twisting or wrenching, bending forward, and even a direct impact on the muscle can set it off. Also, discogenic back pain—from a herniated disk—can cause nerves to fire to lock up the muscles (see page 108).

Other muscle groups can also contribute to back pain. If you have weak or tight hamstrings, core muscles, glutes, or hip flexors, it could affect your body alignment, mechanics, or other factors that could force your back muscles to compensate and overextend themselves.

- **Employ dynamic rest.** Bad back spasms will make you want to lie down for, oh, several years or so. Don't. Don't lie down even for an afternoon. Stay mobile, even if it means taking little shuffle steps around the house. Bed rest during spells of back pain only deconditions your muscles, which is the opposite of what you want to happen. During the acute stage, avoid straining your back, but do simple stretches to loosen your hamstrings, hip flexors, and glutes (see examples below). All of these can help alleviate the spasms.

- **Ice it, then heat it.** Apply ice for 15 minutes 4 to 6 times a day for the first 2 days. After 48 hours, using a heating pad at the same time intervals can help relieve the spasms.

- **Try an NSAID.** An antiinflammatory like ibuprofen or naproxen can help with pain and inflammation.

- **Vary your therapies.** Effective back pain therapies are very individualized.

For example, some of my patients respond well to massage therapy. Acupuncture can also be effective for muscular back pain. Chiropractic can help as well, but for muscular back pain only (not discogenic pain, in my opinion). Also, for chiropractic, your treatment should continue only for a limited time based on the severity of your injury and include a fitness and flexibility component. My point: Try different therapies until you get results. Everyone responds differently to different things.

- **Stretch and strengthen your kinetic chain.** As the pain subsides, start the reconditioning process with basic core strengthening and stretching exercises. Go slow. Stretch your hamstrings, hip flexors, glutes, and core. Do glute bridges and planks, adding reps and intensity as you improve. Once you're pain free, up your kinetic chain conditioning (see "Prevent It" on the following page).

LYING GLUTE STRETCH

Lie faceup on the floor with your knees and hips bent. Cross your left leg over your right so that your left ankle sits across your right thigh. Grab your left knee with both hands and pull it toward the middle of your chest until you feel a comfortable stretch in your glutes. Hold for 30 seconds, then repeat on the opposite side. Repeat twice for a total of three sets—and several times a day if you're really tight.

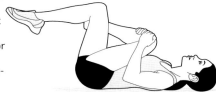

HAMSTRINGS ROLL

Place a foam roller under your right knee, with your leg straight. Cross your left leg over your right ankle. Put your hands flat on the floor for support. Keep your back naturally arched.

Roll your body forward until the roller reaches your glutes. Then roll back and forth. Repeat with the roller under your left knee.
NOTE: If rolling one leg is too difficult, perform the movement with both legs on the roller, as shown.

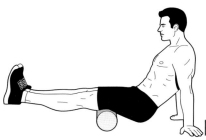

Cont'd on page 106

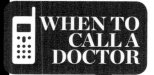

WHEN TO CALL A DOCTOR

In general, muscular back pain doesn't require a doctor's visit, but if your pain is bad, it could be a good idea. Doctors see a lot of back pain cases, so you'll get a thorough going-over to ensure that there is no other underlying issue, such as osteoarthritis or spinal stenosis, to name two.

X-rays can rule out bone issues, and an MRI can illuminate disk issues, though that may not be helpful. Herniated lumbar disks that show up might have nothing to do with your back pain (studies have shown that 30 to 40 percent of folks who have no back pain whatsoever have herniated disks).

A doctor can also prescribe muscle relaxers, which can help alleviate the spasms and allow you to begin rehabbing.

DO YOU NEED SURGERY?

No. Muscular back pain almost always improves with these conservative, home-based measures. One helpful hint: Never forget how painful back spasms can be; it's a great motivator to keep your core in top condition to prevent another flare-up.

LOWER BACK

PREVENT IT

Back pain prevention isn't just about strengthening your back muscles. Your back is working in combination with the rest of your core and your glutes, hip flexors, hamstrings, and quads for optimal performance. If you have weakness or imbalance in one of those areas, you can develop back pain. Your best results come when you target all of those areas. You can increase overall dynamic flexibility by using the Iron Strength workout section of this book (see page 256). But even if you don't use those specific workouts, the stretches and exercises here can be added to any workout.

PLANK

Get into pushup position, but bend your elbows and rest your weight on your forearms. Your body should form a straight line from your shoulders to your ankles. Brace your core and hold. Let your fitness level determine how long you hold the plank, but 30 seconds to a minute is good, while I recommend 3 to 6 minutes total plank time.

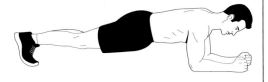

PRONE COBRA

Lie facedown on the floor with your legs straight and your arms next to your sides, palms down.

Contract your glutes and the muscles of your lower back, and raise your head, chest, arms, and legs off the floor.

Simultaneously rotate your arms so that your thumbs point toward the ceiling. At this time, your hips should be the only parts of your body touching the floor. Hold this position for the prescribed time. (Note: If you can't hold it for the entire time, hold for 5 to 10 seconds, rest for 5, and repeat as many times as needed. If the exercise is too easy, you can hold light dumbbells in your hands while you do it.)

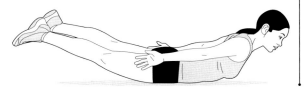

BACK EXTENSION

Position yourself in the back extension station and hook your feet under the leg anchors. Keeping your back naturally arched, place your hands behind your head and lower your upper body as far as you comfortably can. Squeeze your glutes and raise your torso until it's in line with your lower body. Pause, then slowly lower your torso back to the starting position.

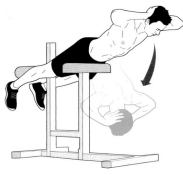

GET SOME CLASS

I highly recommend regular Pilates and yoga classes. The overall effect on your flexibility and core strength will be life-changing. I promise you'll find yourself able to achieve physical feats you couldn't do before. Just hit classes a couple times a week on top of your regular regimen.

SWISS-BALL PIKE

Assume a pushup position with your arms completely straight. Position your hands slightly wider than and in line with your shoulders. Rest your shins on a Swiss ball. Your body should form a straight line from your head to your ankles. Without bending your knees, roll the Swiss ball toward your body by raising your hips as high as you can (push them toward the ceiling). Pause, then return the ball to the starting position by lowering your hips and rolling the ball backward.

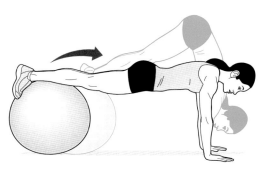

HIP RAISE

Lie faceup on the floor with your knees bent and your feet flat on the floor. Place your arms out to your sides at 45-degree angles, your palms facing up. Raise your hips so your body forms a straight line from your shoulders to your knees. Squeeze your glutes as you raise your hips. Make sure you're pushing with your heels. To make it easier, you can position your feet so that your toes rise off the floor. Pause for 5 seconds in the up position, then lower your body back to the starting position.

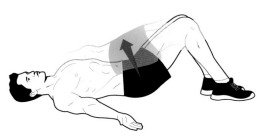

REVERSE HIP RAISE

Lie chest-down on the edge of a bench or Roman chair so that your torso is on the bench but your hips aren't. Keeping your legs nearly straight, lift them until your thighs are in line with your torso. Squeeze your glutes as you lift your hips. Pause, then lower to the starting position. **NOTE:** You can also do this exercise while lying on a Swiss ball with your hands flat on the floor for stability.

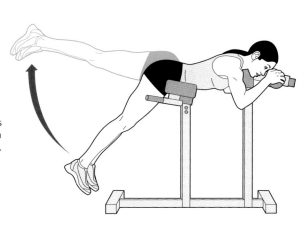

SERIOUS LOWER BACK PROTECTION

Some other intense exercises that build up your core, glutes, hip flexors, quads, and hamstrings—all of which protect your lower back...

- Multidirectional lunges
- Core work, especially with resistance and trunk rotation
- Squats and squat jumps
- Burpees
- Mountain climbers
- Medicine ball slams
- Rowing
- Indoor/outdoor rock climbing

LOWER BACK

107

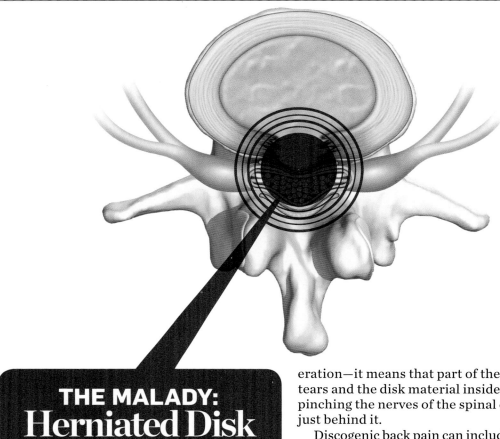

THE MALADY:
Herniated Disk
(slipped disk)

THE SYMPTOMS
Debilitating lower-back pain combined with pain shooting down the backs of the legs (one or both).

WHAT'S GOING ON IN THERE?
Discogenic back pain, aka a slipped or herniated disk, is a more complex issue than simple muscular back pain. The intervertebral disks, which are made of cartilage, are built like marshmallows and sit between the vertebrae for cushioning. When an athlete "slips" a disk—most commonly as the result of a direct impact, a wrenching movement, or degeneration—it means that part of the disk lining tears and the disk material inside bulges out, pinching the nerves of the spinal cord that lie just behind it.

Discogenic back pain can include muscular lower-back pain if the nearby muscles spasm, but a clear signal that the problem's origin is in a disk is pain that shoots down the back of one or both legs. This comes from the irritation of spinal nerves. The biggest nerve in that equation in the lower back is the sciatic nerve, a long, ropelike nerve comprising several nerve roots in the lumbar (lower) spine. For more info, see "Sciatica" on page 110.

Also understand that other muscle groups can contribute to lower-back pain. If you have weak or tight hamstrings, core muscles, glutes, or hip flexors, they could affect your body alignment, mechanics, or other factors that could force your back muscles to compensate and overextend themselves, compromising spinal support and causing injury.

FIX IT

- **Employ dynamic rest.** You'll want to lie down, but minimize the amount of time you spend on your back. Stay mobile, even if it means taking little shuffle steps around the house. Bed rest during spells of back pain only deconditions your muscles, which is the opposite of what you want to happen. During the acute stage, avoid straining your back, but do simple stretches to loosen your hamstrings, hip flexors, and glutes. All of these can help alleviate the spasms.

- **Ice it, then heat it.** Apply ice for 15 minutes 4 to 6 times a day for the first 2 days. After 2 days, using a heating pad at the same time intervals can help relieve the spasms.

- **Try an NSAID.** An antiinflammatory like ibuprofen or naproxen can help with pain and inflammation.

- **Vary your therapies.** Effective pain relief therapies are very individualized. For example, some of my patients respond well to massage therapy. Others swear by acupuncture, though in my experience it works better for muscular, nondiscogenic back pain. My point: Try different therapies until you get results. Everyone responds differently to different things.

- **Stretch and strengthen your kinetic chain.** As the pain subsides, start the reconditioning process with basic core strengthening and stretching exercises. Go slow. Stretch your hamstrings, hip flexors, glutes, and core. Do glute bridges and planks, adding reps and intensity as you improve. Once you're pain free, up your kinetic chain conditioning (see "Prevent It").

PREVENT IT

- **Commit to your kinetic chain.** The more muscles you have supporting your back, the better off your back will be. Therefore, back pain prevention isn't just about strengthening your back muscles. Your back is working in combination with the rest of your core and your glutes, hips, hamstrings, and quads for optimal performance. Your fitness program must include dynamic, compound exercises that target as many of these areas as possible. Workout staples should include multidirectional lunges, core exercises with trunk rotation, squats, squat jumps, burpees, planks, mountain climbers, and more. Plyometric total-body boot-camp-style workouts are terrific (see the workout chapter on page 256 as well as the "Prevent It" section for "Lower Back Spasms" on page 106 for more ideas). I also recommend regularly attending Pilates classes. All of these things focus on strength and flexibility throughout your kinetic chain.

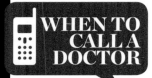

WHEN TO CALL A DOCTOR

If you have pain radiating down the backs of your legs, see a doctor. This is a clear symptom of discogenic back pain and you need to have an MRI to determine the size of the disk herniation and x-rays to reveal any other underlying bone problems.

Once you have this diagnosis, a doctor can give you a cortisone or anesthetic injection to help with the pain.

Physical therapy is also a good idea in these cases, both to reduce the acute muscular pain that often goes along with this problem and to begin reconditioning your kinetic chain to bring muscular stability to the spine. The exercise and stretching ideas I offer here help, but a physical therapist can direct your care and teach you correct form and how many repetitions to do based on your individual case.

DO YOU NEED SURGERY?

It's rarely necessary and is often considered a last resort when nothing else works. Even when surgery is necessary, patients usually fully recover. Still, discogenic back pain usually subsides within a few weeks using these home-based remedies.

LOWER BACK

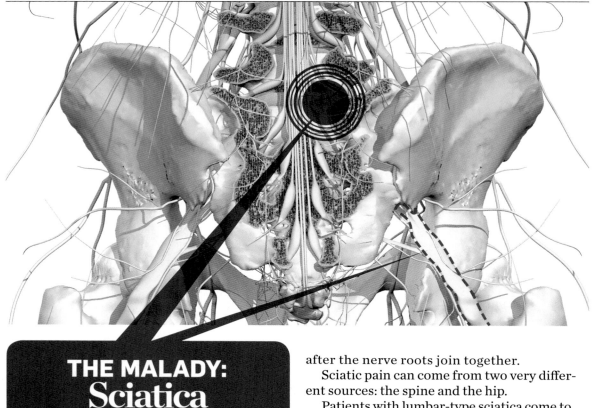

THE MALADY:
Sciatica

THE SYMPTOMS

Lower back pain and shooting pain down the back of one or both legs, sometimes to the toes. It may worsen with sitting or bending forward. With piriformis-based sciatic problems, the pain hits the lower back and/or buttocks, sometimes feeling as if it's deep inside the buttock muscles. It may be too painful to sit on the affected buttock. The pain and/or tingling can radiate down the back of the upper leg as well.

WHAT'S GOING ON IN THERE?

Sciatic pain comes from irritation of the sciatic nerve, a thick, ropelike nerve comprising several nerve roots in the lumbar (lower) spine that merge into one. Technically, sciatic pain is caused by irritation of this nerve

after the nerve roots join together.

Sciatic pain can come from two very different sources: the spine and the hip.

Patients with lumbar-type sciatica come to me describing a shooting pain down the back of one or both legs, sometimes reaching all the way to the toes. Sitting and bending forward make it worse. Nerve roots, which are small branches of the spinal cord that exit at each level of the vertebrae and divide into smaller branches, are often pinched by a bulging or herniated disk in the spine. The nerve is compressed and pain, often excruciating, results. (This is also referred to as discogenic back pain; see "Herniated Disk [Slipped Disk]" on page 108).

Piriformis, or hip, sciatic pain comes from a spot deep within each hip where the piriformis muscle, a hip flexor, crosses over the sciatic nerve. If the muscle is tight or spasms, it can pinch or compress the nerve, causing pain, especially when you're sitting on the affected side (this type of sciatic pain usually hits only one hip). The pain generally doesn't shoot far down the upper leg.

FIX IT

LUMBAR RELATED:

- **Employ dynamic rest.** You'll want to lie down, but minimize the amount of time you spend on your back. Stay mobile, even if it means taking little shuffle steps around the house. Bed rest during spells of back pain only deconditions your muscles, which is the opposite of what you want to happen. During the acute stage, avoid straining your back, but do simple stretches to loosen your hamstrings, hip flexors, and glutes. All of these can help alleviate any accompanying muscle spasms.

- **Ice it, then heat it.** Apply ice for 15 minutes 4 to 6 times a day for the first 2 days. After 2 days, using a heating pad at the same time intervals can help relieve the spasms.

- **Try an NSAID.** An antiinflammatory like ibuprofen or naproxen can help with pain and inflammation.

- **Vary your therapies.** Effective pain relief therapies are very individualized. For example, some of my patients respond well to massage therapy. Others swear by acupuncture. My point: Try different therapies until you get results. Everyone responds differently to different things.

- **Stretch and strengthen your kinetic chain.** As the pain subsides, start the reconditioning process with basic core strengthening and stretching exercises. Go slow. Stretch your hamstrings, hip flexors, glutes, and core. Do glute bridges and planks, adding reps and intensity as you improve. Once you're pain free, up your kinetic chain conditioning (see "Prevent It").

PIRIFORMIS OR HIP RELATED:

See "Piriformis Syndrome" on page 96 for specific remedies.

PREVENT IT

LUMBAR RELATED:

- **Commit to your kinetic chain.** The more muscles you have supporting your back, the better off your back will be. Therefore, back pain prevention isn't just about strengthening your back muscles. Your back is working in combination with the rest of your core and your glutes, hips, hamstrings, and quads for optimal performance. Your fitness program must include dynamic, compound exercises that target as many of these areas as possible. Workout staples should include multidirectional lunges, core exercises

with trunk rotation, squats, squat jumps, burpees, planks, mountain climbers, and more. Plyometric total-body boot-camp-style workouts are terrific (see the workout chapter on page 256 as well as the "Prevent It" section for "Lower Back Spasms" on page 106 for more ideas). I also recommend regularly attending Pilates classes. All of these things focus on strength and flexibility throughout your kinetic chain.

PIRIFORMIS OR HIP RELATED:

See "Piriformis Syndrome" on page 96 for hip-specific conditioning ideas.

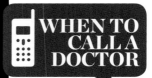

WHEN TO CALL A DOCTOR

If you have pain radiating down the back of one or both legs, see a doctor. This is a clear symptom of discogenic back pain and you need to have an MRI to determine the size of the disk herniation and x-rays to reveal any other underlying bone problems.

A doctor can also give you a cortisone or anesthetic injection to help with the pain. Physical therapy is also a good idea in these cases, both to reduce the acute muscular pain that often goes along with this problem and to begin reconditioning your kinetic chain to bring muscular stability to the spine. The exercise and stretching ideas I offer here help, but a physical therapist can direct your care and teach you the correct form and how many repetitions to do based on your individual case.

DO YOU NEED SURGERY?

It's rarely necessary and is often considered a last resort. Even when surgery is necessary, patients generally recover to full normal activity. Still, discogenic back pain usually subsides within a few weeks using these home-based remedies.

LOWER BACK

ABDOMINALS OBLIQUES & CHEST

When you start talking about pains and strains in the muscles in areas like your abs, sides, and chest, you're talking about the bane of the skill-sport athlete. These muscles are the foundation of high-performance athleticism—every sport from football to golf depends on a healthy torso. Try to twist, reach up, reach out, throw, or swing when one of these areas is injured. It's just not happening, and if you try to force it or play through the pain, the problem will go on and on until something more serious occurs. In this chapter, we'll look at everything from hernias to strained pecs to the dreaded side stitch and fix you up so you can be out there doing what you love to do.

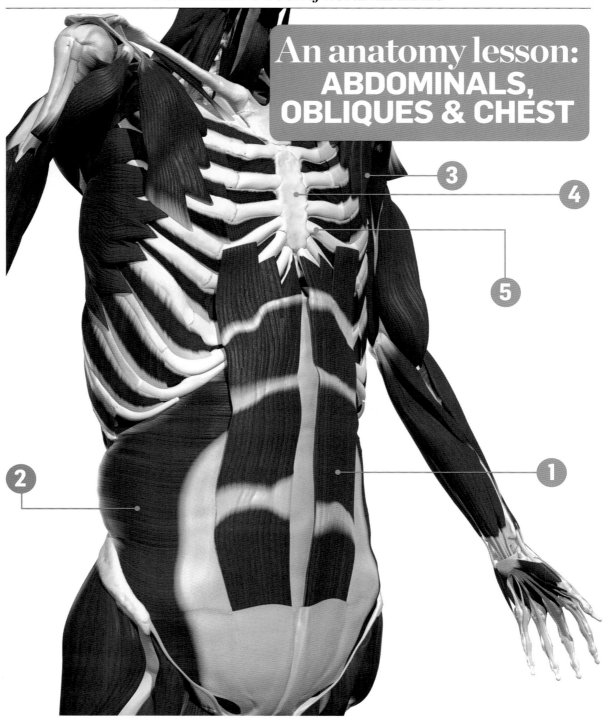

An anatomy lesson: ABDOMINALS, OBLIQUES & CHEST

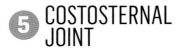 **OBLIQUES**

There are two sets of oblique muscles. The external obliques are closest to the skin and run diagonally to aid with trunk rotation. The deeper, internal obliques also aid in trunk rotation, but they run diagonally in the opposite direction of the external muscles.

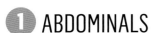 **ABDOMINALS**

There are two sets of abdominal muscles. The rectus abdominis are the more external set, visible beneath the skin as the proverbial "six pack." The transverse abdominis muscles, the deeper muscles, run horizontally beneath the rectus abdominis. These muscles help you bend, and protect your vital organs.

③ PECTORALS

You have two sets of chest muscles. The pectoralis major is the primary chest muscle and attaches at the clavicle, sternum, and ribs. They help pull your upper arms toward the middle of your body. The pectoralis minor is a much smaller muscle beneath the major. It helps pull your shoulders forward.

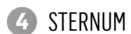 **④ STERNUM**

The breastbone, a flat, t-shaped bone that protects the heart and anchors the upper section of the ribcage in the chest. The clavicles (collarbones) attach to the upper end of the sternum.

⑤ COSTOSTERNAL JOINT

The joints, made of cartilage, where the ribs attach to the sternum. This area can become irritated and cause chest pain that can mimic a heart attack.

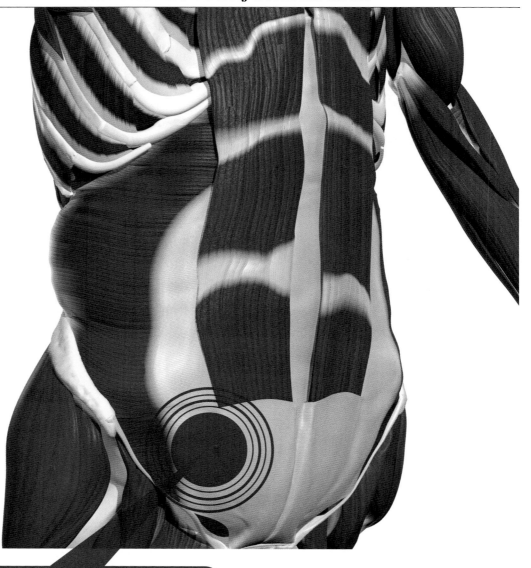

THE MALADY: General Hernia / Sportsman's Hernia

THE SYMPTOMS

Pain in the lower abdomen (a general hernia) or groin (a sportsman's hernia) that worsens with coughing or sneezing. Sometimes pain that appears to be muscular persists for months and turns out to be from a hernia.

WHAT'S GOING ON IN THERE?

A hernia is a tear or weakness in the abdominal wall that allows the intestines or another organ to get pinched in the gap or push outside the abdomen, usually (but not always) causing pain. A general hernia is usually located in the lower abdomen at hip level. The most common kind of hernia, the inguinal hernia, involves the inguinal canal, which runs through the front wall of the abdomen and channels blood and lymph vessels, nerves, the spermatic cord in men, and the round ligament in women from inside the body to closer to the surface. Sections of the intestine or other abdominal organs can poke through at various places along the abdominal wall at the front of the canal, as well as around the inguinal rings at the entrance and exit of the canal.

A sportsman's, or sports hernia, which is named that because it's more common in athletes, occurs lower, near the groin. It's unlike a general hernia because it rarely involves protruding organs. It's a tearing of abdominal muscle, tendon, and/or fascia where it attaches to the pubic bone in the lower pelvis. Your adductors attach here as well, and if they are stronger than the abdominal muscles—as they often are if you under-train your core—they can pull down on the pubic bone, causing the tear. A sports hernia is often mistaken for a chronic groin strain.

As for a general hernia, it's possible to confuse a hernia with an abdominal strain (page 118). If you have pain, try this test: Bear down as if you're having a bowel movement and feel the area where it hurts. Sometimes you can feel a subtle, soft protrusion where the intestine has poked through the abdominal wall. Another signal? Abs strains get better. Hernias don't—unless you have surgery.

FIX IT

• **Let the pros handle it.** Hernias need surgical repair. If you ignore it, you could face serious complications (see "When to Call a Doctor").

PREVENT IT

• **Up your core work.** A strong core is the best prevention for a hernia. In fact, there's no better reason to stay in shape—they're most often caused by weak abs and being overweight. Planks, crunches, and leg raises should be workout staples. Also, I recommend taking a Pilates class a couple times a week.

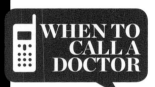

WHEN TO CALL A DOCTOR

As soon as you suspect a hernia. This is also why doctors check for hernias during physicals. If you ignore it, you could have complications:

• **Strangulation.** The tissue that protruded outside the abdominal wall is pinched where it emerges and loses its blood supply. The tissue dies. Then it can turn gangrenous.

• **Testicular damage.** The spermatic cord runs through the inguinal canal, so inguinal hernias can affect the testicles. Some inguinal hernias cause scrotal swelling.

• **Bowel dysfunction and/or obstruction.** If enough of the bowel herniates, you could have intestinal cramping and vomiting. If the bowel is completely obstructed by the pinching, your bowel movements and flatulence will stop.

DO YOU NEED SURGERY?

Yes. Both general and sports hernias require surgery. They are not complicated procedures and athletes usually have a full recovery.

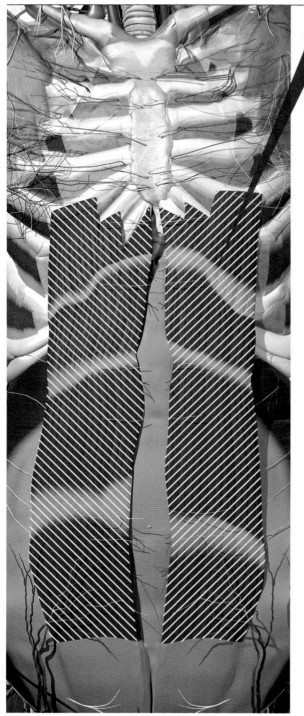

THE MALADY: Abdominal Strain

THE SYMPTOMS

A sharp pain in your torso at the injury site. You'll really feel it during any muscle flexion, including breathing deeply, coughing, sneezing, or laughing.

WHAT'S GOING ON IN THERE?

Your abdominal muscles (which are much more than simply "abs") run in layers across and around your trunk. There are four main components.

- **Transverse abdominis.** This muscle constitutes the deepest layer of abdominals, and it keeps everything that's inside from finding its way outside. Its muscle fibers run horizontally across your front, protect your vital organs, and help you laugh, cough, and sneeze.

- **Internal and external obliques.** These two layers of muscles run diagonally along your sides and help with trunk rotation. For more on them, see "Oblique Strain" on page 122.

- **Rectus abdominis.** These run vertically along your front, closest to the skin. Yes, they form your legendary six-pack. They also aid in trunk flexion.

Like any strain, an abdominal strain comes in three grades, 1 to 3, with 3 being a complete rupture. Grade 1 is pretty straightforward: The area hurts, especially when the muscle is engaged, but you can function. Once you get into grade 2 territory, you could have swelling and bruising, and you find most movements excruciating. Grade 3? You'll be incapacitated and need emergency care.

Any activity requiring explosive trunk rotation or flexion puts you at risk.

FIX IT

- **Employ dynamic rest.** An abdominal strain is a very frustrating injury because the core is so integral to so many movements. Avoid any activity that activates your core. To stay fit, try lower-body workouts that keep muscle flexion below the waist. As long as you can do it pain free, jogging and stationary cycling can work, as well as multidirectional lunges.

- **Ice it.** Apply ice for 15 minutes 4 to 6 times a day for the first 2 days.

- **Try an NSAID.** An antiinflammatory like ibuprofen or naproxen can help with swelling and inflammation.

- **Rehab it.** Once you're pain free, return low-intensity abs work to your workout. Bridges and planks are great for this, but be sure not to overdo it early on. When you're able to return to full activity, be sure to intensify your core work so you'll be stronger than you were when you were injured (see "Prevent It" on the following page).

WHEN TO CALL A DOCTOR

If the pain doesn't improve within 2 weeks, make an appointment. Depending on the severity, abs strains generally heal within 2 to 8 weeks. But you should see some improvement after 2. If not, a doctor can evaluate the severity of your injury and any other underlying factors.

More aggressive treatments include ultrasound therapy, corticosteroid injections, and physical therapy. Also, platelet-rich plasma (PRP) injections are now being used successfully for abdominal strains. The patient's own plasma is injected into the injured area to speed healing. It's new, and may not be covered by insurance, but it's worth investigating if other therapies fail.

DO YOU NEED SURGERY?

Almost never. The most severe ruptures could require surgery—and you'll know it. If you have a full-blown rupture, trust me, you'll want to go to the ER immediately.

PLANK

Get into pushup position, but bend your elbows and rest your weight on your forearms. Your body should form a straight line from your shoulders to your ankles. Brace your core and hold. Let your injury guide you as to how long to hold the plank—but go short to start and be careful not to overdo it.

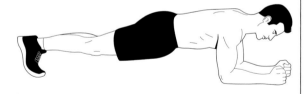

HIP RAISE (BRIDGE)

Lie faceup on the floor with your knees bent and your feet flat on the floor. Place your arms out to your sides at 45-degree angles, your palms facing up. Raise your hips so your body forms a straight line from your shoulders to your knees. Squeeze your glutes as you raise your hips. Make sure you're pushing with your heels. To make it easier, you can position your feet so that your toes rise off the floor. Pause for 5 seconds in the up position, then lower your body back to the starting position. You can hold in the up position for more time as you get stronger.

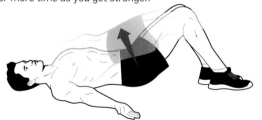

HALF-KNEELING ROTATION

Hold a broomstick or something similar across your back. Kneel down on your left knee and bend your right knee 90 degrees, with your right foot flat on the floor. Keeping your back naturally arched, rotate your left shoulder toward your right knee. Hold that position for 5 seconds, then return to the starting position. That's 1 rep. Start with several reps and raise the number as you get stronger. When finished, switch knee positions and do the same number to your left side.

Cont'd on page 120

119

PREVENT IT

The bottom line: Strains happen because the muscle can't handle what you ask of it. The goal: Stronger and more flexible abs. This isn't about trying to get a six-pack. Core-specific training must be a serious part of your workout regimen. You can increase over-all dynamic flexibility by using the Iron Strength workout section of this book (see page 256)—and there is a good core workout included. But even if you don't use those specific work-outs, the stretches and exercises here can be added to any workout.

CAT CAMEL

Position yourself on your hands and knees. Gently arch your lower back—don't push—then lower your head between your shoulders and raise your upper back toward the ceiling, rounding your spine. That's 1 repetition. Move back and forth slowly, without pushing at either end of the movement.
NOTE: The cat camel may look funny, but slowly flexing and extending your spine in small ranges of motion is a great way to prepare your core for any activity.

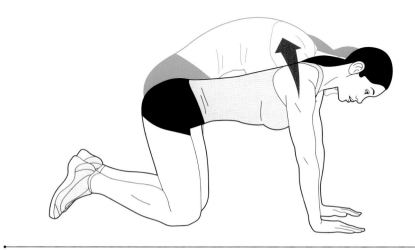

PLANK

Get into pushup position, but bend your elbows and rest your weight on your forearms. Your body should form a straight line from your shoulders to your ankles. Brace your core and hold. Let your fitness level determine how long you hold the plank, but 30 seconds to a minute is good, while I recommend 3 to 6 minutes total plank time.

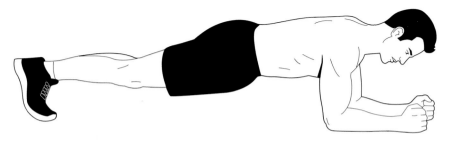

GOOD MOTIVATION
A Canadian study of more than 8,000 people over 13 years found that those with the weakest abdominal muscles had a death rate more than twice that of the people with the strongest midsections.

GET SOME CLASS

I highly recommend regular Pilates and yoga classes. The overall effect on your flexibility and core strength will be life-changing. I promise you'll find yourself able to achieve physical feats you couldn't do before. Just hit classes a couple times a week on top of your regular regimen.

WRIST-TO-KNEE CRUNCH

Lie faceup with your hips and knees bent 90 degrees so that your lower legs are parallel to the floor. Place your fingers on the sides of your head. Lift your shoulders off the floor as if doing a crunch. Twist your upper body to the left while bringing up your left knee to touch your right wrist. Simultaneously straighten your right leg. Return to the starting position and repeat to the other side.

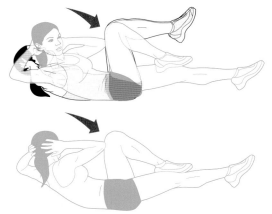

CORE STABILIZATION

Sit on the floor with your knees bent. Hold a weight plate straight out in front of your chest. Your feet should be flat on the floor. Lean back so your torso is at a 45-degree angle to the floor, and brace your core.

Without moving your torso (your belly button should point straight ahead at all times), rotate your arms to the left as far as you can. Pause for 3 seconds. Rotate your arms to the right as far as you can. Pause again, then alternate back and forth. **NOTE:** If you don't have a weight plate, you can substitute a light dumbbell or a basketball, or if you have no object (or need the exercise to be easier), simply clasp your hands together in front of you.

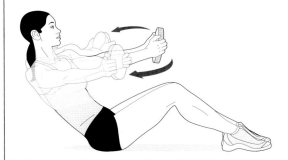

MOUNTAIN CLIMBERS

Get in pushup position with your arms straight (you can use the ground or a bench as your base). This is the starting position. Lift your right foot and raise your knee as close to your chest as you can. Touch the ground with your right foot and then return to the starting position and repeat with your left leg. Go as fast as possible.

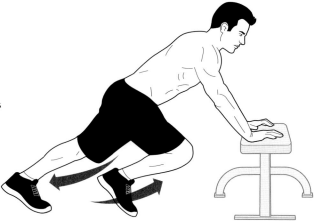

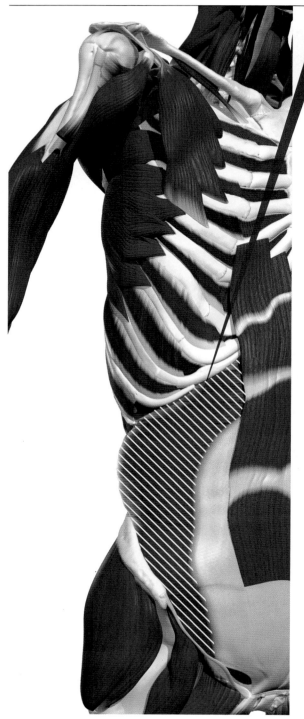

THE MALADY:
Oblique Strain

THE SYMPTOMS

A sharp pain in the side between the lower ribs and the hip. The pain can be severe and increases when the muscle is stretched or contracted by leaning to the left or right (depending on which side is hurt).

WHAT'S GOING ON IN THERE?

The obliques are part of your core and run down each side of your body from your lower ribs to your hips. The internal obliques are at a deeper layer than your external obliques, and they work with your rectus abdominis muscles to help you twist and bend. Whereas the rectus abdominis fibers run vertically and those of the transverse abdominis run horizontally, the oblique fibers run diagonally (opposite to each other). The internal and external obliques on opposite sides complement each other's actions. For example, if you twist your torso to the left, your left internal oblique and right external oblique work together to make it happen. And vice versa if you twist to the right.

Any forceful twisting or overuse can injure your obliques, so baseball and softball players, golfers, tennis players, and athletes playing any other swing-centric sports are at risk. Oblique injuries can be easily aggravated, too, so they can nag if not properly treated.

As with all strains, oblique strains range from grade 1 to 3, with 3 being a complete tear or rupture.

FIX IT

- **Employ dynamic rest.** An oblique strain is a touchy injury because the core is so integral to so many movements and it's very easy to aggravate it. Avoid any activity that activates your core, especially any twisting movements. To stay fit, try lower-body workouts that keep muscle flexion below the waist. As long as you can do it pain free, jogging and stationary cycling can work, as can multidirectional lunges.

- **Ice it.** Apply ice for 15 minutes 4 to 6 times a day for the first 2 days.

- **Try an NSAID.** An antiinflammatory like ibuprofen or naproxen can help with swelling and inflammation.

- **Rehab it.** Once you're pain free, return low-intensity abs work to your workout (see below for examples), but be sure not to overdo it early on. When you're able to return to full activity, intensify your rotational core work so you're stronger than you were when you were injured (see "Prevent It" on the following pages).

WHEN TO CALL A DOCTOR

If the pain doesn't improve within 2 weeks, make an appointment. Depending on the severity, oblique strains generally heal within 2 to 4 weeks. But you should see some improvement after 2. If not, a doctor can evaluate the severity of your injury and any other underlying factors.

More aggressive treatments include ultrasound therapy, corticosteroid injections, and physical therapy.

Another potential therapy is platelet-rich plasma (PRP), which can be tried if the soft tissue doesn't heal in about 5 months. It's new, but a lot of pro athletes have used it and gotten results. In areas of the body that don't have great blood supply, healing is slow. The doctor injects your own PRP into the injured area to promote faster healing. The upside is that it works for most people. The downside is that it's generally not covered by insurance and is expensive.

DO YOU NEED SURGERY?

Almost never. The most severe ruptures could require surgery. If you have a full-blown rupture, you'll want to go to the ER immediately.

PLANK

Get into pushup position, but bend your elbows and rest your weight on your forearms. Your body should form a straight line from your shoulders to your ankles. Brace your core and hold. Let your injury guide you as to how long to hold the plank—but go short to start and be careful not to overdo it.

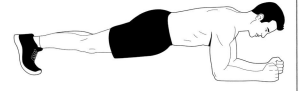

SIDE PLANK

Lie on your side and use your forearm to support your body. Raise your hips until your body forms a straight line from shoulder to ankles. Hold for 5 to 10 seconds, increasing the time as you get stronger. Repeat the same number of seconds and reps for the other side.

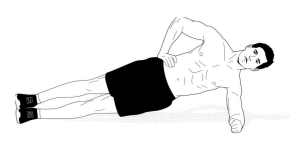

HALF-KNEELING ROTATION

Hold a broomstick or something similar across your back. Knee down on your left knee and bend your right knee 90 degrees, with your right foot flat on the floor. Keeping your back naturally arched, rotate your left shoulder toward your right knee. Hold that position for 5 seconds, then return to the starting position. That's 1 rep. Start with several reps and raise the number as you get stronger. When finished, switch knee positions and do the same number to your left side.

Cont'd on page 124

PREVENT IT

The bottom line: Strains happen because the muscle can't handle what you ask of it. The goal: Stronger and more flexible obliques. Core-specific training with trunk rotation must be a serious part of your workout regimen. You can increase over-all dynamic flexibility by using the Iron Strength workout section of this book (see page 256)—and there is a good core workout included. But even if you don't use those specific workouts, the stretches and exercises here can be added to any workout.

CAT CAMEL

Position yourself on your hands and knees. Gently arch your lower back—don't push—then lower your head between your shoulders and raise your upper back toward the ceiling, rounding your spine. That's 1 repetition. Move back and forth slowly, without pushing at either end of the movement.

NOTE: The cat camel may look funny, but slowly flexing and extending your spine in small ranges of motion is a great way to prepare your core for any activity.

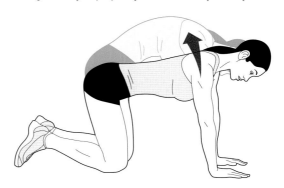

ROLLING SIDE PLANK

Start by performing a side plank with your right side down. Hold for 1 or 2 seconds, then roll your body over onto both elbows—into a traditional plank—and hold for 1 or 2 seconds. Next, roll all the way up onto your left elbow so that you're performing a side plank facing the opposite direction. Hold for another second or two. That's 1 repetition. Make sure to move your whole body as a single unit each time you roll.

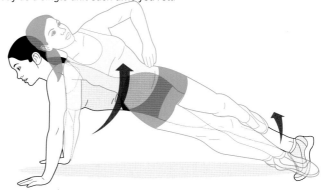

A BIG BONUS

Four out of five adults will experience severe lower-back pain at least once in their lives. Multiple studies have shown that regular core workouts don't just reduce the instance of back injuries, but also reduce the amount of pain an injured person experiences.

GET SOME CLASS

I highly recommend regular Pilates and yoga classes. The overall effect on your flexibility and core strength will be life-changing. I promise you'll find yourself able to achieve physical feats you couldn't do before. Just hit classes a couple times a week on top of your regular regimen.

WRIST-TO-KNEE CRUNCH

Lie faceup with your hips and knees bent 90 degrees so that your lower legs are parallel to the floor. Place your fingers on the sides of your head. Lift your shoulders off the floor as if doing a crunch. Twist your upper body to the left while bringing up your left knee to touch your right wrist. Simultaneously straighten your right leg. Return to the starting position and repeat to the other side.

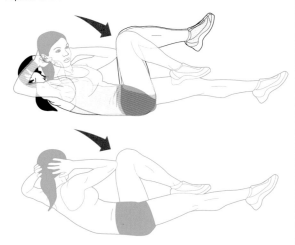

CORE STABILIZATION

Sit on the floor with your knees bent. Hold a weight plate straight out in front of your chest. Your feet should be flat on the floor. Lean back so your torso is at a 45-degree angle to the floor, and brace your core.

Without moving your torso (your belly button should point straight ahead at all times), rotate your arms to the left as far as you can. Pause for 3 seconds. Rotate your arms to the right as far as you can. Pause again, then continue to alternate back and forth.

NOTE: If you don't have a weight plate, you can substitute a light dumbbell, a basketball, a rock, or if you have no object (or need the exercise to be easier), simply clasp your hands together in front of you.

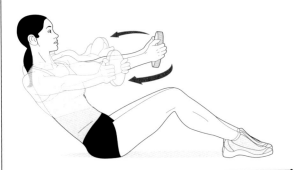

SINGLE-LEG SIDE PLANK

Lie on your side and use your forearm to support your body. Raise your hips until your body forms a straight line from shoulder to ankles. Then raise your top leg as high as you can and hold it that way for the duration of the exercise. Halfway through the prescribed time, switch sides.

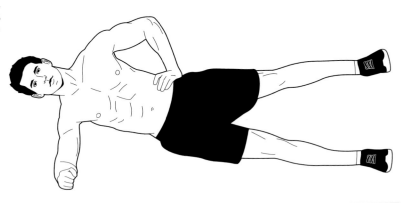

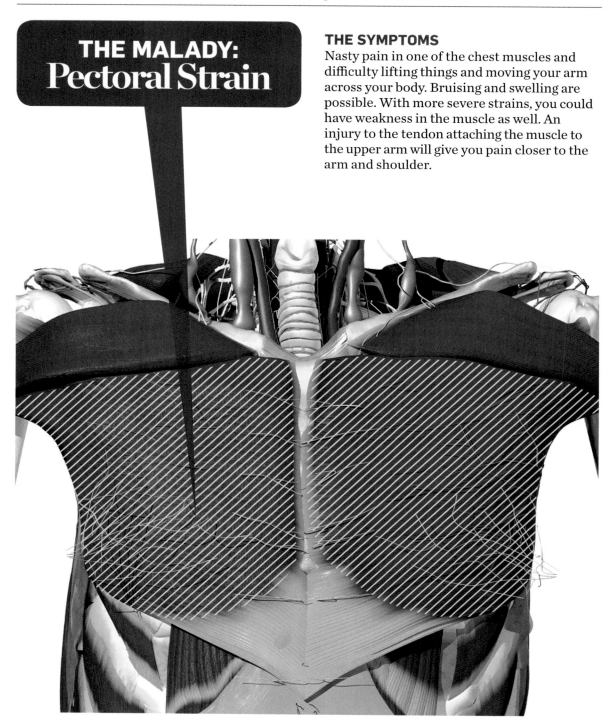

THE MALADY:
Pectoral Strain

THE SYMPTOMS

Nasty pain in one of the chest muscles and difficulty lifting things and moving your arm across your body. Bruising and swelling are possible. With more severe strains, you could have weakness in the muscle as well. An injury to the tendon attaching the muscle to the upper arm will give you pain closer to the arm and shoulder.

WHAT'S GOING ON IN THERE?

The primary chest muscles are the pectoralis major and minor. The pectoralis major is the big muscle running from your sternum to your upper arm (the humerus bone). It's one powerful muscle, and it's the foundation of any arm movement. The pectoralis minor is a smaller muscle, but it's also strong and dense. It runs on the side of your chest from the ribs to the shoulder blade (the scapula).

Pec strains aren't as common as, say, hamstring strains, but when they happen, they take you out of the game because they take your arms out of the equation. Moving your arms and lifting things will be painful.

The most common source of pec strains, not surprisingly, is weight lifting, especially doing bench presses. Contact-sport athletes (football, hockey, wrestling) are also at risk from a direct impact on the muscle, an explosive movement, or overuse.

FIX IT

- **Employ dynamic rest.** Get out from under that barbell and avoid any activity that fires your pecs. And there are a lot of them: Any lifting or fast arm movements can aggravate the injury. Avoid core work—it's just too easy to engage your chest, even involuntarily. Use lower-body workouts to stay fit. As long as you can do it pain free (by not engaging your arms), jogging and stationary cycling can work.

- **Ice it.** Apply ice for 15 minutes 4 to 6 times a day for the first 2 days.

- **Try an NSAID.** An antiinflammatory like ibuprofen or naproxen can help with swelling and inflammation.

- **Rehab it.** Once you're pain free, start with stretching and light resistance activities like pushups, building up the number of reps over several weeks. Once you have the full range of motion and better strength, incorporate light bench presses into your workouts and gradually build back up to your pre-injury level. Also add more dynamic exercises to your routine (see "Prevent It" on the following page). Don't go too hard, too fast. You'll certainly want to, but you'll risk reinjury.

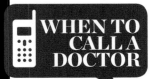

WHEN TO CALL A DOCTOR

If your pain doesn't improve within a couple of weeks, see a doctor. Also, make an appointment for a more severe strain. The pectoral muscles are so important to not just sports performance, but everyday movements like lifting. Tears in the muscle or tendon should be evaluated to ensure that the injured area returns to full function and health.

DO YOU NEED SURGERY?

Grade 3 strains—full ruptures—can require surgery. In some cases, athletes never fully recover their strength, power, or range of motion. This is one main reason to back off activity at the first sign of any grade of pec strain. You don't want to risk the worst-case scenario here.

ABDOMINALS, OBLIQUES & CHEST

Cont'd on page 126

PREVENT IT

Pushups and bench press are obviously great chest exercises, but if you want to build a strong, dynamic upper body, you need to expand your repertoire. You can increase overall dynamic flexibility by using the Iron Strength workout section of this book (see page 256). But even if you don't use those specific workouts, the stretches and exercises here can be added to any workout.

DOORWAY STRETCH

Bend your right arm 90 degrees (the "high-five" position) and place your forearm against a door frame. Stand in staggered stance, your right foot in front of your left. Rotate your chest to your right until you feel a comfortable stretch in your chest and the front of your shoulder. Hold for 30 seconds. Switch arms and legs and repeat for your other side. Repeat for a total of 3 reps for each side.

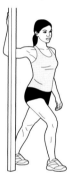

DIP

Grasp the bars of a dip station and lift yourself so your arms are perfectly straight. Cross your ankles behind you. Slowly lower yourself by bending your elbows until your upper arms dip just below your elbows. Keep your elbows tucked close to your body. Pause, then push back up to the starting position.

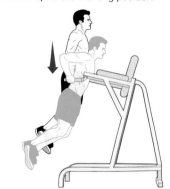

PRONE COBRA

Lie facedown on the floor with your legs straight and your arms next to your sides, palms down.

Contract your glutes and the muscles of your lower back, and raise your head, chest, arms, and legs off the floor.

Simultaneously rotate your arms so that your thumbs point toward the ceiling. At this time, your hips should be the only parts of your body touching the floor. Hold this position for the prescribed time. (Note: If you can't hold it for the entire time, hold for 5 to 10 seconds, rest for 5, and repeat as many times as needed. If the exercise is too easy, you can hold light dumbbells in your hands while you do it.)

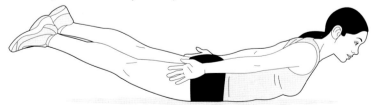

PREVENT A MUSCLE IMBALANCE

If you work your chest more than you work the muscles of your upper back, you're a candidate for poor posture and you increase your injury risk. If you do 10 reps of a pushing exercise (like a pushup or bench press), be sure to also do 10 reps of a pulling exercise (such as an inverted row) to keep your muscles in balance.

TRICK OUT YOUR PUSHUP

Mix in these variations on a classic to surprise your muscles and build a more action-ready body.

- **Decline Pushup.** Place your feet on a box or bench as you perform a pushup; this increases the amount of weight you have to lift.

- **Single-Leg Decline Pushup.** Place one foot on a box or bench and hold the other in the air. If you feel strain in your lower back, you're not keeping your core tight. To make your core work even harder, do this exercise with your feet on a Swiss ball.

- **Spiderman Pushup.** As you lower your body to the floor, lift your right foot off the floor, swing your right leg out sideways, and try to touch your knee to your elbow. Alternate legs on each pushup.

- **Staggered-Hands Pushup.** Place one hand in standard pushup position and your other hand a few inches farther forward. This increases the challenge to your core and shoulders.

- **Diamond Pushup.** Place your hands close enough together to make a triangle with your thumbs and forefingers.

TRIPLE-STOP BARBELL BENCH PRESS

Perform a standard bench press but pause for 10 seconds at each stop. First stop: a couple inches below the starting position. Second stop: halfway down. Third stop: just above your chest. Then push back to the starting position.

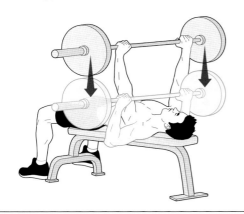

INVERTED ROW

Grab the bar above you with an overhand, shoulder-width grip. Hang with your arms completely straight and your hands positioned directly above your shoulders. Your body should form a straight line from your ankles to your head. Initiate the movement by pulling your shoulder blades back, then continue the pull with your arms to lift your chest to the bar. Pause, then slowly lower your body back to the starting position.

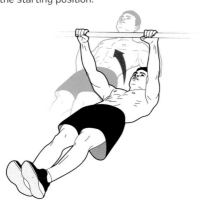

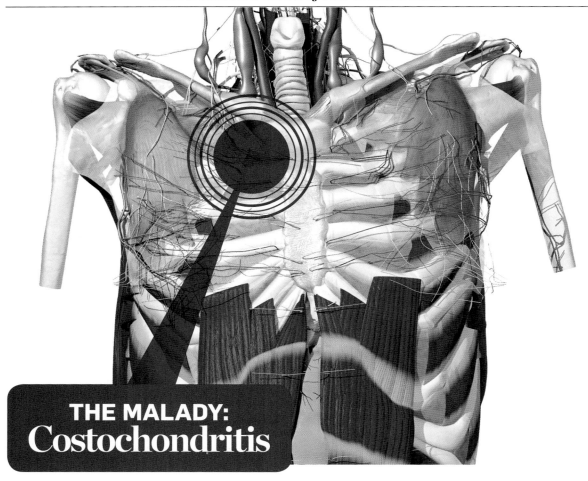

THE MALADY:
Costochondritis

THE SYMPTOMS

Pain, sharp or dull, where your ribs attach to the sternum (aka the breastbone). The spot is usually tender to the touch. You can also have pain when you cough or sneeze.

WHAT'S GOING ON IN THERE?

Your ribs and breastbone are connected by cartilage at the costosternal joint, and when that cartilage becomes inflamed, you have costochondritis.

In most folks, there seems to be no discernible cause of costochondritis, but in athletes, a blow to the chest, as well as heavy lifting or strenuous exercise, can bring it on. Other possible causes include an infection in the costosternal joint, heavy coughing, or sneezing.

The tricky thing about costochondritis: You may think you're having a heart attack. The pain is centered in your chest, right above your heart, and in some cases it hurts to breathe. Chest pain and shortness of breath are classic heart attack symptoms.

A related condition, Tietze syndrome, features the symptoms of costochondritis along with swelling in the affected costosternal joint. There's no telling how long the condition will last—some cases last a few days, others a few months.

FIX IT

- **Employ dynamic rest.** Avoid any activity that involves using your chest, especially lifting. No contact sports, either. Use lower-body workouts to stay fit. As long as you can do it pain free, jogging and stationary cycling can work.

- **Try an NSAID.** An antiinflammatory like ibuprofen or naproxen can help with swelling and inflammation.

- **Ice it.** Apply ice for 15 minutes 4 to 6 times a day for the first 2 days.

- **Try a heating pad.** After icing the area for the first 2 days, applying low heat several times a day can help.

PREVENT IT

- **Build a strong chest.** There is no definitive way to prevent costochondritis, but having a stronger chest can certainly help. If all you're doing is bench presses and pushups, expand your repertoire to include more dynamic exercises. Change up your hand positions for pushups and pullups (widened, narrowed, staggered). Add in dumbbell and inclined bench press moves. Also adopt compound lifts. Try the death crawl: Get in the pushup position, supporting yourself with your hands gripping dumbbells. Do 2 pushups. Then do 2 rows with the right dumbbell, then 2 with the left. Now, while remaining in the pushup position, perform a "walking plank" for about 6 feet, taking small steps with the dumbbells and your toes.

  After 6 feet, repeat the pushups and rows. Then go another 6 feet. After 3 complete reps, do the same thing but backward until you're back where you started. Through all of this, keep your body rigid and do not break from the pushup position. The point is to find new ways to challenge your pecs so they can take what's dished out.

- **And don't forget your back.** Make sure you don't have a muscle imbalance between your chest and back muscles. Chest muscles that overpower your back can draw your shoulders forward and cause them to slump. Maintain good posture and be sure to balance "push" exercises (pushup, bench press) with equal reps of pull exercises (rows, pullups).

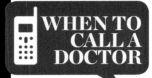

WHEN TO CALL A DOCTOR

Chest pain can be crazy scary, so get medical help immediately. Pain in the center of your chest—sharp, dull, gentle, nasty—can be many things, and only a pro can determine what it is. Even if it turns out to be something as simple as costochondritis, having all the scarier propositions ruled out will give you peace of mind.

As far as more aggressive treatments for costochondritis go, your doctor may prescribe a long-term course of antiinflammatory medicine. A corticosteroid injection might help if the home-based care listed here doesn't work.

DO YOU NEED SURGERY?

Almost never. In very rare cases, when all of the other therapies have been exhausted, surgery to remove the inflamed cartilage is an option. But in the vast majority of cases, the condition clears up on its own.

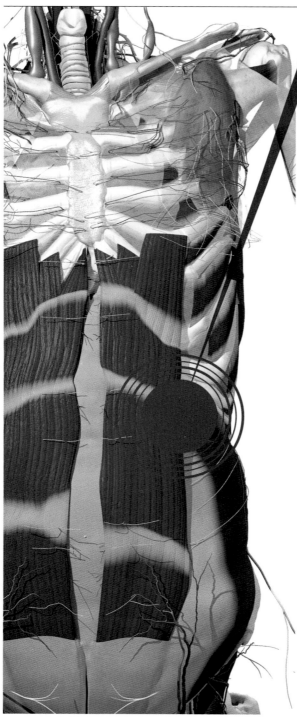

THE MALADY: Side Stitch

THE SYMPTOMS

A sharp pain in the side while running or otherwise exerting, sometimes severe enough to force you to stop.

WHAT'S GOING ON IN THERE?

The dreaded side stitch can be caused by several things. The most common cause is a diaphragm spasm—especially for runners who are just starting out with a program or pushing a run beyond their current capability.

The diaphragm is the muscle that separates the lungs and chest cavity from the abdominal cavity, and it expands and contracts with every breath. When it has to work too hard it can spasm, causing a pain that feels like a knife in your side.

Another common scenario: The diaphragm is working fine, but the breathing effort is excessive due to panting and puffing, and the accessory muscles of breathing, the obliques, spasm.

Other causes that are less common include exercise-induced bronchospasm and anatomical problems with the lungs.

Triathletes face a cause specific to their sport: the stress of transitioning from cycling to running. If the core muscles aren't stretched after a long bike leg, they may spasm.

FIX IT

- **Stretch it.** First, try to relieve the side stitch without stopping your activity. Raise your arm on the side that hurts and place that hand on the back of your head. Continue the activity. The idea is to allow those side muscles to stretch, hopefully relieving the spasm and, of course, the pain. Try this for 30 to 60 seconds. Repeat if the side stitch returns or doesn't abate.

  If this is ineffective, take a break and stretch those side muscles as you rest. This is a two-pronged attack. One, you stretch the spasming muscles. And two, you rest your diaphragm and obliques, which should solve the problem.

PREVENT IT

- **Strengthen your core.** Since the most common causes of side stitches are muscle related, increasing core strength with exercises like planks and crunches—especially with rotation— often fixes the problem. (See "Prevent It" for "Oblique Strain" on page 124 for more suggestions.)

- **Try Pilates.** I'm a big fan of Pilates classes for core reconditioning. Adding just two sessions a week to your normal regimen will give you incredible results. No more side stitches is one benefit, but the benefits to your sports performance will be even bigger.

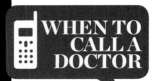

WHEN TO CALL A DOCTOR

If you get chronic side stitches and none of these basic measures work, see a sports doctor. Your side stitches could be lung related, such as exercise-induced bronchospasm or anatomical problems with the lungs. If one of those is your diagnosis, your doctor will most likely prescribe an inhaler, which is usually effective in these cases. (However, your author-doctor says with a smile, it's still a good idea to keep your core strong. Planks and core rotation, kids!)

DO YOU NEED SURGERY?
No.

ABDOMINALS, OBLIQUES & CHEST

NECK & SHOULDERS

Why does the shoulder chapter start with the neck? Because so many of the shoulder problems I see are actually referred pain coming from the neck. They go together better than peanut butter and jelly. Look at all the moving parts in this area of the body: the cervical vertebrae that make up the upper portion of your spine, which houses your spinal cord and the nerve roots that allow your entire upper body to function; your shoulder joints, which are ball-and-socket mechanisms surrounded by muscles, tendons, and cartilage; and support structures like the scapulas (shoulder blades) and clavicles (collarbones). There are so many ways this area can break down, and if you play an overhead sport like baseball, swimming, tennis, or volleyball, you're particularly vulnerable. In this section I'll show you how to ID and fix some of the most common and painful problems—and reveal some simple preventive tips that will keep you in the game.

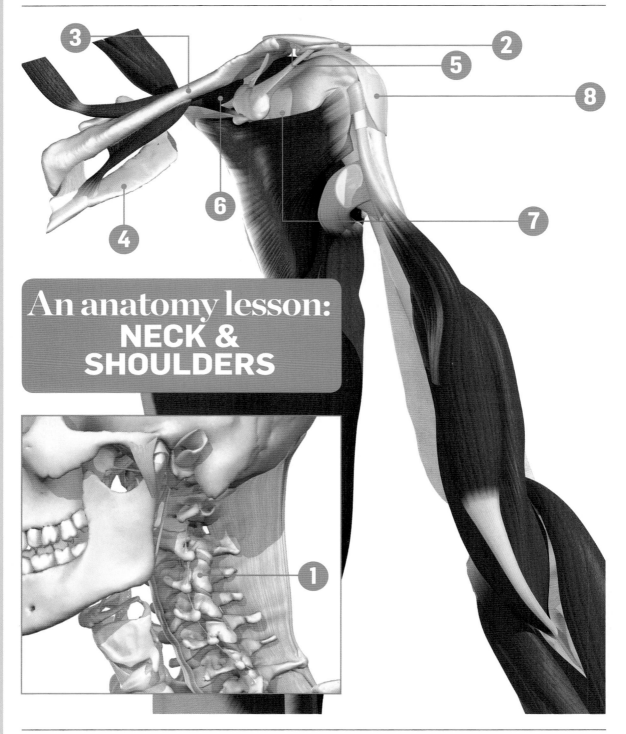

An anatomy lesson:
NECK & SHOULDERS

2 ACROMION

A long, protruding portion of bone in the upper scapula. You can feel your acromion as the bone at the top of your shoulder just above your deltoid muscle. If the acromion digs into or pinches the rotator cuff, you have a shoulder impingement.

1 CERVICAL VERTEBRAE

The vertebrae in the upper section of the spine (the thoracic and lumbar being the middle and lower sections, respectively). Each vertebra has its own designation from C1 to C7 and most nerve-based neck and shoulder pain originates from one or more of these points.

3 CLAVICLE, A.K.A. THE COLLARBONE

A long bone running from the sternum to the acromion on the scapula. It helps with shoulder stability and movement.

4 SCAPULA, A.K.A. THE SHOULDER BLADE

A triangular bone in the upper back that connects to the clavicle and upper end of the humerus. It helps protect the shoulder joint.

5 ACROMIOCLAVICU-LAR JOINT, A.K.A. THE A.C. JOINT

The joint in the upper shoulder where the clavicle and acromion meet. It allows you to raise your arm above your head. A "separated shoulder" occurs when the ligaments attaching these bones are injured.

6 ROTATOR CUFF

A group of muscles in the back of the shoulder – the supraspinatus, infraspi-natus, teres minor, and subscapularis -- that help hold the ball of the humerus in the shoulder socket and allow arm rotation.

8 SUBACROMIAL BURSA

Bursa (or bursae) are fluid-filled sacs that act as shock absorbers between a bone and muscle, tendon, or skin. The subacromial bursa lies under the acromion of the shoulder blade and above the head of the humerus. This location makes it susceptible to pinch-ing or irritation.

7 LABRUM

A thick rim of cartilage around the ball of the humerus that deepens the shoulder socket and allows the joint to move freely. The biceps ligament in the shoulder attaches to the labrum.

NECK & SHOULDERS

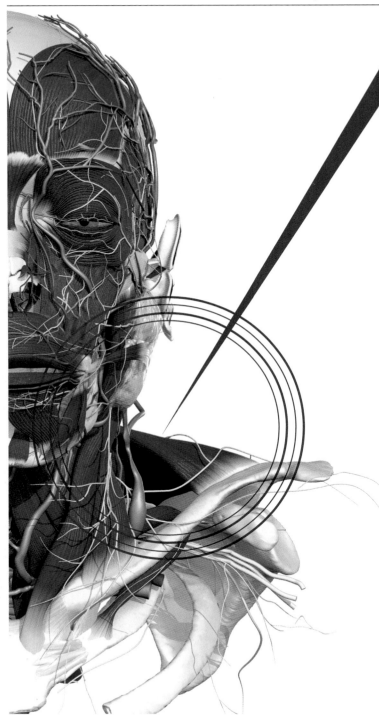

THE MALADY: Muscular Neck Pain

THE SYMPTOMS

Pain, sometimes severe, in the neck muscles that can cause a spasm or a "locking up" sensation.

WHAT'S GOING ON IN THERE?

The human body has a set of muscles that run along both sides of your spine all the way from your tailbone to the back of your head. That's a lot of muscle. And that's why muscular pain is the most common type of neck pain.

Localized pain is the main give-away that your problem is muscular, which is a much simpler issue to treat than something related to your cervical spine (the part of the spine in the neck). When you get muscle spasms on the sides of your neck, the pain tends not to radiate down into your fingers the way it would with a cervical disk or nerve problem (see "Nerve-Based Neck Pain [Cervical Radiculopathy]" on page 142). The pain is in the muscles on one or both sides of your spine and that's it.

The causes are usually classic: asking too much of an unprepared or fatigued muscle, overuse, or even sleeping on it wrong.

FIX IT

- **Employ dynamic rest.** Avoid activities that engage the neck and shoulders. Use lower-body workouts to maintain fitness.

- **Ice it.** Apply ice to the neck for 15 minutes 4 to 6 times a day for the first 2 days.

- **Try an NSAID.** An antiinflammatory like ibuprofen or naproxen can help with swelling and inflammation.

- **Go for a massage.** Massaging the neck muscles can help a lot. A professional massage therapist will be trained in addressing this type of pain.

- **Reestablish range of motion.** As pain improves, try these exercises to help recondition your neck and shoulders. Once you're pain free, move on to more aggressive neck and shoulder conditioning to help prevent the problem from recurring. (See "Prevent It" on the following page.)

NECK STRETCHES. Stand with your hands behind your neck. Bend your neck back and look at the ceiling. Squeeze your shoulder blades together. Hold for a moment and return to the starting position.

Work up to 10 reps. Also, try basic head rotation to the left and right, as well as tilting your head to the left and right, for up to 10 reps each.

BASIC RESISTANCE. Do the same movements just described, but change them to resistance exercises by using your hand to prevent your head from moving, i.e., by putting your hand on the right side of your head and trying to tilt your head to the right while your hand prevents it. Hold for 5 seconds. Do this for tilting your head left and right, turning your head left and right, and bending your head forward and backward. Do 10 reps of each movement.

SHOULDER REHAB. Shoulder shrugs, holding at the top for 5 seconds, are effective. Another good exercise: Stand with your arms at your sides and elbows bent at 90-degree angles. Shrug your shoulders backward in a circular motion as you squeeze your shoulder blades together. Hold for 5 seconds and return to the starting position. Do 10 reps.

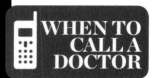

WHEN TO CALL A DOCTOR

Muscular neck pain doesn't usually require a doctor visit. In most cases, pain resolves within 1 to 2 weeks with conservative care, depending on the severity of the problem. But if your pain isn't responding to home-based care within a couple of weeks, schedule an appointment with a sports doctor to see if there are other issues to address. Your doctor may suggest other conservative measures that could help, such as acupuncture. Also, if you have a desk job, consider consulting a physical therapist about ergonomic adjustments you can make to your office chair and desk that could help.

DO YOU NEED SURGERY?
No.

UPPER-BACK ROLL

Lie faceup with a foam roller under your mid-back, at the bottom of your shoulder blades. Clasp your hands behind your head and pull your elbows toward each other. Raise your hips off the floor slightly.

Slowly lower your back downward, so that your upper back bends over the foam roller. Raise back to the start and roll forward a couple of inches—so that the roller sits higher under your upper back—and repeat. Roll forward one more time and do it again. That's 1 rep.

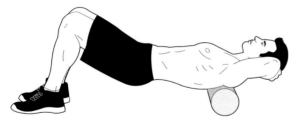

Cont'd on page 140

NECK & SHOULDERS

PREVENT IT

Properly conditioned neck and shoulder muscles are crucial, especially in sports that require swinging and throwing. Your regular upper-body workout should include lots of overhead shoulder work. You can increase overall dynamic flexibility by using the Iron Strength workout section of this book (see page 256). But even if you don't use those specific workouts, the stretches and exercises here can be added to any workout.

BARBELL SHRUG

Grab a barbell with an overhand grip that's just beyond shoulder-width apart, and let the bar hang at arm's length in front of your waist. Keeping your back naturally arched, lean forward slightly at your hips. Shrug your shoulders as high as you can, as if raising the tops of your shoulders toward your ears. Keep your arms straight. Pause, then reverse the movement back to the starting position.

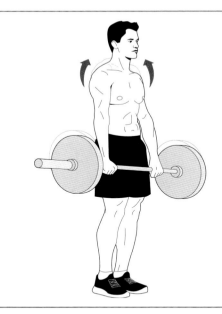

INVERTED ROW

Grab the bar above you with an overhand, shoulder-width grip. Hang with your arms completely straight and your hands positioned directly above your shoulders. Your body should form a straight line from your ankles to your head. Initiate the movement by pulling your shoulder blades back, then continue the pull with your arms to lift your chest to the bar. Pause, then slowly lower your body back to the starting position.

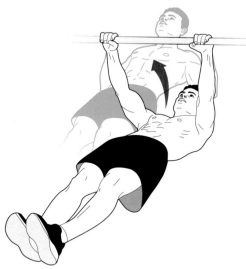

WATCH YOUR POSTURE
Most people spend hours each day in an office chair, and lousy posture can contribute to neck problems. When you're sitting, imagine that there's a straight line from your ears down to your hips. Your shoulders should be back and open, feeling as if they're resting on your shoulder blades. This keeps your body aligned and also promotes good breathing. Also, get up, move around, and stretch at least once an hour.

DON'T SHRUG OFF THE SHRUG

Shrugs are one of the best exercises for your neck and upper back. One of the primary muscles in this transaction is the levator scapula, which runs down the back of your neck and attaches to the inside edge of your shoulder blade. It works with your upper trapezius to help shrug your shoulder, which is why you can strengthen it with barbell and dumbbell shrugs.

REAR LATERAL RAISE

Grab a pair of dumbbells and bend forward at your hips until your torso is nearly parallel to the floor. Set your feet shoulder-width apart. Let the dumbbells hang straight down from your shoulders, your palms facing each other. Without moving your torso, raise your arms straight out to your sides until they're in line with your body. Pause, then slowly return to the starting position.

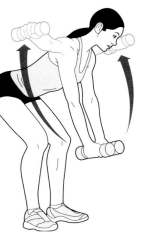

SERRATUS CHAIR SHRUG

Sit upright on a chair or bench and place your hands flat on the sitting surface next to your hips. Completely straighten your arms. Allow your shoulders and back muscles to relax so your torso lowers between your shoulders. Your hips should just be off the edge of the bench. Press your shoulders down as you lift your upper body. Your torso should rise between your shoulders. Pause for 5 seconds, then lower your body back to the starting position.

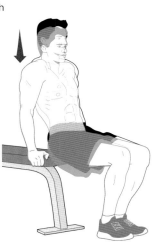

FLOOR Y-T-I RAISES
NOTE: Do one full set of each letter.

Y RAISE

Lie facedown on the floor. Allow your arms to rest on the floor, completely straight and at a 30-degree angle to your body, your palms facing each other (thumbs up). Your body should resemble the letter Y. Raise your arms as high as you can, pause, then slowly lower back to the starting position.

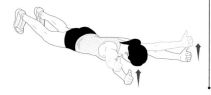

T RAISE

Lie facedown on the floor. Move your arms so they're out to your sides—perpendicular to your body with the thumb sides of your hands pointing up—and raise them as high as you can. Pause, then slowly lower back to the starting position.

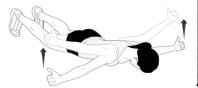

I RAISE

Lie facedown on the floor. Position your arms straight above your shoulders so your body forms a straight line from your feet to your fingertips. Your palms should be facing each other, thumbs pointing up. Raise your arms as high as you can, pause, then slowly lower back to the starting position.

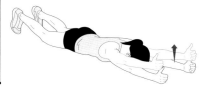

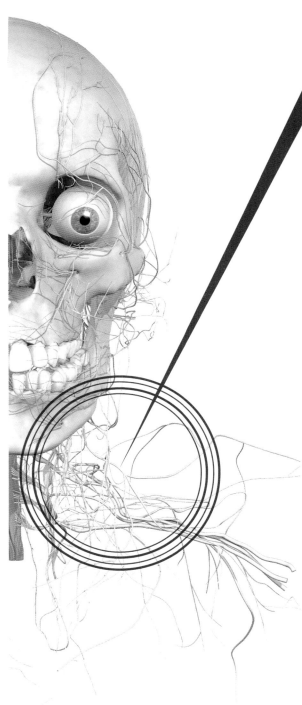

THE MALADY:
Nerve-Based Neck Pain
(cervical radiculopathy)

THE SYMPTOMS

Sharp pain radiating into the shoulder and sometimes into the arm and hand, especially when lifting and/or turning your head. Variations include numbness, tingling, and weakness.

WHAT'S GOING ON IN THERE?

Cervical radiculopathy is more common than you think and confuses a lot of athletes. This condition causes pain in the shoulder and/or arm, and athletes think something is wrong with either one or both when the problem is actually neither. The issue is in the neck.

Your cervical spine (the part in your neck) houses your spinal cord, which has nerve roots that branch off to supply motor and sensory function to your upper arms. When you raise your head and/or twist your neck, the nerve roots can be pinched where they exit the cervical spine. *Voilà,* you have pain in the nerves down the line, in the shoulder or arm.

This is called referred pain, which is pain that comes from a different part of the body from where you feel it. Statistically, the most common origin of referred pain in the upper extremities is the neck, and the most common site of the referred pain is the shoulder or arm. I see this a lot, especially in cyclists and swimmers.

So what causes the problem? Your neck vertebrae being out of alignment, or having a degenerative condition like arthritis or bone spurs, but the most common cause in young and middle-aged athletes is having a herniated cervical disk that's compressing a nerve root.

FIX IT

- **See a doctor.** It's smart to see a doctor for this radiating arm or shoulder pain because a proper diagnosis usually requires some detective work. See "When to Call a Doctor."

- **Employ dynamic rest.** Avoid any activities that engage the neck and shoulders. Use lower-body workouts to maintain fitness.

- **Ice it.** Apply ice to the neck for 15 minutes 4 to 6 times a day for the first 2 days.

- **Try an NSAID.** An antiinflammatory like ibuprofen or naproxen can help with swelling and inflammation.

- **Reestablish range of motion.** As pain improves, try these exercises to help recondition your neck and shoulders. Once you're pain free, move on to more aggressive neck and shoulder conditioning to help prevent the problem from recurring.

NECK STRETCHES. Stand with your hands behind your neck. Bend your neck back and look at the ceiling. Squeeze your shoulder blades together. Hold for a moment and return to the starting position. Work up to 10 reps. Also, try basic head rotation to the left and right, as well as tilting your head to the left and right, for up to 10 reps each.

BASIC RESISTANCE. Do the same movements just described, but change them to resistance exercises by using your hand to prevent your head from moving, i.e., by putting your hand on the right side of your head and trying to tilt your head to the right while your hand prevents it. Hold for 5 seconds. Do this for tilting your head left and right, turning your head left and right, and bending your head forward and backward. Do 10 reps of each movement.

SHOULDER REHAB. Shoulder shrugs, holding at the top for 5 seconds, are effective. Another good exercise: Stand with your arms at 90-degree angles in front of your body. Rotate them to the sides as you squeeze your shoulder blades together. Hold for 5 seconds and return to the starting position. Do 10 reps.

PREVENT IT

- **Recondition your neck and shoulders.** Having properly conditioned muscles in your neck and shoulders can help keep everything in its place. The stronger and more flexible the muscles, the more support your spine has, which can prevent nerve compression. Your regular upper-body workout should include lots of overhead shoulder work, as well as the resistance exercises mentioned in "Fix It" that specifically target your neck. I also recommend regularly doing yoga and Pilates workouts for overall kinetic chain conditioning. (See "Prevent It" for "Muscular Neckpain" on page 140 for more suggestions.)

- **Watch your posture.** Most people spend hours each day in an office chair, and lousy posture can contribute to neck problems. While sitting, imagine that there's a straight line from your ears down to your hips. Your shoulders should be back and open, feeling as if they're resting on your shoulder blades. This keeps your body aligned and also promotes good breathing. Also, get up, move around, and stretch at least once an hour.

WHEN TO CALL A DOCTOR

A physical exam of the neck and upper body can help offer clues as to which movements cause the pain. X-rays of the neck can show if bones are out of alignment, and an MRI can reveal cervical disc herniation.

Over-the-counter antiinflammatories (ice along with ibuprofen or naproxen) are generally effective against cervical radiculopathy pain. A sports doc can also use more aggressive therapies to ease symptoms. For intense pain, a short course of oral steroids can be used, and if pain persists, the doctor can inject corticosteroids directly into the area. Physical therapy is also a mainstay of initial treatment, with a focus on cervical traction.

DO YOU NEED SURGERY?

Rarely. With the basic therapies listed here, most patients are asymptomatic within 2 to 4 weeks.

NECK & SHOULDERS

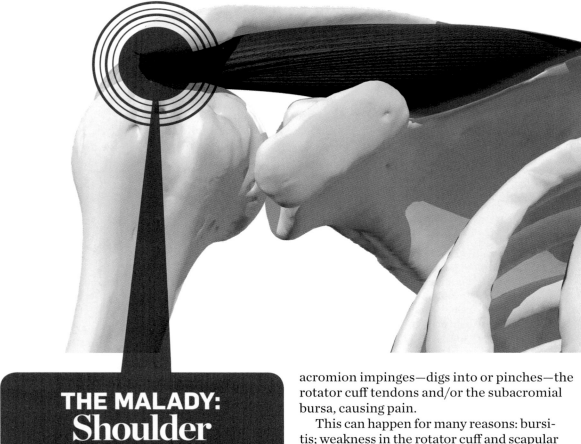

THE MALADY:
Shoulder Impingement

THE SYMPTOMS

A pinching sensation, pain, and possible weakness when you lift your arms above your head.

WHAT'S GOING ON IN THERE?

The rotator cuff is a collection of muscles that surround the shoulder joint and help hold the humerus bone of your upper arm in the shoulder socket. Impingement happens when the arm lifts and a bone in the shoulder called the acromion impinges—digs into or pinches—the rotator cuff tendons and/or the subacromial bursa, causing pain.

This can happen for many reasons: bursitis; weakness in the rotator cuff and scapular (shoulder blade) stabilizing muscles; an injury to the tendon attaching the rotator cuff to the humerus, especially when there is tendinitis; poor athletic mechanics; and a shoulder shape that predisposes you to injury.

Baseball, tennis, weight lifting, swimming, volleyball, and even competitive sailing put you at risk.

NOTE: Also beware "frozen shoulder," which can come on spontaneously or after an impingement when the shoulder isn't being used. The joint tightens, or "freezes," especially at night. Women tend to be more prone to this. See a doctor, as early diagnosis and treatment—usually with a cortisone injection—is key.

- **See a doctor.** The shoulder is a complex and important joint, so see a sports doc at the first sign of shoulder pain. See "When to Call a Doctor" for more details.

- **Employ dynamic rest.** Lay off the upper-body work (including swimming), and use lower-body workouts to maintain fitness.

- **Ice it.** Ice applied to the shoulder for 15 minutes several times a day can help reduce inflammation.

- **Try an NSAID.** An antiinflammatory like ibuprofen or naproxen can help with the pain.

- **Start rehabbing.** As the pain improves, do some rotator cuff exercises to help strengthen your shoulder. Here are three.

SHOULDER SQUEEZE #1. Lie facedown on an exercise bench. Hold your arms out to your sides parallel to the floor, bent at 90 degrees with your thumbs pointing toward the ceiling. Now try to raise your elbows toward the ceiling and feel your shoulder blades squeezing together. Hold for a moment and return to the starting position. Do 10 to 20 reps depending on your strength.

SHOULDER SQUEEZE #2. While lying facedown on the bench, hold your arms along your sides with your palms up. Keeping your arms straight, lift your palms toward the ceiling, again feeling your shoulder blades squeeze together. Hold for a moment and return to the starting position. Again, do 10 to 20 reps.

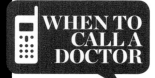

WHEN TO CALL A DOCTOR

Always see a sports doctor at the first sign of shoulder pain. A proper diagnosis is critical in not just fixing the problem, but also in preventing the problem from getting worse because you don't know what it is.

Once diagnosed, the first step is usually physical therapy. Your doctor may give you a corticosteroid injection to help relieve the pain enough to start rehabbing. The therapist will test you for underlying strength deficiencies and imbalances. Then you'll begin a strengthening program for your shoulder. This usually solves the problem.

If this doesn't work, an MRI can look for underlying soft-tissue injuries such as a torn rotator cuff tendon or labrum, the cartilage in the shoulder.

DO YOU NEED SURGERY?
Sometimes. It is possible if you have a significant rotator cuff tear, or if you've developed a bone spur that irritates the connective tissue. Arthroscopic surgery can handle bone spurs and smaller tears. Larger tears require open surgery. Results are usually good, but the severity of the injury and your age will determine if you return to your preinjury performance level.

PERFORM EXTERNAL ROTATIONS

Use a light weight to do this classic rotator cuff exercise. Why is it so important? It helps cure shoulder muscle imbalances. The rotator cuff muscles attach to the outside of the upper arm. Your lats and pecs, however, attach to the inside of your upper arm. If the opposing sets are out of balance, you're more prone to injury as well as lousy posture. The following is a basic external rotation exercise. You can also do this exercise while standing using a cable station.

SEATED DUMBBELL EXTERNAL ROTATION

Grab a dumbbell in your right hand and sit on a bench. Place your right foot on the bench with your knee bent. Bend your right elbow 90 degrees and place the inside portion of it on your right knee. Use your free hand for support. Without changing the bend in your elbow, and while keeping your wrist straight, rotate your upper arm and forearm up and back as far as you can. Pause, then return to the starting position. Perform the prescribed number of repetitions with your right arm, then switch and perform the same number with your left arm.

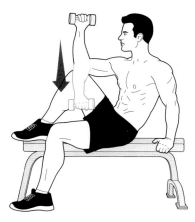

Cont'd on page 146

PREVENT IT

Having a strong, balanced shoulder resists this type of injury because well-conditioned muscles reduce the load on the rotator cuff. That means that shoulder work must be a staple of your upper-body workouts, and you must work opposing muscle groups to avoid an imbalance (for every push exercise like a pushup, do an equal amount of a pulling exercise like rows). You can increase overall dynamic flexibility by using the Iron Strength workout section of this book (see page 256). But even if you don't use those specific workouts, the stretches and exercises here can be added to any workout.

SLEEPER STRETCH

Lie on the floor on your left side with your left upper arm on the floor and your elbow bent 90 degrees. Adjust your torso so that your right shoulder is slightly behind your left, not directly over it. Your fingers on your left hand should point toward the ceiling. Gently push your left hand toward the floor until you feel a comfortable stretch in the back of your left shoulder. Hold for 30 seconds, then roll over and repeat the stretch for your right shoulder. Perform 2 to 3 times a day to improve flexibility, or 3 times a week to maintain flexibility.

PULLUP

Grab the pullup bar with a shoulder-width, overhand grip. Hang at arm's length. You should return to this position—known as a dead hang—each time you lower your body back down. Cross your ankles behind you. Pull your chest to the bar as you squeeze your shoulder blades together. Once the top of your chest touches the bar, pause, then slowly lower your body back to a dead hang.

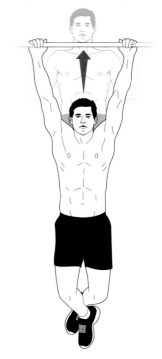

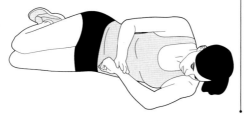

AVOID UPRIGHT ROWS
Research shows that roughly two-thirds of men are at high risk for shoulder impingement when performing upright rows. It's a popular exercise where, for example in the case of the barbell variety, you stand holding the barbell in front of you with an overhand grip and lift the weight up the front of your body until you're holding the bar just under your chin. Impingement most often occurs when your upper arms are simultaneously at shoulder level or higher and rotated inward—the exact position they're in at the top of the upright row.

SWIMMERS, IMPROVE YOUR MECHANICS

The key to healthy swimming is good coaching. Learning proper technique straight out of the gate is the best way to start. If you're already a dedicated water rat, a good swim coach can spot and correct any mechanical flaws you have that could cause injury. So consult with a good local coach—the worst that can happen is that you improve.

SERRATUS CHAIR SHRUG

Sit upright on a chair or bench and place your hands flat on the sitting surface next to your hips. Completely straighten your arms. Allow your shoulders and back muscles to relax so your torso lowers between your shoulders. Your hips should just be off the edge of the bench. Press your shoulders down as you lift your upper body. Your torso should rise between your shoulders. Pause for 5 seconds, then lower your body back to the starting position.
NOTE: You can do this exercise at your desk or your couch while you watch TV.

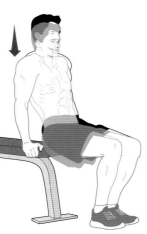

INVERTED SHOULDER PRESS

Assume a pushup position, but place your feet on a bench or chair and push your hips up so that your torso is nearly perpendicular to the floor. Your hands should be slightly wider than your shoulders, and your arms should be straight.

Without changing your body posture, lower your body until your head nearly touches the floor. Pause, then return to the starting position by pushing your body back up until your arms are straight.

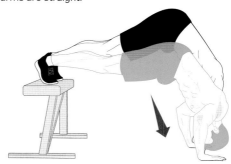

FLOOR Y-T-I RAISES

NOTE: Do one full set of each letter.

Y RAISE

Lie facedown on the floor. Allow your arms to rest on the floor, completely straight and at a 30-degree angle to your body, your palms facing each other (thumbs up). Your body should resemble the letter Y. Raise your arms as high as you can, pause, then slowly lower back to the starting position.

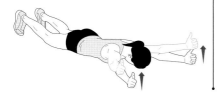

T RAISE

Lie facedown on the floor. Move your arms so they're out to your sides—perpendicular to your body with the thumb sides of your hands pointing up—and raise them as high as you can. Pause, then slowly lower back to the starting position.

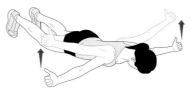

I RAISE

Lie facedown on the floor. Position your arms straight above your shoulders so your body forms a straight line from your feet to your fingertips. Your palms should be facing each other, thumbs pointing up. Raise your arms as high as you can, pause, then slowly lower back to the starting position.

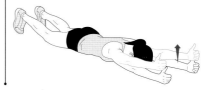

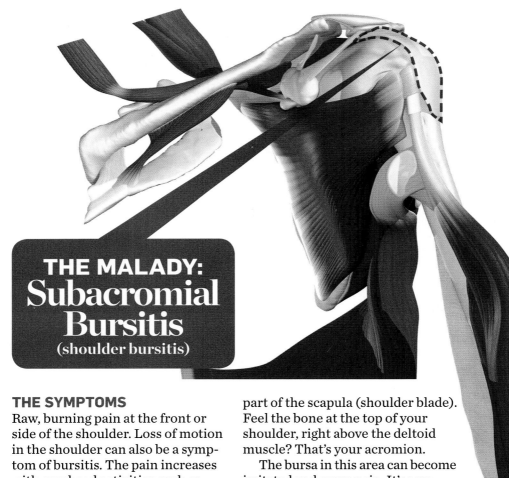

THE MALADY:
Subacromial Bursitis
(shoulder bursitis)

THE SYMPTOMS

Raw, burning pain at the front or side of the shoulder. Loss of motion in the shoulder can also be a symptom of bursitis. The pain increases with overhead activities such as throwing, swimming, etc. The pain may also increase if you lean on your elbow.

WHAT'S GOING ON IN THERE?

Bursae are fluid-filled shock absorbers located between a bone and a muscle, tendon, or skin. In the shoulder's case, the subacromial bursa interacts with the rotator cuff and the surrounding bones, especially the acromion, which is part of the scapula (shoulder blade). Feel the bone at the top of your shoulder, right above the deltoid muscle? That's your acromion.

The bursa in this area can become irritated and cause pain. It's common for subacromial bursitis (a.k.a. shoulder bursitis, meaning bursitis under the acromion) to accompany shoulder impingement (see page 144) or rotator cuff strain (see page 152), but it can have a variety of causes. The most typical ones for athletes are rotator cuff weakness, shoulder instability, a shoulder impact, and overuse, especially in overhead sports like baseball, tennis, swimming, and volleyball.

FIX IT

- **See a doctor.** The shoulder is a complex and important joint, so see a sports doc at the first sign of shoulder pain. See "When to Call a Doctor" for more details.

- **Employ dynamic rest.** Lay off the upper-body work (including swimming), and use lower-body workouts to maintain fitness.

- **Ice it.** Ice applied to the shoulder for 15 minutes several times a day can help reduce inflammation.

- **Try an NSAID.** An antiinflammatory like ibuprofen or naproxen can help with the pain.

- **Start rehabbing.** As the pain improves, do some rotator cuff exercises to help strengthen your shoulder. Here are two.

SHOULDER SQUEEZE #1 Lie facedown on an exercise bench. Hold your arms out to your sides parallel to the floor, bent at 90 degrees with your thumbs pointing toward the ceiling. Now try to raise your elbows toward the ceiling and feel your shoulder blades squeezing together. Hold for a moment and return to the starting position. Do 10 to 20 reps depending on your strength.

SHOULDER SQUEEZE #2 While lying facedown on the bench, hold your arms along your sides with your palms up. Keeping your arms straight, lift your palms toward the ceiling, again feeling your shoulder blades squeeze together. Hold for a moment and return to the starting position. Again, do 10 to 20 reps.

PREVENT IT

- **Work the shoulder both ways.** Having a strong, balanced shoulder is the best injury-prevention strategy—strong muscles take the strain off tendons, cartilage, bones, and of course bursae. Even better here: The muscles in and around the shoulder respond well to exercise. Shoulder work must be a staple of your upper-body workouts, and you must work opposing muscle groups to avoid an imbalance. That means, for example, that if you do a pushing exercise (such as bench presses or overhead presses), you need to do an equivalent amount of a pulling movement (like rowing or pullups). Also, add in some rotator cuff exercises like the ones in "Fix It," especially if you're in an overhead sport. (Also see "Prevent It" for Shoulder Impingement on page 146 for more suggestions.)

- **Swimmers, improve your mechanics.** The key to healthy swimming is good coaching. Learning proper technique straight out of the gate is the best way to start. If you're already a dedicated water rat, a good swim coach can spot and correct any mechanical flaws you have that could cause injury. So consult with a good local coach—the worst that can happen is that you improve.

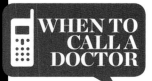

WHEN TO CALL A DOCTOR

It's always a good idea to see a sports doctor for shoulder pain. In the case of bursitis, it's common for it to accompany shoulder impingement and/or rotator cuff tendinitis. A proper diagnosis will catch any and all of these issues, plus any underlying problems that might exist.

Conservative, home-based care is generally enough to resolve bursitis, but if the pain doesn't improve within a week or if the pain is severe, your doctor may give you a corticosteroid injection and prescribe physical therapy. Note, however, that I won't do an injection when rotator cuff tendinitis is present. In general, however, you should be pain free within a couple of weeks. Proper shoulder conditioning can then prevent any further issues from developing.

DO YOU NEED SURGERY?

Extreme cases that don't respond to normal treatment can benefit from surgical intervention, but these are rare.

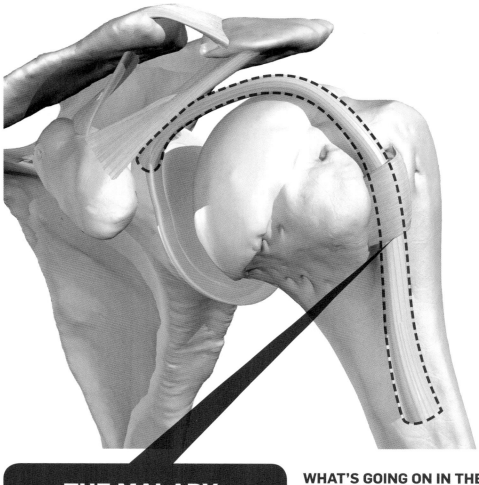

THE MALADY:
Biceps
Tendinitis

THE SYMPTOMS

Pain at the front of the shoulder, several inches below the collarbone, that gets worse when lifting or during overhead exertion.

WHAT'S GOING ON IN THERE?

A big part of the socket in your ball-and-socket shoulder joint is the labrum, a thick rim of cartilage that surrounds the ball of the humerus and helps keep it in place. The labrum also happens to be the anchor point for the upper biceps tendon. So that tendon is close to moving bone, rotator cuff muscles, and other connective tissues—that's a lot going on in a small area, which means a lot of things can irritate and strain the biceps tendon.

The most common issue is overuse. But other shoulder maladies also can affect the biceps tendon, such as rotator cuff problems (see page 152), shoulder impingement (see page 144), and shoulder dislocation (see page 160).

Don't ignore this pain or try to play through it. Chronic irritation of the biceps tendon can lead to a rupture—and you'll know it when that happens. You generally hear an audible pop or tearing sound, and the biceps can ball up under the skin. Obviously, this is not good. Address the pain as soon as you feel it.

Athletes who play overhead sports like baseball, tennis, swimming, gymnastics, volleyball, and even rowing and kayaking are most at risk for biceps tendinitis.

FIX IT

- **Employ dynamic rest.** Avoid lifting and overhead exertion. Use lower-body and core workouts to maintain fitness.

- **Ice it.** Apply ice to the area for 15 minutes 4 to 6 times a day for the first 2 days.

- **Try an NSAID.** An antiinflammatory like ibuprofen or naproxen can help with swelling and inflammation.

- **Rebuild the area.** Basic exercises that work the biceps and shoulder muscles will help get you back to preinjury form. Here are three you can try. Be conservative with the number of sets and reps you do, depending on the severity of your injury.

ROTATOR CUFF ROTATION. With your elbow against your side and your arm bent at 90 degrees, apply light resistance with your other hand (or rubber resistance bands) as you bring your forearm across your belly and then return to the starting position. Be sure to change the direction of the resistance as you change the direction of the movement so you work the muscle with both pushing and pulling.

BICEPS STRETCH. Stand facing a wall that is about 6 inches away. Lift your arm straight out to the side and put the side of your thumb against the wall, palm down. Keeping your arm straight, turn away from the outstretched arm (keeping your hand against the wall) until you feel a stretch in the biceps and shoulder. Hold for 20 to 30 seconds, breathing normally.

BICEPS CURL. Start doing this movement with no weight and move on to light weights as you get stronger.

PREVENT IT

- **Build strong and supple muscles.** Powerful and flexible arms and shoulders relieve connective tissues like tendons of a massive amount of stress. Make sure your upper-body regimen employs balanced resistance training that includes both pushing (pushups, bench presses) and pulling (pullups, rowing) movements.

- **Perfect your form.** Lousy form can cause an injury. If you're in an overhead sport, always consult with your coach about how to maintain proper form, especially when throwing. Everyone's body type is different, which means proper form needs to be achieved individually. Work on it.

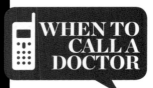

WHEN TO CALL A DOCTOR

Biceps tendinitis usually heals by itself over several weeks. However, if your pain is severe, and especially if you have pain in other areas of the shoulder, see a doctor to reveal the extent of the tendinitis and any complications.

Physical therapy can help. A doctor can also administer corticosteroid injections to help with pain and inflammation, but injections need to be precisely placed—injecting directly into the tendon can bring on a rupture.

Some facilities now offer ultrasound-guided injections, in which the doctor uses an ultrasound image to guide the needle. This is incredibly helpful in situations where accuracy counts. If your doctor is talking injection, ask about this new development.

DO YOU NEED SURGERY?

Not likely. If conservative, home-based care doesn't improve your symptoms within 6 months, surgery could be an option, depending on what's causing your tendinitis. Nerve decompression and removal of irritating parts of bone are two surgical possibilities. Your doctor will discuss all of this with you.

NECK & SHOULDERS

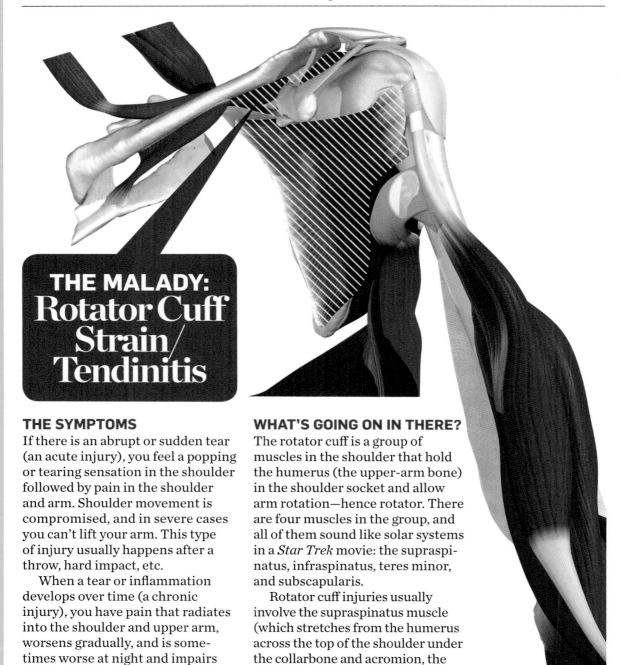

THE MALADY: Rotator Cuff Strain/Tendinitis

THE SYMPTOMS

If there is an abrupt or sudden tear (an acute injury), you feel a popping or tearing sensation in the shoulder followed by pain in the shoulder and arm. Shoulder movement is compromised, and in severe cases you can't lift your arm. This type of injury usually happens after a throw, hard impact, etc.

When a tear or inflammation develops over time (a chronic injury), you have pain that radiates into the shoulder and upper arm, worsens gradually, and is sometimes worse at night and impairs sleep. Weakness is common.

WHAT'S GOING ON IN THERE?

The rotator cuff is a group of muscles in the shoulder that hold the humerus (the upper-arm bone) in the shoulder socket and allow arm rotation—hence rotator. There are four muscles in the group, and all of them sound like solar systems in a *Star Trek* movie: the supraspinatus, infraspinatus, teres minor, and subscapularis.

Rotator cuff injuries usually involve the supraspinatus muscle (which stretches from the humerus across the top of the shoulder under the collarbone and acromion, the upper part of the scapula) and/or the infraspinatus muscle (which reaches across the back of the shoulder blade to meet the humerus).

The two most common rotator cuff injuries? A tear in a muscle or tendon (a strain) and inflammation of a tendon (tendinitis). Other conditions, such as shoulder impingement (see page 144) and subacromial bursitis (see page 148) can accompany a rotator cuff injury.

Another issue in this area is the scapula (shoulder blade) and the muscles surrounding it.

When those muscles aren't strong enough to keep the scapula tracking the way it should, you get a condition called scapular dyskinesis. That can put too much load on the rotator cuff muscles and cause tendinitis or bursitis.

Any overhead activity can injure the rotator cuff, so baseball, tennis, swimming, volleyball, cricket, and even less obvious sports like kayaking and sailing put you at risk.

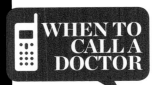

WHEN TO CALL A DOCTOR

Immediately, especially for an acute injury. You don't want to mess with shoulder pain, especially if you suspect a rotator cuff injury. They generally heal successfully over weeks or months depending on the severity, but x-rays and MRIs are helpful in pinpointing the injury and identifying any additional issues like shoulder impingement, bone spurs, and so on.

If conservative, home-based care doesn't help, a doctor can inject antiinflammatory corticosteroids into the area and also prescribe physical therapy. I'd say about 90 percent of cases respond to these approaches.

DO YOU NEED SURGERY?

Not all rotator cuff tears need surgery. Younger adults who want to continue their athletic careers are generally better candidates. Complete tears require reconstruction. Surgery is also a possibility for folks who see no improvement within 8 to 12 weeks or so with conservative care. Recovery is long—at least 6 months—but the outcome is usually good.

FIX IT

- **See a doctor.** Any shoulder pain—especially that from an acute injury—needs to be evaluated by a sports doctor. See "When to Call a Doctor" for more details.

- **Employ dynamic rest.** Lay off the upper-body work (including swimming), and use lower-body workouts to maintain fitness.

- **Ice it.** Ice applied to the shoulder for 15 minutes several times a day can help reduce inflammation.

- **Try an NSAID.** An antiinflammatory like ibuprofen or naproxen can help with the pain.

- **Start rehabbing.** As the pain improves, do some rotator cuff exercises to help strengthen your shoulder. Here are two (see "Prevent It" on the following page for more suggestions).

SHOULDER SQUEEZE. Lie facedown on an exercise bench. Hold your arms out to your sides parallel to the floor, bent at 90 degrees with your thumbs pointing toward the ceiling. Now try to raise your elbows toward the ceiling, feeling your shoulder blades squeeze together. Hold for a moment and return to the starting position. Do 10 to 20 reps depending on your strength.

SEATED DUMBBELL EXTERNAL ROTATION

Grab a dumbbell in your right hand and sit on a bench. Place your right foot on the bench with your knee bent. Bend your right elbow 90 degrees and place the inside portion of it on your right knee. Use your free hand for support. Without changing the bend in your elbow, and while keeping your wrist straight, rotate your upper arm and forearm up and back as far as you can. Pause, then return to the starting position. Perform the prescribed number of repetitions with your right arm, then switch and perform the same number with your left arm.

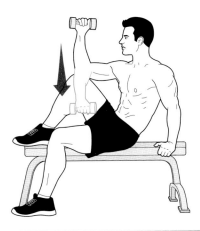

Cont'd on page 154

PREVENT IT

Having a strong, balanced shoulder is the best injury-prevention strategy. Even better here: The muscles in and around the shoulder respond well to exercise. That means that shoulder work must be a staple of your upper-body workouts, and you must work opposing muscle groups to avoid an imbalance (for every push exercise like a pushup, do an equal amount of a pulling exercise like rows). You can increase overall dynamic flexibility by using the Iron Strength workout section of this book (see page 256). But even if you don't use those specific workouts, the stretches and exercises here can be added to any workout.

SLEEPER STRETCH

Lie on the floor on your left side with your left upper arm on the floor and your elbow bent 90 degrees. Adjust your torso so that your right shoulder is slightly behind your left, not directly over it. Your fingers on your left hand should point toward the ceiling. Gently push your left hand toward the floor until you feel a comfortable stretch in the back of your left shoulder. Hold for 30 seconds, then roll over and repeat the stretch for your right shoulder. Perform 2 to 3 times a day to improve flexibility, or 3 times a week to maintain flexibility.

PULLUP

Grab the pullup bar with a shoulder-width, overhand grip. Hang at arm's length. You should return to this position—known as a dead hang—each time you lower your body back down. Cross your ankles behind you. Pull your chest to the bar as you squeeze your shoulder blades together. Once the top of your chest touches the bar, pause, then slowly lower your body back to a dead hang.

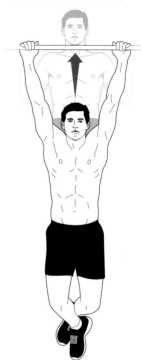

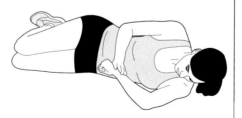

A SHOULDER FITNESS TEST
Hold your arm so that your elbow is bent at a right angle and your upper arm is parallel to the floor, as if you're giving a high-five. Without changing the position of your upper arm or moving your shoulder, rotate your forearm as far as you can forward and down, and then reverse the movement in the other direction. You want to be able to rotate your forearm 180 degrees. If you fall short, use the sleeper stretch to improve your flexibility.

STOP RUSHING

Proper warmup is crucial for your shoulders, especially if you're in a sport that requires wrenching, full-force shoulder action. Listen to your coaches' advice about proper mechanics and warmup procedures and don't skimp on or rush through them. Sport-specific procedures like these have been tested over time and keep athletes healthy. Ignore them at your own risk.

CABLE DIAGONAL RAISE

Attach a stirrup handle to the low pulley of a cable station. Standing with your left side toward the weight stack, feet shoulder-width apart, grab the handle with your right hand and position it in front of your left hip, with your elbow slightly bent. Imagine you're about to pull a sword from a scabbard. Without changing the bend in your elbow, pull the handle up and across your body until your hand is above your head. Lower the handle to the starting position. Complete the prescribed number of repetitions with your right arm, then immediately do the same number with your left arm.

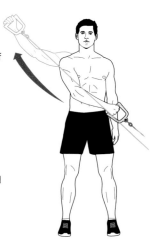

BARBELL SHRUG

Grab a barbell with an overhand grip that's just beyond shoulder-width apart, and let the bar hang at arm's length in front of your waist. Keeping your back naturally arched, lean forward slightly at your hips. Shrug your shoulders as high as you can, as if raising the tops of your shoulders toward your ears. Keep your arms straight. Pause, then reverse the movement back to the starting position.

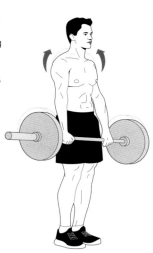

REAR LATERAL RAISE

Grab a pair of dumbbells and bend forward at your hips until your torso is nearly parallel to the floor. Set your feet shoulder-width apart. Let the dumbbells hang straight down from your shoulders, your palms facing each other. Without moving your torso, raise your arms straight out to your sides until they're in line with your body. Pause, then slowly return to the starting position.

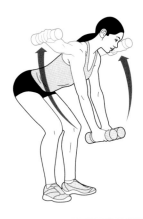

SCAPTION

Standing with your feet shoulder-width apart, hold a pair of dumbbells at arm's length next to your sides. Your palms should be facing each other and your elbows slightly bent. Without changing the bend in your elbows, raise your arms at a 30-degree angle to your body (so that they form a Y) until they're at shoulder level. The thumb sides of both hands should be facing up. Pause, then slowly lower the weights back to the starting position.

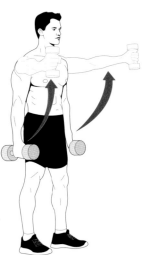

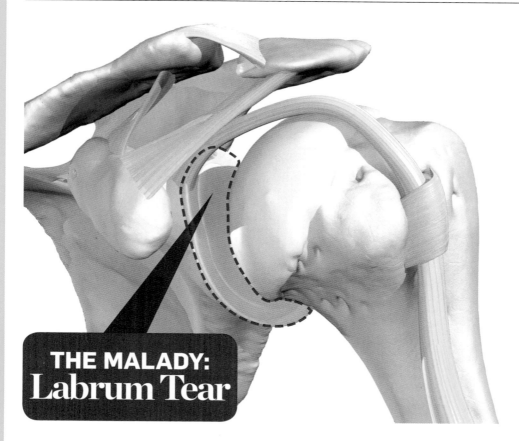

THE MALADY:
Labrum Tear

THE SYMPTOMS

Pain in the shoulder, especially with overhead exertion; a clicking or grinding sensation, and possibly locking of the joint; and weakness and/or joint instability.

WHAT'S GOING ON IN THERE?

The ball-and-socket joint that joins the humerus and the scapula actually has a very shallow socket (called the glenoid socket). The socket is deepened by a thick rim of cartilage, called the labrum, that surrounds and protects the ball of the humerus and allows the joint to move freely. Articular cartilage—cartilage that covers parts of bone within a joint where movement takes place—on the end of the humerus works with the labrum to give you a smooth-

functioning joint. Certain tendons, like the biceps tendon, attach to the labrum as well.

There are different kinds of labrum tears. Fraying of the labrum can occur with overuse and is generally asymptomatic. A tear above the midpoint of the glenoid socket is a superior labrum tear; a tear below the midpoint is an inferior tear. A superior tear that involves the biceps ligament is a SLAP (superior labrum from anterior to posterior) lesion.

What causes labrum tears? Repetitive motion (think baseball pitchers); a sudden pull on the arm, such as when lifting a heavy weight; an explosive reaching motion; a direct impact to the shoulder; a fall on an outstretched arm. Dislocated shoulders commonly come with labrum tears as well.

FIX IT

- **See a doctor.** Any shoulder pain—especially when caused by an acute injury—needs to be evaluated by a sports doctor. See "When to Call a Doctor" for more details.

- **Employ dynamic rest.** Lay off the upper-body work and use lower-body workouts to maintain fitness.

- **Ice it.** Ice applied to the shoulder for 15 minutes several times a day can help reduce inflammation.

- **Try an NSAID.** An antiinflammatory like ibuprofen or naproxen can help with the pain.

- **Start rehabbing.** As the pain improves, do some rotator cuff exercises to help strengthen your shoulder. Here are two.

SHOULDER SQUEEZE #1. Lie facedown on an exercise bench. Hold your arms out to your sides parallel to the floor, bent at 90 degrees with your thumbs pointing toward the ceiling. Now try to raise your elbows toward the ceiling and feel your shoulder blades squeezing together. Hold for a moment and return to the starting position. Do 10 to 20 reps depending on your strength.

SHOULDER SQUEEZE #2. While lying facedown on the bench, hold your arms along your sides with your palms up. Keeping your arms straight, lift your palms toward the ceiling, again feeling your shoulder blades squeeze together. Hold for a moment and return to the starting position. Again, do 10 to 20 reps.

PREVENT IT

- **Work the shoulder both ways.** Having a strong, balanced shoulder is the best injury-prevention strategy, and the muscles in and around the shoulder respond well to exercise. Shoulder work must be a staple of your upper-body workouts, and you must work opposing muscle groups to avoid an imbalance. That means, for example, that if you do a pushing exercise (such as bench presses or overhead presses), you need to do an equivalent amount of pulling movements (rowing, pullups). Also, add in some rotator cuff exercises like the ones in "Fix It," especially if you're in an overhead sport. See "Prevent It" for Rotator Cuff Strain on page 154 for more suggestions.

- **Reconsider that dive.** Professional athletes are expected to sacrifice their bodies for the game. Weekend warriors—especially those who may not be properly conditioned—have a choice. Making a diving catch in a softball game is a wonderful moment, but dislocating your shoulder and tearing your labrum, which could keep you out of work and affect your earning power (especially if you work with your hands), may not be worth it. Prioritize with your common sense, not your ego.

WHEN TO CALL A DOCTOR

See a sports doctor immediately for any shoulder pain. Labrum tears show up on MRIs, but having one doesn't necessarily mean surgery. In fact, I'd say that more people with labrum tears avoid surgery than have it. The key is to make your symptoms go away. If they go away, you can exist just fine with a labrum tear, and generally, conservative, home-based therapies can relieve symptoms.

DO YOU NEED SURGERY?

If conservative methods fail, pain persists, or the joint is unstable, surgery may be recommended. If you need surgery, the extent of it depends on the type of tear. A basic tear of the labrum rim requires removal or repair of the tear. If the biceps tendon is involved (in a SLAP lesion), the tendon needs to be repaired or reattached. You can generally return to sport-specific exercises 6 weeks after surgery and see full recovery in 3 to 4 months.

NECK & SHOULDERS

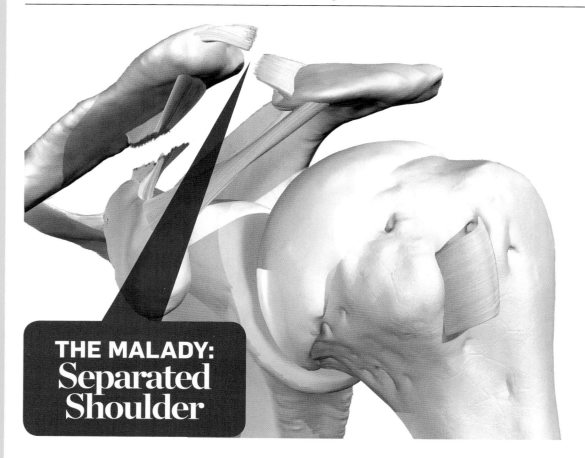

THE MALADY:
Separated Shoulder

THE SYMPTOMS

Shoulder pain, especially when you bring your arm across your body. You could have some bruising and swelling in the area, and maybe even a bump at the top of your shoulder. Joint weakness and loss of movement are also common.

WHAT'S GOING ON IN THERE?

People often confuse a separated shoulder with a dislocated shoulder. They're not even close. A dislocated shoulder occurs when the ball of the humerus dislocates from the socket joint of the scapula. A separated shoulder involves the acromioclavicular joint (a.k.a. the AC joint), where the collarbone and the long,

protruding portion of the upper scapula meet. This long, protruding section is called the acromion. You can feel the acromion when you rub the bone at the top of your shoulder just above your deltoid muscle.

The end of the collarbone attaches to the acromion via two ligaments that stabilize the AC joint. One is the acromioclavicular ligament and the other is the coracoclavicular ligament. If one or both of these ligaments is overstretched or torn, you have a separated shoulder.

The most common causes are sustaining a direct impact to or falling on the shoulder. So playing any full-contact sport puts you at risk. Less obvious sports that present an increased risk include skiing, gymnastics, and volleyball.

FIX IT

- **See a doctor.** Any shoulder pain—especially when caused by an acute injury—needs to be evaluated by a sports doctor. See "When to Call a Doctor" for more details.

- **Employ dynamic rest.** Lay off the upper-body work and use lower-body workouts to maintain fitness. Use a sling to help immobilize your arm during your daily activities.

- **Ice it.** Ice applied to the shoulder for 15 minutes several times a day can help reduce inflammation.

- **Try an NSAID.** An antiinflammatory like ibuprofen or naproxen can help with the pain.

- **Start rehabbing.** As the pain improves, do some rotator cuff exercises to help strengthen your shoulder. Here are two.

SHOULDER SQUEEZE. Lie facedown on an exercise bench. Hold your arms out to your sides parallel to the floor, bent at 90 degrees with your thumbs pointing toward the ceiling. Now try to raise your elbows toward the ceiling and feel your shoulder blades squeeze together. Hold for a moment and return to the starting position. Do 10 to 20 reps depending on your strength.

SEATED DUMBBELL EXTERNAL ROTATION

Grab a dumbbell in your right hand and sit on a bench. Place your right foot on the bench with your knee bent. Bend your right elbow 90 degrees and place the inside portion of it on your right knee. Use your free hand for support. Without changing the bend in your elbow, and while keeping your wrist straight, rotate your upper arm and forearm up and back as far as you can. Pause, then return to the starting position. Perform the prescribed number of repetitions with your right arm, then switch and perform the same number with your left arm.

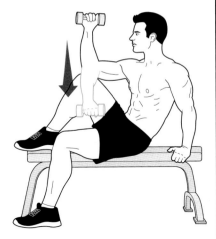

PREVENT IT

- **Work the shoulder both ways.**
  Having a strong, balanced shoulder is the best injury-prevention strategy, and the muscles in and around the shoulder respond well to exercise. Shoulder work must be a staple of your upper-body workouts, and you must work opposing muscle groups to avoid an imbalance.

That means, for example, that if you do a pushing exercise (such as bench presses or overhead presses), you need to do an equivalent amount of pulling movements (like rowing or pullups). See "Prevent It" for Rotator Cuff Strain on page 154 for more suggestions.

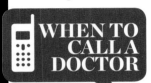

WHEN TO CALL A DOCTOR

See a sports doctor for any shoulder pain. A physical examination and an x-ray can diagnose a separated shoulder. Unless it's a severe separation, the problem generally heals with conservative, home-based therapies like the ones listed here. You should see a doctor because a separated shoulder can be accompanied by complications such as a fracture or rotator cuff injury.

The key to getting back to activity and preventing injury is regaining strength and full function. That makes shoulder conditioning a huge priority for you going forward. The stronger the muscles around the joint are, the fewer problems you'll have.

DO YOU NEED SURGERY?

Not for a basic separated shoulder. In general, time and the conservative remedies listed here are enough to relieve the initial pain, and patients usually have full shoulder function back after several weeks. However, severe shoulder separation can involve completely torn ligaments and a dislocated or broken collarbone. Surgery might be needed in these cases to fix the ligaments and set the bone, and it is usually successful.

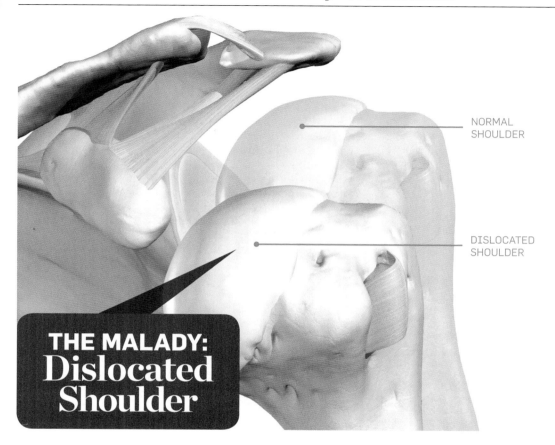

NORMAL
SHOULDER

DISLOCATED
SHOULDER

THE MALADY:
Dislocated
Shoulder

THE SYMPTOMS

Incredible pain and a shoulder joint that looks out of whack (that's a medical term). You can also have bruising and swelling, and possibly numbness, tingling, and weakness in your neck or down your arm.

WHAT'S GOING ON IN THERE?

Don't confuse a dislocated shoulder with a separated shoulder. A separated shoulder involves overstretched or torn ligaments in the acromioclavicular joint (a.k.a. the AC joint), where the collarbone and shoulder blade meet. A dislocated shoulder, in contrast, involves the ball-and-socket joint of the shoulder. To be specific, the ball of the humerus pops out of the socket joint of the scapula. A dislocated shoul-

der is a more extensive injury than a separated shoulder, and the shoulder is the most commonly dislocated joint.

The easiest way to dislocate your shoulder is to dive and land on your outstretched arm. A direct impact can also dislocate a shoulder. As you can imagine, playing football, hockey, gymnastics, and all sports that can cause a wicked fall put you at risk.

Your shoulder can also be "partially" dislocated, meaning that the bone isn't quite in or out of the socket. This is called a subluxation.

NOTE: Once you dislocate your shoulder, you'll always be more susceptible to dislocation. This makes shoulder conditioning crucial as you recover and move forward (see "Prevent It").

FIX IT

- **Don't try to "pop it back in"!** Sling the arm, apply ice to help with the swelling, and see a doctor immediately. If you try to pop it back in yourself, you could really mess up nerves, ligaments, cartilage, muscles, and bones that may be messed up already. Let a medical pro relocate the shoulder.

- **Employ dynamic rest.** Lay off the upper-body work and use lower-body workouts to maintain fitness. Use a sling to immobilize your arm during your daily activities until the pain improves.

- **Ice it.** Ice applied to the shoulder for 15 minutes several times a day can help reduce inflammation and swelling.

- **Try an NSAID.** An antiinflammatory like ibuprofen or naproxen can help with the pain.

- **Start rehabbing.** After several days, and as pain allows, begin range-of-motion exercise without resistance. Here are two basic ones. After 2 weeks, add resistance with an exercise band or light dumbbell.

STANDING EXTERNAL ROTATION. While standing, bend your arm to 90 degrees and lay your forearm across your belly. As you hold the 90-degree angle, move your arm outward until your hand is pointing in the opposite direction. Return to the starting position. Do 10 to 20 reps. (When you add in resistance, be sure to apply it in each direction to maintain muscle balance.)

STANDING ELBOW RAISE. While standing, bend your arm to 90 degrees and lift your elbow up and to the side until your arm is level with your shoulder and parallel to the floor. Holding the 90-degree angle, raise your hand until your forearm is vertical. Return to the starting position. Do 10 to 20 reps. (Add resistance with an exercise band and apply it in both directions to maintain muscle balance.)

PREVENT IT

- **Work the shoulder both ways.** Having a strong, balanced shoulder is the best injury-prevention strategy, and the muscles in and around the shoulder respond well to exercise. Shoulder work must be a staple of your upper-body workouts, and you must work opposing muscle groups to avoid an imbalance. That means, for example, that if you do a pushing exercise (such as bench presses or overhead presses), you need to do an equivalent amount of pulling movements (rowing, pullups). Also, add in some shoulder exercises like the ones in "Fix It," especially if you're in an overhead sport.

- **Reconsider that dive.** Professional athletes are expected to sacrifice their bodies for the game. Weekend warriors—especially those who may not be properly conditioned—have a choice. Making a diving catch in a softball game is a wonderful moment, but dislocating your shoulder and tearing your labrum, which could keep you out of work and affect your earning power (especially if you work with your hands), may not be worth it. Prioritize with your common sense, not your ego.

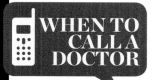

WHEN TO CALL A DOCTOR

See a doctor immediately. An ER doctor can help with initial care, but I also recommend seeing a sports doctor for a complete examination as soon as possible. In addition to the intense pain that a dislocated shoulder can cause, the complications that can go with it are too numerous to ignore. Torn labrum cartilage is a classic, but you can also tear ligaments, damage nerves, and break bones during a dislocation. A doctor can do a full array of diagnostic tests— x-ray, MRI, etc.—to see the extent of the damage.

A doctor can also prescribe pain meds if warranted and send you to physical therapy. Basic dislocations heal up in a few weeks, but you definitely need to recondition your shoulder going forward.

DO YOU NEED SURGERY?

For most people with a first-time dislocation, no. It's possible, however, if you have repeated dislocations or your connective tissues need to be repaired. Surgery may also be an option if you have nerve or blood vessel damage.

UPPER ARMS & ELBOWS

An eagle can't fly with a broken wing. And that's exactly how you feel when you hurt your elbow. You can't grip. You can't lift. You can't throw. Even everyday activities become a challenge. And what's worse is that some of our most popular sports carry an elevated risk of injuring an elbow: baseball, softball, football, golf, tennis, and more. And know this: Elbow injuries linger or get worse if you ignore them. So don't. Here are some of the most common injuries I see and treat, and how I help all those wounded eagles get back up in the sky where they belong.

An anatomy lesson:
UPPER ARMS & ELBOW

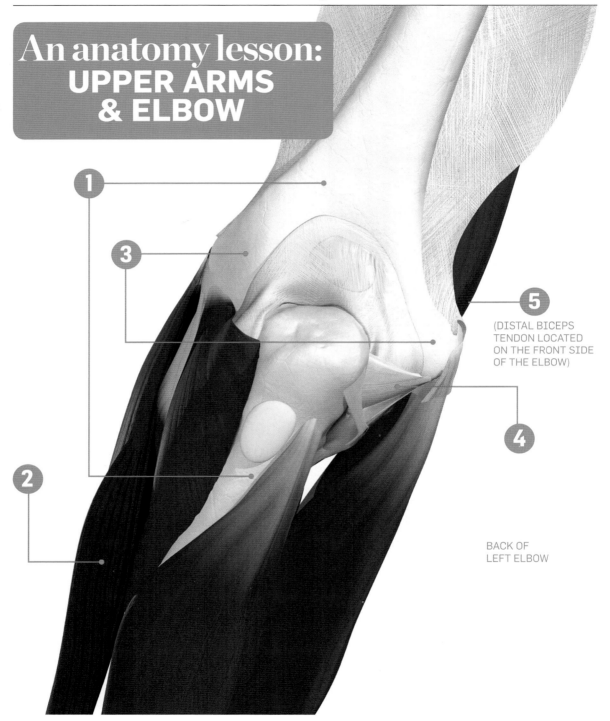

5
(DISTAL BICEPS
TENDON LOCATED
ON THE FRONT SIDE
OF THE ELBOW)

BACK OF
LEFT ELBOW

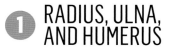 ## RADIUS, ULNA, AND HUMERUS

The bones of the upper and lower arm. The radius and ulna attach to the humerus at the elbow, forming a hinge joint.

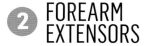 ## FOREARM EXTENSORS

A group of muscles on the lateral (outer) side of the forearm that help you move your hand at the wrist and grip objects. The tendons for these muscles come together at the lateral epicondyle of the elbow.

③ EPICONDYLES

Points on either side of the humerus, near the elbow, where forearm tendons attach. The forearm extensor tendons attach on the lateral (outer) epicondyle, while other forearm tendons and the ulnar collateral ligament attach at the medial (inner) epicondyle.

④ ULNAR COLLATERAL LIGAMENT, A.K.A. MEDIAL COLLATERAL LIGAMENT

Connects the ulna to the humerus on the medial (inner) side of the elbow. When you hear sportswriters talk about "Tommy John" surgery, this is the ligament that's being replaced.

⑤ DISTAL BICEPS TENDON

The lower tendon of the biceps that attaches to the radius in the forearm near the elbow. This connection allows you to flex and extend your elbow and rotate your forearm.

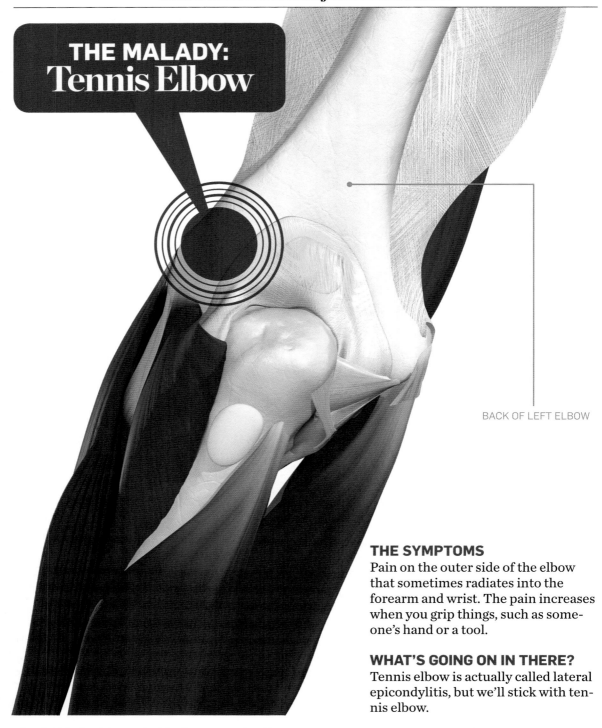

THE MALADY:
Tennis Elbow

BACK OF LEFT ELBOW

THE SYMPTOMS
Pain on the outer side of the elbow that sometimes radiates into the forearm and wrist. The pain increases when you grip things, such as someone's hand or a tool.

WHAT'S GOING ON IN THERE?
Tennis elbow is actually called lateral epicondylitis, but we'll stick with tennis elbow.

The condition is a classic overuse injury, but it can also be caused by asking too much of an unprepared muscle. The forearm has a series of muscles on the lateral (outer) side called the extensors. You use these muscles to straighten, raise, and lower your wrist, and they're engaged when you're gripping something (like a racket or a hammer).

The tendons for these extensor muscles come together and attach on a lower protrusion of the humerus (the upper-arm bone) called the lateral epicondyle—again, lateral because it's on the outer side of the bone. (The inner side of the bone is the medial side; see Golfer's Elbow on page 170.)

When these tendons become irritated or strained by a repetitive wrist motion and/or gripping something, you have tennis elbow. That the name includes the word *tennis* is a nod to how common this injury is in tennis players, but really, anyone who grips and swings something is at risk.

FIX IT

- **Employ dynamic rest.** Avoid activities that engage the elbow and forearm, which includes hard gripping. Use lower-body workouts to maintain fitness.

- **Ice it, then heat it.** Apply ice to the area for 15 minutes 4 to 6 times a day for the first 2 days. After that, applying heat on the same schedule can boost bloodflow to the tendon, which is crucial to healing.

- **Try an NSAID.** An antiinflammatory like ibuprofen or naproxen can help with swelling and inflammation.

- **Try a strap.** An elbow strap or brace can help stabilize the tendons in the elbow and keep the condition from getting worse (or prevent it in the first place).

- **Recondition your forearm.** As the pain improves, you can do some simple exercises to rehab your arm and get yourself back to your normal activities. Here are three suggestions.

TENNIS BALL SQUEEZE. Squeeze a tennis ball in your hand. Hold for several seconds and release. Start with a few reps and increase the number as pain allows. If you feel pain, back off.

ARM ROTATIONS. Hold your arm straight out in front of you parallel to the floor and palm up. Make a fist. Turn your fist over as if you're flipping a pancake. Add reps as the pain allows. As you get stronger, add weight to your fist by holding a light dumbbell, then a hammer, and eventually a racket.

WRIST EXTENSION AND FLEXION.
Extension: With your arm straight out in front of you parallel to the floor and your palm down, bend your wrist downward. Hold for several seconds. Return to the starting position and repeat.
Flexion: With your arm straight out in front of you parallel to the floor and your palm up, lift your wrist upward. Hold for several seconds. Return to the starting position and repeat. You can also add a light dumbbell to these exercises as you get stronger.

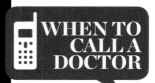

WHEN TO CALL A DOCTOR

If your pain doesn't improve within a week or two with home-based remedies, see a doctor. It could be a severe case of tennis elbow, or you could have another underlying issue. A doctor can send you for an MRI to see what the trouble is.

Physical therapy is a good option here. Your doctor can also use corticosteroid injections, though that treatment's falling out of favor because in the short term it helps, but in the long term, the pain can return and having multiple injections can cause the tendons in the joint to degenerate.

Platelet-rich plasma (PRP) is a new approach being used in patients with tennis elbow to help regenerate the tendons. In areas of the body that don't have great blood supply, healing is slow. The doctor injects your own PRP into the injured area to promote faster healing. The upside is that it works for most people. The downside is that it's generally not covered by insurance and is expensive.

DO YOU NEED SURGERY?

Doubtful. Only in severe cases that don't respond to conservative care for months or even a year would surgery become an option.

Cont'd on page 168

PREVENT IT

If you play a "gripping" sport that requires you to swing a racket, bat, or club, or any activity that requires a strong grip, you have to condition your arms, especially your forearms. The stronger and more supple your extensor muscles, the less stress you put on the connective tissue in your elbow. You can increase overall dynamic flexibility by using the Iron Strength workout section of this book (see page 256). But even if you don't use those specific workouts, the stretches and exercises here can be added to any workout.

WRIST CURL

Grab a barbell with an underhand, shoulder-width grip. Kneel in front of a bench. Place your forearms on the bench so that your palms are facing up and your hands are hanging off the bench. Allow your wrists to bend backward from the weight of the barbell. Curl your wrists upward by raising your palms toward your body. The movement should occur only from your wrists. Reverse the movement to return to the starting position.

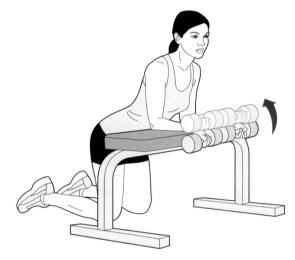

WRIST EXTENSION

Grab a barbell with an overhand, shoulder-width grip. Kneel in front of a bench. Place your forearms on the bench so that your palms are facing down and your hands are hanging off the bench. Allow your wrists to bend forward from the weight of the barbell. Extend your wrist upward by raising the backs of your hands toward your body. Don't raise your forearms off the bench. Reverse the movement to return to the starting position.

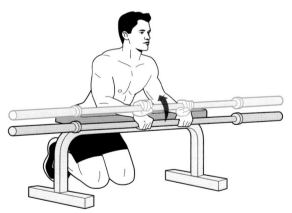

DEVELOP A CRUSHING GRIP

A strong grip is a measurement of overall strength, but it will also help keep your arms and elbows healthy. A great exercise that challenges not just your grip, but your whole body is the Farmer's Walk. It's simple: Grab a pair of heavy dumbbells and let them hang naturally at arm's length at your sides. Use a firm grip. Walk forward for as long as you can while holding the dumbbells. If you can walk for longer than 60 seconds, use a heavier weight.

DO A SMARTER PUSHUP

Pushups are known as a chest exercise, but they work just about your entire upper body, including your forearms and triceps. Mix in these variations on a classic to surprise your muscles and build a more action-ready body.

- **Diamond Pushup.** Place your hands close enough together to make a triangle with your thumbs and forefingers.

- **Decline Pushup.** Place your feet on a box or bench as you perform a pushup; this increases the amount of weight you have to lift.

- **Single-Leg Decline Pushup.** Place one foot on a box or bench and hold the other in the air. If you feel strain in your lower back, you're not keeping your core tight. To make your core work even harder, do this exercise with your feet on a Swiss ball.

- **Spiderman Pushup.** As you lower your body to the floor, lift your right foot off the floor, swing your right leg out sideways, and try to touch your knee to your elbow. Alternate legs on each pushup.

- **Staggered-Hands Pushup.** Place one hand in standard pushup position and your other hand a few inches farther forward. This increases the challenge to your core and shoulders.

TRY A STRAP

An elbow strap or brace—both of which are widely available in sporting goods stores, or check your local pharmacy—can help prevent injury. Give one a try.

STANDING DUMBBELL CURL (REVERSE GRIP)

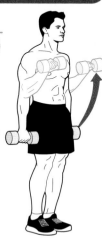

Grab a pair of dumbbells and let them hang at arm's length next to your sides. Turn your arms so that your palms face behind you (this is the "reverse grip," which puts more emphasis on your forearms during the lift). Without moving your upper arms, bend your elbows and curl the dumbbells as close to your shoulders as you can. Pause, then slowly lower the weights back to the starting position. Each time you return to the starting position, completely straighten your arms.

TRICEPS PRESSDOWN

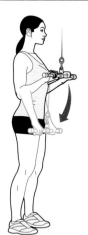

Attach a straight bar to the high pulley of a cable station. Bend your arms and grab the bar with an overhand grip, your hands shoulder-width apart. Tuck your upper arms next to your sides. Without moving your upper arms, push the bar down until your elbows are locked. Slowly return to the starting position.

PERFECT YOUR FORM

Tennis elbow commonly results from lousy form, especially on the backhand. If tennis elbow is a problem for you, consult with a coach to evaluate and adjust your form. A bonus: Your game will improve!

THE MALADY:
Golfer's Elbow

THE SYMPTOMS
Pain in the inner side of your elbow, sometimes radiating into your forearm or hand. Gripping something or making a fist can make it worse.

BACK OF LEFT ELBOW

WHAT'S GOING ON IN THERE?
Golfer's elbow, like tennis elbow, is slang for a much more flowery term, medial epicondylitis. It's also referred to as pitcher's elbow and climber's elbow, which shows you that more than one sport puts stress on this particular area of the elbow.

The forearm muscles that flex your wrist, fingers, and thumb come together on the inner side of your elbow (medial refers to the inner side, lateral to the outer), where the tendons attach to a part of the humerus called the medial epicondyle.

These tendons are stressed whenever you swing something like a golf club or a baseball bat or throw a ball. If they become strained or irritated, you have golfer's elbow.

FIX IT

- **Employ dynamic rest.** Avoid activities that engage the elbow and forearm, which includes hard gripping. Use lower-body workouts to maintain fitness.

- **Ice it, then heat it.** Apply ice to the area for 15 minutes 4 to 6 times a day for the first 2 days. After that, applying heat on the same schedule can boost bloodflow to the tendon, which is crucial to healing.

- **Try an NSAID.** An antiinflammatory like ibuprofen or naproxen can help with swelling and inflammation.

- **Try a strap.** An elbow strap or brace can help stabilize the tendons in the elbow and keep the condition from getting worse (or prevent it in the first place).

- **Recondition your forearm.** As the pain improves, you can do some simple exercises to rehab your arm and get yourself back to your normal activities. Here are three suggestions.

TENNIS BALL SQUEEZE. Squeeze a tennis ball in your hand. Hold for several seconds and release. Start with a few reps and increase the number as pain allows. If you feel pain, back off.

ARM ROTATIONS. Hold your arm straight out in front of you parallel to the floor and palm up. Make a fist. Turn your fist over as if you're flipping a pancake. Add reps as the pain allows. As you get stronger, add weight to your fist by holding a light dumbbell, then a hammer, and eventually a racket.

WRIST EXTENSION AND FLEXION.
Extension: With your arm straight out in front of you parallel to the floor and your palm down, bend your wrist downward. Hold for several seconds. Return to the starting position and repeat.
Flexion: With your arm straight out in front of you parallel to the floor and your palm up, lift your wrist upward. Hold for several seconds. Return to the starting position and repeat. You can also add a light dumbbell to these exercises as you get stronger.

PREVENT IT

- **Train for your sport.** If you play a "gripping" sport where you swing a club, bat, or racket, or any sport or activity that requires a strong grip, you have to condition your arms, especially your forearms. The stronger and more supple your extensors, the less stress you put on the tendons and elbows. Target your forearms as part of a sport-specific training program. (See "Prevent It" for Tennis Elbow on page 168 for more suggestions.)

- **Perfect your form.** Lousy form can cause injury. Whatever your game, consult with a coach to evaluate your swing. You could have bad habits you aren't aware of, and simple adjustments can make a difference. A bonus: Your game will improve!

- **Strap it.** An elbow strap or brace can help prevent injury. Give one a try.

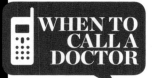

WHEN TO CALL A DOCTOR

If your pain doesn't improve within a week or two with home-based remedies, see a sports doctor. It could be a severe case of golfer's elbow, or you could have another underlying issue (such as a fracture or arthritis).

Physical therapy is a good option here. Your doctor can also use corticosteroid injections, though that treatment's falling out of favor because in the short term it helps, but in the long term, the pain can return and having multiple injections can cause the tendons in the joint to degenerate.

Platelet-rich plasma (PRP) is a new approach being used in patients with golfer's elbow to help regenerate the tendons. In areas of the body that don't have great blood supply, healing is slow. The doctor injects your own PRP into the injured area to promote faster healing. The upside is that it works for most people. The downside is that it's generally not covered by insurance and is expensive.

DO YOU NEED SURGERY?
Doubtful. Only in severe cases that don't respond to conservative care for months or even a year would surgery become an option.

UPPER ARMS & ELBOWS

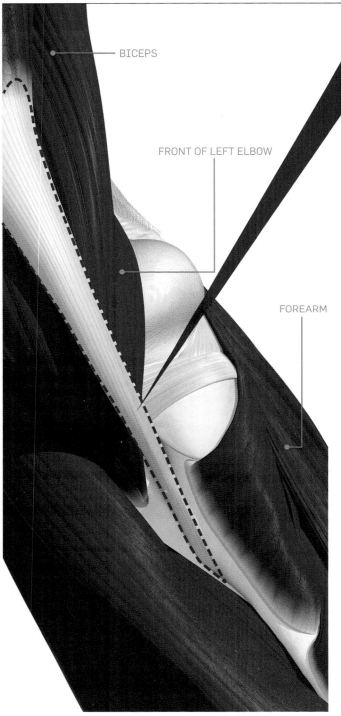

BICEPS

FRONT OF LEFT ELBOW

FOREARM

THE MALADY: Distal Biceps Tendinitis

THE SYMPTOMS

Pain at the front of the elbow, just above the joint, that gets worse when extending or flexing your elbow or when turning your palm from the down to the up position.

WHAT'S GOING ON IN THERE?

Your biceps is more than just a big vanity muscle; it also flexes and extends your elbow and rotates your forearm. It's attached to the radial tuberosity, a part of the radius (the smaller lower-arm bone) near your elbow, by the distal biceps tendon, meaning the lower one. (The proximal, or upper, biceps tendon attaches to the labrum in the shoulder joint.) If this tendon is overused or traumatized by a sudden movement, it can tear, causing irritation and pain.

Don't ignore this pain or try to play through it. Chronic irritation of the biceps tendon can lead to a rupture—and you'll know it if it happens. You generally hear an audible pop or tearing sound and the biceps can ball up under the skin. Obviously, this is not good. Address the pain as soon as you feel it.

Most athletes are at risk for distal biceps tendinitis, but lifting too much weight is a primary cause. It can happen when you lift something that is too heavy and your arm straightens, putting stress on the extended biceps and tendon.

FIX IT

- **Employ dynamic rest.** Avoid lifting, especially any biceps stress. Use lower-body and core workouts to maintain fitness.

- **Ice it.** Apply ice to the area for 15 minutes 4 to 6 times a day for the first 2 days.

- **Try an NSAID.** An antiinflammatory like ibuprofen or naproxen can help with swelling and inflammation.

- **Rebuild the area.** Basic exercises that work the biceps will help get you back to pre-injury form. Here are three to try. Be conservative with the number of sets and reps you do based on the severity of your injury.

FOREARM SUPINATION. With your elbow bent to 90 degrees, hold your forearm out in front of you, palm down. Turn your palm up. This directly works the biceps. Gradually add weight, like a hammer or a can of beans, and add reps as you get stronger.

BICEPS STRETCH. Stand facing a wall that is about 6 inches away. Lift your arm straight out to the side and put the side of your thumb against the wall, palm down. Keeping your arm straight, turn away from the outstretched arm (keeping your hand against the wall) until you feel a stretch in the biceps, elbow, and shoulder. Hold for 20 to 30 seconds, breathing normally.

BICEPS CURL. Start doing this movement with no weight and move on to light weights as you get stronger.

PREVENT IT

- **Build strong and supple muscles.** Powerful and flexible arms and shoulders relieve connective tissues like tendons of a massive amount of stress. Make sure your upper-body regimen includes balanced resistance training that has both pushing (pushups, bench presses) and pulling (pullups, rowing) movements.

- **Perfect your form.** Lousy form can cause an injury. If you lift weights, never break form. If you can't maintain proper form, use a lighter weight. Work on it.

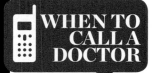

WHEN TO CALL A DOCTOR

Biceps tendinitis usually heals by itself over several weeks, depending on the severity. If your pain improves with home-based care, you should be fine. However, if your pain is severe, see a doctor. Examinations and MRIs can reveal the extent of the tendinitis and any complications that are tagging along.

Physical therapy can help. A doctor can sometimes administer a corticosteroid injection to help with pain and inflammation, but injections in this area need to be precisely placed—injecting directly into the tendon can bring on a rupture—so conservative remedies are always the first option. Many facilities now offer ultrasound-guided injections that use an ultrasound image to put the needle right where it needs to be.

DO YOU NEED SURGERY?

If you rupture the distal biceps tendon, that requires immediate surgery. It's never pretty; your biceps detaches from the bone and rolls up in a ball under the skin. Trust me, you'll know it if that happens.

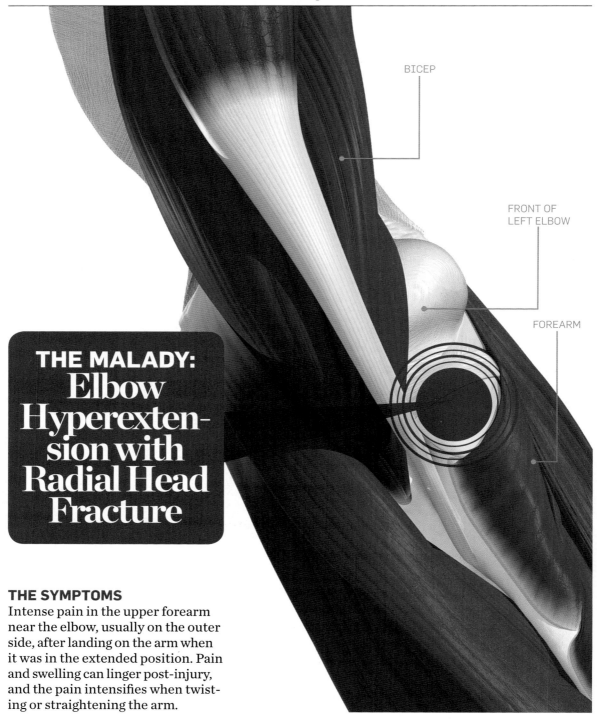

BICEP

FRONT OF
LEFT ELBOW

FOREARM

THE MALADY:
Elbow Hyperextension with Radial Head Fracture

THE SYMPTOMS

Intense pain in the upper forearm near the elbow, usually on the outer side, after landing on the arm when it was in the extended position. Pain and swelling can linger post-injury, and the pain intensifies when twisting or straightening the arm.

WHAT'S GOING ON IN THERE?

When the elbow is extended farther than normal—hyperextended—the bones, muscles, and connective tissues around and in the elbow are traumatized, which can result in sprained ligaments, strained tendons, and bruised or fractured bones.

A hyperextension injury caused by a direct load on the wrist is most commonly seen with a radial head fracture. The smaller bone in your forearm is the radius, and the radial head is the disc-shaped part at the end of that bone near the elbow. The protruding bone near your funny bone is the radial head. It aids in all movements of the elbow—flexion, extension, and rotation.

Athletes in high-impact sports, or in any sport where you can land on an extended arm or wrist, are at risk—think football, gymnastics, martial arts, rugby, and even falling off a bicycle.

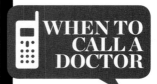

WHEN TO CALL A DOCTOR

I recommend a doctor visit for any elbow injury. A physical exam and x-rays are used for diagnosis, and a doctor can confirm or rule out complications like a radial head fracture. A simple hyperextension should heal up in a few days to a week. More severe cases could take 6 to 8 weeks. A basic nondisplaced radial head fracture can usually heal up just fine with splinting. A doctor can also determine if physical therapy is necessary.

DO YOU NEED SURGERY?

Not for a simple hyperextension. A displaced radial head fracture could need surgery to stabilize the bone so it can heal.

FIX IT

- **Employ dynamic rest.** Even if the swelling comes without pain, avoid using the elbow until it subsides. Trade upper-body exercises for intense lower-body and core work.

- **Ice it.** Apply ice for 15 minutes 4 to 6 times a day for the first 2 days of the swelling. Elevating it as you ice it can also help reduce the swelling.

- **Try an NSAID.** An antiinflammatory like ibuprofen or naproxen can help with the pain and inflammation.

- **Sling it.** Using a sling or brace to prevent your elbow from fully extending can help with the pain of a more severe hyperextension.

- **Rebuild strength.** When you're pain free, begin arm exercises with light resistance, such as biceps curls and triceps extensions. Go slow and concentrate on the extension of the elbow. Build up the number of sets and reps as your condition improves. How many will depend on how severe your injury is and how far you need to go to regain normal strength and range of motion.

PREVENT IT

- **Build strength.** It may not be possible to prevent an elbow hyperextension (such as when you're in the middle of a rugby scrum, for example). But it's a simple fact that the stronger your arms, the more impact they can handle. If you're not training for your sport, your injury risk skyrockets. Do the upper-body work.

- **Wear a brace.** If you've had hyperextension before, or any kind of elbow injury, wearing a protective brace during play can help prevent another.

UPPER ARMS & ELBOWS

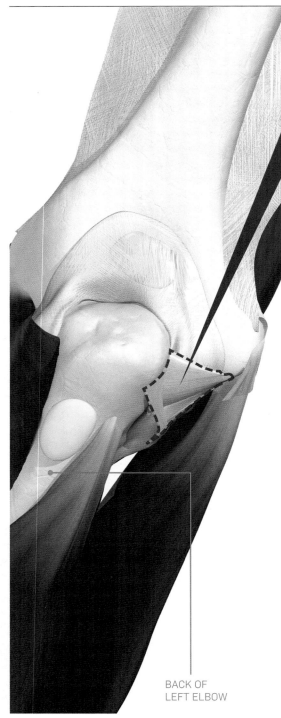

BACK OF
LEFT ELBOW

THE MALADY:
Ulnar Collateral Ligament Sprain
(a.k.a. medial collateral ligament)

THE SYMPTOMS

If the sprain happens suddenly, you feel a popping sensation and acute pain in the inner side of the elbow during a throw or when making another overhead forward motion.

When a sprain develops over time, you have recurring or chronic pain in the inner side of the elbow, especially when throwing or performing another overhead forward motion. The pain can make throwing difficult. It's also painful to make a fist.

WHAT'S GOING ON IN THERE?

The elbow has several ligaments joining the humerus (the upper-arm bone) to the ulna and radius (the lower-arm bones): The radial collateral ligament joins the radius and the humerus on the lateral, or outer, side of your elbow; the annular ligament of the radius joins that bone to the ulna; and the ulnar collateral ligament connects the ulna to the humerus on the medial, or inner, side of the elbow.

If you're a baseball fan, you're probably familiar with the ulnar collateral ligament (UCL), which is also called the medial collateral ligament. If a player, especially a pitcher, has a UCL injury, it's a big problem. This ligament is responsible for the majority of the elbow's stability. It has three bands: the anterior (which provides the most stability), posterior, and transverse.

Forceful overhead acceleration, called medial elbow overload, puts the most stress on the UCL. Throwing a ball and serving in tennis are two examples. The forearm lags behind the elbow as you accelerate the throw, and your UCL is basically the only thing keeping your elbow joint from flying apart. So you see just how much stress something like pitching can put on one band of tissue. Eventually the repeated force causes overstretching and microtears in the ligament that can get worse over time. Repetitive throwing is the most common cause of UCL injury, but anyone who engages in forceful overhead motions is at risk.

NOTE: When kids have medial elbow overload, the ligament generally doesn't tear. Instead, the ligament tears the growth plate, which is softer, off the bone. This is called Little Leaguer's elbow.

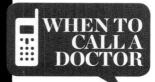

WHEN TO CALL A DOCTOR

When you have this kind of specific elbow pain, see a doctor. Even a mild UCL injury can eventually get much worse with continued stress. For a basic UCL sprain, conservative remedies generally do the trick over a period of weeks or months, depending on the severity of the injury. If your doctor thinks it's appropriate, you could have an MRI to see, if the ligament has been injured.

DO YOU NEED SURGERY?

It's possible. Acute injuries with significant tears and UCLs damaged by overuse could require "Tommy John surgery," in which a tendon from your wrist is used to replace the damaged UCL. The recovery is long (it takes a pro-level pitcher at least 12 months to return to game action), but the results are generally good. However, this is not always the case, so the best strategy is to try to prevent this injury from ever happening. Unfortunately, we are seeing these types of ligament tears in athletes at younger and younger ages. See the following page for ways to prevent it.

FIX IT

- **Get it checked out.** Don't mess with elbow pain. See "When to Call a Doctor."

- **Employ dynamic rest.** Stop any activity that hurts. Avoid lifting and overhead exertion. Use lower-body and core workouts to maintain fitness.

- **Ice it.** Apply ice to the area for 15 minutes 4 to 6 times a day for the first 2 days.

- **Try an NSAID.** An antiinflammatory like ibuprofen or naproxen can help with swelling and inflammation.

- **Rehab it.** Here are three basic range-of-motion exercises. If you feel pain when doing them, back off. The point is to get to a pain-free state and then rebuild your strength so you can return to throwing.

WRIST EXTENSION AND FLEXION.

Extension: With your arm straight out in front of you parallel to the floor and your palm down, bend your wrist downward. Hold for several seconds. Return to the starting position and repeat.

Flexion: With your arm straight out in front of you parallel to the floor and your palm up, lift your wrist upward. Hold for several seconds. Return to the starting position and repeat. You can add a light dumbbell to these exercises as you get stronger.

ARM ROTATION. Hold your arm straight out in front of you parallel to the floor and palm up. Make a fist. Turn your fist over as if you're flipping a pancake. Add reps as the pain allows. As you get stronger, add weight to your fist by holding a light dumbbell, then a hammer, and eventually a racket.

ROTATOR CUFF ROTATION. This is one way to introduce very light resistance to the UCL. With your elbow against your side and your arm bent to 90 degrees, apply light resistance with your other hand as you bring your forearm across your belly and then return to the starting position. For muscle balance, be sure to change the direction of the resistance when you change the direction of the movement so you work the muscle for both pushing and pulling.

Cont'd on page 178

UPPER ARMS & ELBOWS

PREVENT IT

When people see someone throw a ball hard, they say, "Good arm." Not necessarily. Throwing, especially pitching, involves the entire body, particularly the hips, legs, glutes, and core. If you're in an overhead sport, you must train your entire body so you can execute and maintain proper throwing mechanics. There's no way around this. If you stress your elbow without proper conditioning, you will get hurt. That's why the exercises on this page are designed to train your entire body for your little ol' elbow. You can increase overall power and dynamic flexibility by using the Iron Strength workout section of this book (see page 256). But even if you don't use those specific workouts, the exercises here can be added to any workout.

BODYWEIGHT JUMP SQUATS

Place your fingers on the back of your head and pull your elbows back so that they're in line with your body. Perform a bodyweight squat until your thighs are parallel to the floor, then explosively jump as high as you can (imagine you're pushing the floor away from you as you leap). When you land, immediately squat and jump again. Hold dumbbells at your side to make it more challenging.

SINGLE-ARM DUMBBELL SWING

Hold a dumbbell at arm's length in front of your waist. Without rounding your lower back, bend at your hips and knees and swing the dumbbell between your legs. Keeping your arm straight, thrust your hips forward and swing the dumbbell to shoulder level as you rise to a standing position. Swing the weight back and forth. Halfway through your time, switch arms.

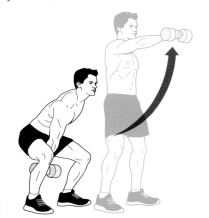

DUMBBELL ROWS FROM PLANK

Get into pushup position gripping hexagonal dumbbells in your hands as a base. Do a single arm row, pulling the dumbbell toward your chest. Halfway through your prescribed time, switch arms.

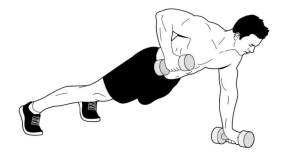

MASTER YOUR MECHANICS

Whether you're throwing a baseball or a javelin or trying to serve a tennis ball at 120 mph, proper body mechanics are crucial to staying healthy. Warm up properly. Focus on each throw. Listen to your coaches. If you pitch, listen to your catcher if he or she points out a mechanical flaw. If you have pain in another part of your body, such as your knee, you may be compromising your mechanics as you compensate for that pain. Mechanics are a major part of your game, and equally as important as how hard you throw.

MOUNTAIN CLIMBERS

Get in pushup position with your arms straight. This is the starting position. Lift your right foot and raise your knee as close to your chest as you can. Touch the ground with your right foot and then return to the starting position and repeat with your left leg. Go as fast as possible.

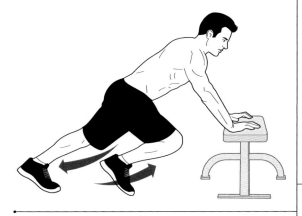

DUMBBELL PUSH PRESS

Stand holding a pair of dumbbells just outside your shoulders, with your arms bent and palms facing each other. Stand with your feet shoulder-width apart and knees slightly bent. Dip your knees and explosively push up with your legs as you press the weights straight over your shoulders. Lower the dumbbells back to the starting position and repeat.

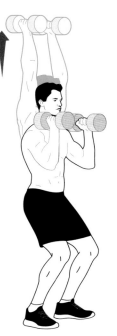

PISTOL SQUAT (WITH OPTIONAL PLYO)

Stand holding your arms straight out in front of your body at shoulder level, parallel to the floor. Raise your right leg off the floor and hold it there. Keeping your right leg straight, push your hips back and lower your body as far as you can without breaking form. As you do this, raise your right leg so that it doesn't touch the floor, and keep your torso as upright as possible. Pause, then push your body back to the starting position. Halfway through the prescribed time, switch legs.

For a bigger challenge, as you rise out of the squat, add in a jump off your plant leg.

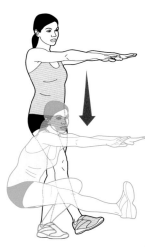

SIDE PLANK

Lie on your side and use your forearm to support your body. Raise your hips until your body forms a straight line from shoulder to ankles. Hold and repeat for other side.

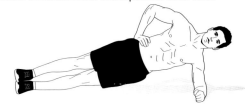

BURPEES

Stand with your feet shoulder-width apart and arms at your sides. Lower your body into as deep a squat as you can. Now kick your legs backward so that you're in pushup position. Do a pushup, then quickly bring your legs back into the squat position. Stand up quickly and jump. That's 1 rep.

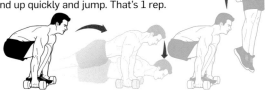

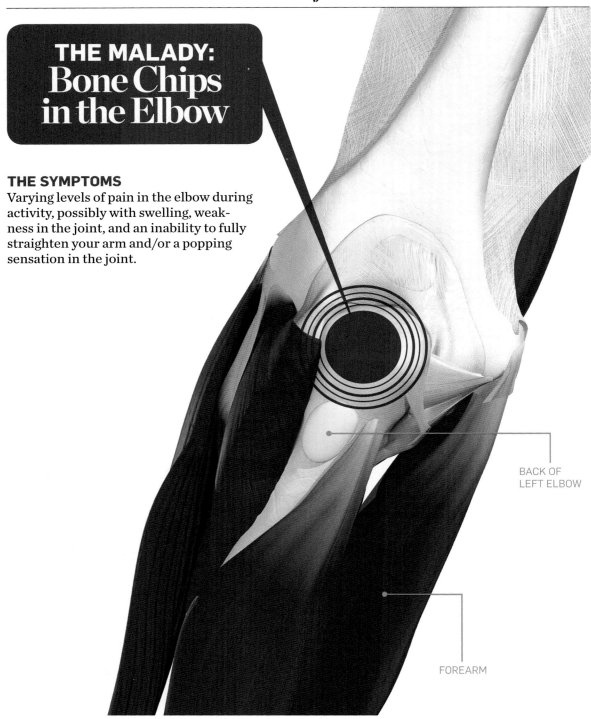

THE MALADY: Bone Chips in the Elbow

THE SYMPTOMS
Varying levels of pain in the elbow during activity, possibly with swelling, weakness in the joint, and an inability to fully straighten your arm and/or a popping sensation in the joint.

BACK OF LEFT ELBOW

FOREARM

WHAT'S GOING ON IN THERE?

The fancy name for bone chips in a joint is osteochondritis dissecans. Picture the end of, say, your humerus in the elbow. An injury to the elbow or, more commonly, a series of microtraumas (basically, overuse) can decrease bloodflow to the tip of the bone. Subsequent overuse can cause a small piece of cartilage and the bone beneath it to chip off the end of the bone.

The severity of the problem worsens over time because it is a degenerative process. A bone chip in its early stages hasn't had a chance to become fully detached and remains in the joint. If you catch it at this stage, with proper care it generally heals itself. Full-blown bone chips become loose bodies in the joint and can cause other issues such as joint instability and locking.

Bone chips can show up in ankles, knees, and hips as well. Elbow bone chips are a classic baseball injury, but any sport that involves heavy arm use puts you at risk. Bone chips put you at risk for osteoarthritis later in life.

This problem is seen in adolescents as well as adults. Since children are still growing and their bodies can replace damaged bone, they generally recover better than adults do.

FIX IT

- **Get it checked out.** See "When to Call a Doctor."

- **Employ dynamic rest.** Avoid hard exertion of the elbow joint. Use lower-body and core workouts to maintain fitness.

- **Ice it.** Apply ice to the area for 15 minutes 4 to 6 times a day to help with swelling.

- **Try an NSAID.** An antiinflammatory like ibuprofen or naproxen can help with swelling and inflammation.

PREVENT IT

- **Train your body for your elbow.**
  When people see someone throw a ball hard, they say, "Good arm." Not necessarily. Throwing, especially pitching, involves the entire body, especially the hips, legs, glutes, and core. If you're in an overhead sport, you must train your entire body—the upper body, lower body, and especially your core—so you can execute and maintain proper throwing mechanics. There's no way around this. If you stress your elbow without proper conditioning, you will get hurt. See "Prevent It" for Ulnar Collateral Ligament Sprain on page 178 for more suggestions.

- **Master your mechanics.**
  Whether you're throwing a baseball or trying to serve a tennis ball at 120 mph, proper body mechanics are crucial to staying healthy. Warm up properly. Focus on each throw. Listen to your coaches. If you pitch, listen to your catcher if he or she points out a mechanical flaw. If you have pain in another part of your body, such as your knee, you may be compromising your mechanics as you compensate for that pain. Mechanics are a major part of your game, and equally as important as how hard you throw.

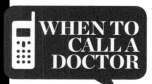

WHEN TO CALL A DOCTOR

I suggest a doctor visit for any elbow pain. An x-ray will show what stage the injury (called a lesion on the bone) is in, and an MRI can show more detail and perhaps whether or not it has the potential to heal on its own. Your doctor could take x-rays of both of your elbows to compare them. In some cases where the piece of bone is fully displaced, your doctor may even be able to feel the chip under the skin.

Conservative treatment includes allowing the problem to heal on its own. If you are symptom free and have full range of movement within a few weeks, you should be able to return to your sport. But be sure to get clearance from your doctor first.

DO YOU NEED SURGERY?

Possibly. If conservative treatments don't help within 3 months or the bone chip gets caught in the moving parts of the joint, a surgeon can go in and clean up or reattach the bone fragments. Surgery is generally successful, but it's possible that you could lose some of the normal range of motion in the joint.

FOREARMS WRISTS & HANDS

From football to golf, virtually every sport requires you to use your forearms, wrists, and hands. Even soccer requires you to put your hands on the ball occasionally, and how would you break a fall without hands? What's worse, if you have pain or an injury in these areas, it doesn't just affect your athletic performance, it hits home in the rest of your life even more because virtually every occupation, from construction to computers, requires a good set of hands. Not to worry. I'll show you how to identify your problem and what to do about it.

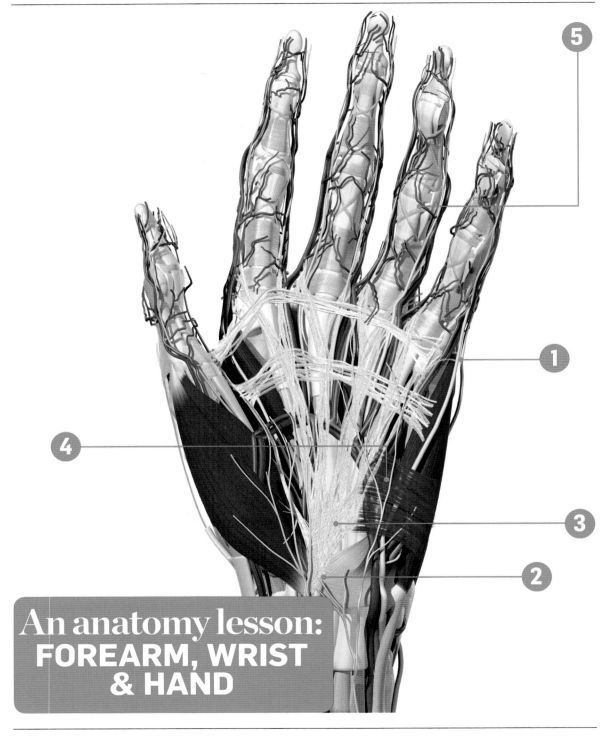

An anatomy lesson:
FOREARM, WRIST & HAND

2 CARPAL TUNNEL

A narrow pathway in the center of the wrist where the median nerve, as well as a group of tendons, pass through from the forearm into the hand. If the pathway narrows from genetics or inflammation, and the median nerve is compressed, carpal tunnel syndrome results.

1 ULNAR NERVE

A large nerve running through the forearm near the ulna into the hand, where it runs on the lateral (outer) side. When you hit your "funny bone," your ulnar nerve supplies the weird feeling.

3 MEDIAN NERVE

A large nerve running down the arm on the medial (inner) side. At the wrist, it runs through the carpal tunnel into the hand. If the nerve becomes compressed or irritated, this causes carpal tunnel syndrome.

4 GUYON'S CANAL, A.K.A. THE ULNAR CANAL

The part of the wrist where the ulnar nerve and ulnar artery pass from the forearm into the hand. Ulnar nerve compression here ir in the hand can cause numbness.

5 PROXIMAL INTERPHALANGEAL JOINT, A.K.A. THE PIP JOINT

The middle joint of a finger. This is the most commonly injured joint in sprained, jammed, or dislocated fingers.

FOREARMS, WRISTS & HANDS

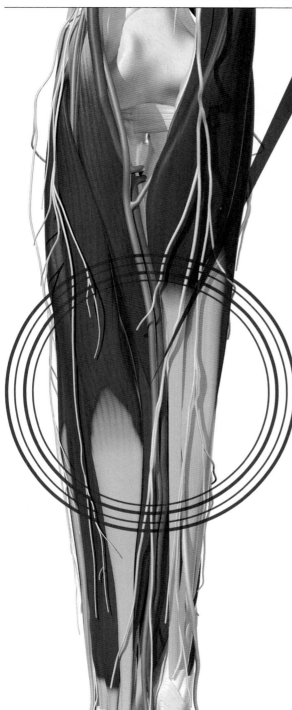

THE MALADY:
Forearm Strain

THE SYMPTOMS

Pain in the forearm during activity, especially hand movements, and possibly at night. The muscles of the forearm feel stiff and there could be some swelling. Severe strains involve more pain and loss of strength. Pain can come on gradually (as a chronic problem) or suddenly from a forceful movement (as an acute injury).

WHAT'S GOING ON IN THERE?

The forearm has a lot more "moving parts," so to speak, than you think. Along with the radius and ulna, you have more than a dozen muscles and tendons stretching between your elbow and wrist. In the same way that the lower leg deals directly with the foot, ankle, and knee, all of the forearm's parts work in conjunction with the hand, wrist, and elbow. The forearm muscles support constant wrist pronation (rotation so the palm faces down) and supination (rotation so the palm faces up), as well as extension and flexion of the elbow.

Because of that, you can strain a muscle or tendon with overuse over time or abruptly with a forceful movement. Forearm tendinitis is also common with overuse.

Like all strains, forearm strains are graded from 1 to 3. Grade 1 is mild and involves no loss of strength. Grade 2 involves more severe pain and loss of strength. Grade 3 is a muscle-tendon rupture and requires surgery.

IMPORTANT: Another forearm injury that could be at fault when your forearm hurts is pronator syndrome, which is compression of the median nerve by muscles in the forearm, especially the pronator muscle. This is less common than carpal tunnel syndrome, which is caused by compression of the median nerve in the wrist. A key symptom of pronator syndrome is forearm weakness that makes it difficult for you to make an okay sign with your thumb and index finger. The remedies presented in "Fix It" for a forearm strain can also help with pronator syndrome.

FIX IT

- **Employ dynamic rest.** Avoid activities that engage the elbow and forearm, which includes hard gripping. Use lower-body workouts to maintain fitness.

- **Ice it.** Apply ice to the area for 15 minutes 4 to 6 times a day for the first 2 days.

- **Try an NSAID.** An antiinflammatory like ibuprofen or naproxen can help with swelling and inflammation.

- **Massage.** A massage technique called myofascial release can help relieve symptoms. Every muscle is encased in a tough, fibrous sheath called the fascia, which can tighten and constrict the muscle. Regular forearm massage can loosen the fascia, allowing the muscle to relax.

- **Recondition your forearm.** As the pain improves, you can do some simple exercises to rehab your arm and get yourself back to your normal activities. Here are three.

TENNIS BALL SQUEEZE. Squeeze a tennis ball in your hand. Hold for several seconds and release. Start with a few reps and increase the number as pain allows. If you feel pain, back off.

ARM ROTATIONS. Hold your arm straight out in front of you parallel to the floor and palm up. Make a fist. Turn your fist over as if you're flipping a pancake. Add reps as the pain allows. As you get stronger, add weight to your fist by holding a light dumbbell, then a hammer, and eventually a racket.

WRIST EXTENSION AND FLEXION. **Extension:** With your arm straight out in front of you parallel to the floor and your palm down, bend your wrist downward. Hold for several seconds. Return to the starting position and repeat. **Flexion:** With your arm straight out in front of you parallel to the floor and your palm up, lift your wrist upward. Hold for several seconds. Return to the starting position and repeat. You can also add a light dumbbell (or even a can of beans) to these exercises as you get stronger.

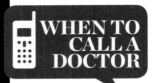

WHEN TO CALL A DOCTOR

Most forearm strains or cases of tendinitis don't require a doctor visit, but for more severe strains you'll want to go. A doctor can help find out just how badly injured you are and if there are any other injuries or complications that go along with it.

Mild strains usually heal up in a week or two. Grade 2 problems can linger for 6 weeks. Grade 3 strains are a different story (see below). The key with forearm strains is to let them heal completely. They tend to hang around or to come back if you don't give them enough time to heal and rehab properly. Be mindful of pain as you return to activity and back off when you need to.

DO YOU NEED SURGERY?

Almost never, but if the strain is severe enough, yes. Ruptures need to be repaired. Recovery and rehab will last for months. And in the very rare cases of pronator syndrome that don't heal with conservative measures, nerve decompression surgery could be an option.

Cont'd on page 188

FOREARMS, WRISTS & HANDS

PREVENT IT

If you play a "gripping" sport that requires you to swing a racket, bat, or club, or any sport or activity that requires a strong grip, you have to condition your arms, especially your forearms. The stronger and more supple your extensor muscles, the less chance you have of pulling a muscle from a sudden force or longer-term overuse. You can increase over-all dynamic flexibility by using the Iron Strength workout section of this book (see page 256). But even if you don't use those specific workouts, the stretches and exercises here can be added to any workout.

WRIST CURL

Grab a barbell with an underhand, shoulder-width grip. Kneel in front of a bench. Place your forearms on the bench so that your palms are facing up and your hands are hanging off the bench. Allow your wrists to bend backward from the weight of the barbell. Curl your wrists upward by raising your palms toward your body. The movement should occur only from your wrists. Reverse the movement to return to the starting position.

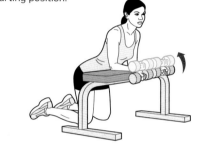

WRIST EXTENSION

Grab a barbell with an overhand, shoulder-width grip. Kneel in front of a bench. Place your forearms on the bench so that your palms are facing down and your hands are hanging off the bench. Allow your wrists to bend forward from the weight of the barbell. Extend your wrist upward by raising the backs of your hands toward your body. Don't raise your forearms off the bench. Reverse the movement to return to the starting position.

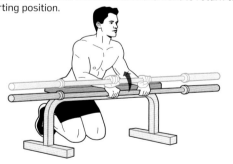

STANDING DUMBBELL CURL (REVERSE GRIP)

Grab a pair of dumbbells and let them hang at arm's length next to your sides. Turn your arms so that your palms face behind you (this is the "reverse grip" which puts more emphasis on your forearms during the lift). Without moving your upper arms, bend your elbows and curl the dumbbells as close to your shoulders as you can. Pause, then slowly lower the weights back to the starting position. Each time you return to the start-ing position, completely straighten your arms.

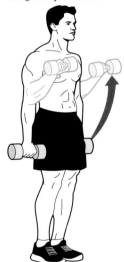

SUPERCHARGE YOUR FOREARMS, WRISTS, AND HANDS
Wrap a towel around each spot where you grasp a barbell or dumbbell. This increases the diameter of the bar, which forces you to work harder to grip it (some gyms may have thick-grip barbells). You can use this strategy with just about any forearm exercise on this page—as well as any other movement you can think of, from barbell rows to dumbbell curls.

ACHIEVE A KUNG-FU GRIP

A strong grip is a measurement of overall strength, but it will also help keep your arms and elbows healthy. Here's a simple exercise: Grab the top of a hex dumbbell with each hand (you can also work each hand separately). Hold the dumbbell for as long as you can. For maximum strength, choose the heaviest weight you can hold for about 20 seconds. To build more muscle, choose the heaviest weight you can hold for 60 seconds.

CABLE OVERHEAD TRICEPS EXTENSION

Attach a rope handle to the high pulley of a cable station. Grab the rope and stand with your back to the weight stack. Stand in a staggered stance, one foot in front of the other, your knees slightly bent. Bend at your hips until your torso is nearly parallel to the floor. Hold an end of a rope in each hand behind your head, with your elbows bent 90 degrees. Without moving your upper arms, push your forearms forward until your elbows are locked. Allow your palms to turn downward as you completely straighten your arms. Pause, then return to the starting position.

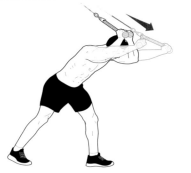

TRICEPS PRESSDOWN

Attach a straight bar to the high pulley of a cable station. Bend your arms and grab the bar with an overhand grip, your hands shoulder-width apart. Tuck your upper arms next to your sides. Without moving your upper arms, push the bar down until your elbows are locked. Slowly return to the starting position.

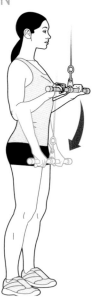

INCHWORM

Stand tall with your legs straight and bend over and touch the floor. Keeping your legs straight, walk your hands forward (if you can't reach the floor with your legs straight, bend your knees just enough so you can; as your flexibility improves, try to straighten them a little more). Keeping your core braced, walk your hands out as far as you can without allowing your hips to sag.

  Then take tiny steps to walk your feet back to your hands. That's 1 repetition. Do 5 forward and then 5 more in reverse.
NOTE: This is a good total-body exercise, but as you "walk with your hands," you'll feel the effectiveness in your forearms and hands.

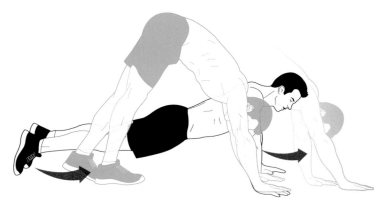

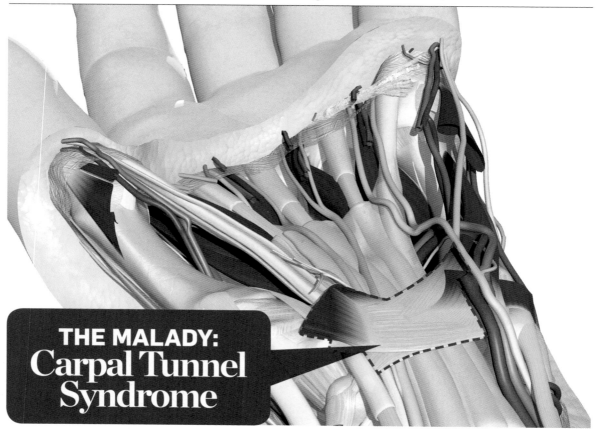

THE MALADY:
Carpal Tunnel Syndrome

THE SYMPTOMS

Burning, tingling, and/or numbness in the fingers and hand, possibly with shooting pain in the wrist, hand, and forearm—all of which come and go. Loss of grip strength. Symptoms start gradually and worsen if the condition isn't addressed.

WHAT'S GOING ON IN THERE?

The carpal tunnel is a narrow, rigid passage between bones and ligaments in the wrist. The median nerve, a large nerve that runs through your forearm and into your hand via the carpal tunnel, can get compressed in the tunnel by irritated tendons or other swelling. Since the median nerve is responsible for the feeling and movement in most of your hand (excluding the pinky), this causes all sorts of havoc in the hand in the forms of pain, tingling, numbness, and possibly weakness.

Carpal tunnel syndrome isn't thought of as a sports injury per se, but many athletes who depend on grip for their games—cyclists, pitchers, golfers, tennis players, and more—are candidates for it. Any injury to the wrist or overuse can cause swelling that compresses the median nerve.

There are other causes of carpal tunnel syndrome as well: a genetic predisposition for a narrow carpal tunnel, for example, that makes the condition easier to develop, or a health condition that affects the joints, such as rheumatoid arthritis or hypothyroidism. Sometimes there's no discernible cause at all.

FIX IT

- **Get it checked out.** See "When to Call a Doctor."

- **Employ dynamic rest.** Avoid activities that engage the wrist, especially hard gripping. Using a wrist brace to immobilize the joint until your symptoms improve is a good idea. Use lower-body workouts to maintain fitness.

- **Ice it.** Applying ice to the area for 15 minutes 4 to 6 times a day can help relieve swelling in the wrist.

- **Try an NSAID.** An antiinflammatory like ibuprofen or naproxen can help with swelling and inflammation.

- **Stretch out.** As the pain improves, you can do some simple stretches to rehab your wrist and get yourself back to normal activities. The idea here is to increase flexibility in the hand and wrist to take pressure off the median nerve in the carpal tunnel.

HOOK, BOW, CLENCH. Hold your hand out with your wrist and fingers straight. Do the following moves without moving your wrist: Bend your fingers into hooks (by bending the top two knuckles), hold for several seconds, then straighten your fingers. Bend your fingers from their base at the third knuckle (as if they're taking a bow), hold for several seconds, then straighten your fingers. Make a fist. Hold for several seconds, then straighten your fingers. Increase the number of reps as your condition improves.

DOWNWARD WALL STRETCH. Stand facing a wall with your arm straight out in front of you, palm up and thumb out to the side. Press your fingers and palm against the wall to stretch your fingers downward. Hold this stretch for 10 seconds and release. Increase the number of reps as your condition improves. Bonus: While holding the stretch, use your free hand to gently pull your outstretched thumb back toward you so you feel a stretch in the base of your thumb and hand.

FIST/WRIST STRETCH. Stand with your arm straight out in front of you, palm down. Make a fist. Bend your wrist toward the floor and hold for 10 seconds, then release the fist. Increase the number of reps as your condition improves.

WHEN TO CALL A DOCTOR

I suggest making a trip to a doctor as soon as you have carpal tunnel symptoms. The condition will worsen if you try to play through it or ignore it. It's a pretty simple diagnosis, and your doctor will be able to judge how severe your case is. If the basic therapies found here don't improve your symptoms and it's warranted, a doctor can administer corticosteroid injections.

DO YOU NEED SURGERY?

It's possible. If your condition doesn't improve within 6 months with conservative treatment, you could be a candidate for a carpal tunnel release procedure in one or both hands. The surgery is fairly common and is performed with a local anesthetic. Recovery can take months, but this usually cures the problem.

PREVENT IT

- **Train for forearm and grip strength.** If you play a "gripping" sport that requires you to swing a racket, bat, or club, or do any sport or activity that requires a strong grip (like football), you have to condition your arms, especially your forearms. There are two goals here: to have well-conditioned arms, wrists, and fingers that take stress off the connective tissues and keep the median nerve from being compressed; and to stay in shape so you might be able to prevent a wrist injury that could lead to swelling and compression of the median nerve. Any weight training involving your hands, especially that done with kettlebells, will help your grip strength. For your forearms and hands, the old-school approach works, too: Some professional pitchers over the decades were famous for rolling a pair of large stainless steel ball bearings in their hands or churning their hands deep in a barrel of rice. Unconventional for sure, but that it works the forearm is undeniable.

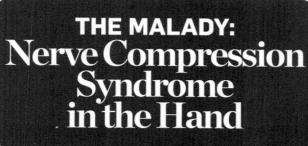

THE MALADY:
Nerve Compression Syndrome in the Hand

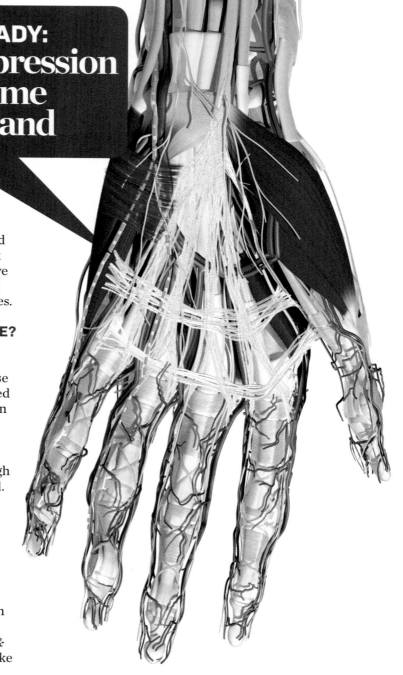

THE SYMPTOMS

Loss of feeling and function in the fingers, usually the pinky and ring finger. Your fingers can lock up and look like Mr. Spock's "Live long and prosper" sign. It's most common in cyclists and triathletes.

WHAT'S GOING ON IN THERE?

Cyclists and triathletes spend many hours training on bikes, which can lead to specific overuse injuries. The symptoms described above signal a nerve compression injury.

The ulnar nerve runs just beneath the skin on the lateral, or outer, side of the hand, through a small area called Guyon's canal. The problem comes from the pressure the bike's handlebars put on that part of the hand during a long ride.

The primary symptom is numbness in that outer part of the hand. Sometimes muscular function can be disrupted, which leaves the rider looking like Mr. Spock (or Mork from *Mork & Mindy*, depending on how you like your science fiction).

FIX IT

- **Remove the pressure.** Normal function should return to your hand soon after a long ride. During a long ride, however, change hand positions every 15 minutes or so to prevent excessive pressure on the ulnar nerve. Rotate between every grip option on your handlebars (use your drops and hoods), and even alternate riding one-handed every now and then to keep the pressure off the nerve.

PREVENT IT

- **Strengthen your core.** A more powerful core can reduce some of the pressure your body weight puts on your hands and handlebars. Increased core strength is always a plus, anyway. Add some extra core work to your training regimen, especially planks.

- **Lower your saddle.** A lower saddle may take some weight off your hands. Experiment with your fit, or ask the folks at your local bike shop to help you out.

- **Try gloves.** Cycling gloves add some padding between the handlebar and your ulnar nerve.

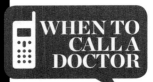

WHEN TO CALL A DOCTOR

Resting and relieving the pressure on the ulnar nerve is usually enough to fix the problem. If you have persistent numbness or loss of muscle function even after you've removed the pressure, see a doctor to make sure something else isn't affecting the area.

DO YOU NEED SURGERY?

Rarely. Conservative remedies should fix the problem, though a small percentage of patients require nerve decompression surgery.

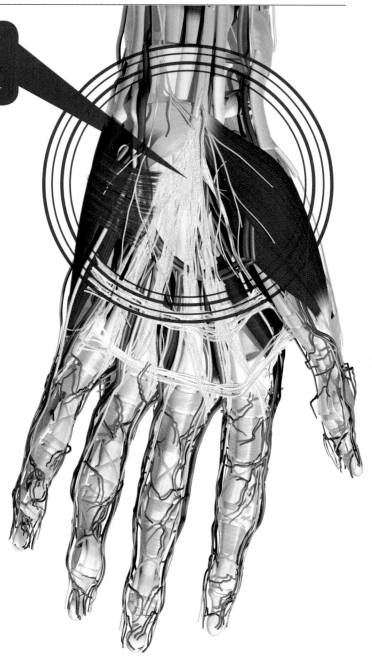

THE MALADY:
Wrist Effusion

THE SYMPTOMS
Swelling of the wrist that can also (but not necessarily) include pain, stiffness, and limitation of the range of motion.

WHAT'S GOING ON IN THERE?
Effusion is a fancy word for swelling. The question is, Why is the wrist swollen? Find the answer to that by asking another question: When did it swell up?

Within an hour or two of an activity: Swelling that occurs soon after an activity is much more serious than swelling that shows up, say, the next day. Example: You take a big cut with a baseball bat and the wrist swells up. This is a sign of bleeding within the wrist, or hemarthrosis. Basically, something has been torn or broken. Sudden-onset effusion is a sign that something serious is going on.

Hours later or the day after an activity: Swelling that arrives later is generally caused by excess synovial fluid (the lubricant in the joints), much like too much oil in a car. Overuse or an underlying medical condition is usually the cause. Something in there is irritated or being rubbed during activity and the body responds by overlubricating the wrist to compensate. Osteoarthritis is one of the most common causes, but far less common maladies can also be the culprits, such as rheumatoid arthritis, infection, gout, bursitis, and Lyme disease. Advancing age raises your risk.

FIX IT

- **See a doctor.** Anytime you have a swollen joint, you should see a doctor (check out "When to Call a Doctor" for more). This is especially true with sudden-onset effusion.

- **Employ dynamic rest.** Even if the swelling comes without pain, avoid using the wrist until the swelling subsides. Trade upper-body exercises for intense lower-body and core work.

- **Ice it.** Apply ice for 15 minutes 4 to 6 times a day for the first 2 days of swelling. Elevating the wrist as you ice it can also help reduce the swelling.

- **Try an NSAID.** Even if you have no pain, ibuprofen or naproxen could help with swelling due to inflammation.

PREVENT IT

- **Strengthen your arms.** Strong arms and hands protect your wrists. Make sure your upper-body regimen includes balanced resistance training with both pushing (pushups, bench presses) and pulling (pullups, rowing) movements. Working out with iron, especially kettlebells, is great for improving grip and hand strength. You may not be able to prevent a wrist effusion caused by health issues, but properly trained arms can only help your wrist recover in the long run no matter what the issue turns out to be. See "Prevent It" for Forearm Strain on page 188 for more suggestions.

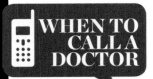

WHEN TO CALL A DOCTOR

My philosophy is that anytime you have joint swelling, you should see a doctor because you need to figure out what the problem is. Try to pinpoint when the effusion began in relation to your athletic activities, especially if your wrist has swollen up with no discernible cause such as an overt injury and you have no other symptoms that suggest a related illness.

Also, if the wrist is swollen but has some bonus symptoms like redness or warmth of the skin and/or you have a fever, it could signal an infection. Get to an ER pronto.

WILL YOU NEED SURGERY?
There's no way to tell until you see a doctor. The biggest issue with wrist swelling is figuring out the cause. A physician can help shed light on the mystery, whether by physical exam or review of images such as MRIs or x-rays.

FOREARMS,
WRISTS &
HANDS

195

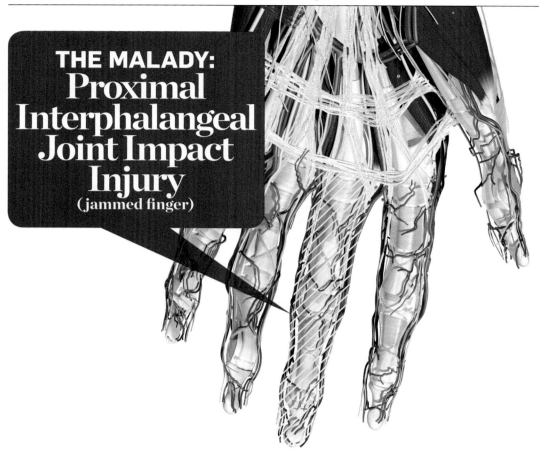

THE MALADY:
Proximal Interphalangeal Joint Impact Injury
(jammed finger)

THE SYMPTOMS

Pain, swelling, and weakness or instability in the middle joint of a finger after a direct impact "jams" the finger back into itself.

WHAT'S GOING ON IN THERE?

There are two ways to go here. When it happens, you can say that you suffered an impact injury to your proximal interphalangeal joint. Or you can say you jammed your finger.

This is a common injury, especially in basketball and football. The proximal interphalangeal (PIP) joint is the middle joint of a finger. When there's an impact on the tip of your finger that drives it back into your hand, like when you try to intercept a pass in basketball, the PIP joint takes the brunt of the impact. This type of impact can also cause hyperextension of the PIP joint. And it hurts like crazy.

Several different injuries can happen when you jam your finger. The PIP joint, like your elbow and knee, has ligaments, tendons, and cartilage that give the joint stability and range of motion. One of these structures is called the volar plate; it's cartilage where it connects to the middle bone of your finger, but a ligament where it connects to the first (or proximal) finger bone. An impact that causes volar plate "disruption" will give you swelling and pain in the joint. You can also overstretch or tear ligaments or tendons in the joint.

FIX IT

- **Check your rotation.** Bend all of your fingers toward your palm at the third knuckle (the base of your fingers), as if your fingers are taking a bow. If the injured finger crosses over one of its neighbors, you have what's called rotational deformity and you need to see a doctor immediately to see how extensive your injury is.

- **Take a break.** If you jam your finger during a game, hit the sidelines for a bit until you can determine how badly you're hurt. If you've got a lot of pain, swelling, and joint instability, you're out; see "When to Call a Doctor." If your pain improves and you have a full range of motion and normal hand strength, you can get back in the game, but you should...

- **Buddy tape it.** Do this whether you're going back in the game or to see a doctor. It's an easy way to give your injured finger support and protect it from accidental banging or bending.

For a basic jam, tape the injured finger to the finger next to it, one strip above and one below the injured joint. A strip of foam padding between the two fingers can add extra protection.

- **Employ dynamic rest.** If your injury is bad enough to require time to heal, avoid activities that aggravate the PIP joint. Use the time off to jack up your running, swimming, and lower-body workouts not just to keep fit, but also to get in even better shape.

- **Ice it.** Applying ice to the area for 15 minutes 4 to 6 times a day for the first 2 days can help relieve swelling in the PIP joint. Wet and freeze a washcloth to use for the icing; once it thaws a bit, you can wrap your whole finger in it. Submerging your finger or hand in cold water also works well.

- **Try an NSAID.** An antiinflammatory like ibuprofen or naproxen can help with swelling and inflammation.

PREVENT IT

- **Prepare.** That's shorthand meaning get in the best shape you can, use proper form, and keep your eyes, ears, and brain in the game at all times. The fact is, jammed fingers are common and sometimes things just happen. But if you're in top shape and fully aware

of what's happening in the game at all times, you might catch that basketball instead of jamming your finger against it or block that linebacker instead of jamming your finger on his shoulder pad as he spins past you.

WHEN TO CALL A DOCTOR

A simple jammed finger is painful, but not necessarily a big deal. However, if you have extreme pain, swelling, and joint weakness or instability, see a sports doctor. Also see a doctor if what you think is a simple jammed finger doesn't improve within a couple of days or the swelling and pain get worse. X-rays and MRIs will show fractures and connective tissue tears.

In many cases, splinting the PIP joint and giving it time to heal does the trick. Do not splint your finger on your own and assume everything will be peachy. There are different ways to splint different injuries, and you don't want to get it wrong. Leave it to your doctor.

DO YOU NEED SURGERY?

It depends on the severity of your injury. Full ruptures of connective tissues could require reconstruction. You won't know until you consult with a doctor.

FOREARMS, WRISTS & HANDS

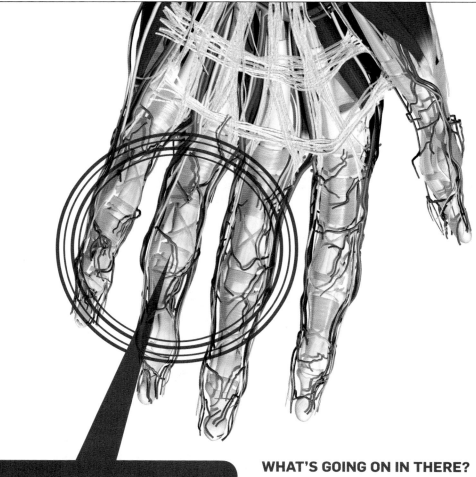

THE MALADY:
Sprained Finger

THE SYMPTOMS

For mild (grade 1) finger sprains, pain and swelling in the injured joint. For more severe (grade 2 or 3) sprains, greater pain and swelling, and perhaps bruising, along with a limited range of motion and joint weakness and/or instability. The pain is worse when you try to bend the finger.

WHAT'S GOING ON IN THERE?

Your finger joints are very much like your elbows and knees in that they have a set of ligaments holding the bones together. If they become overstretched and/or torn, you have a sprain.

Also like your elbows and knees, each finger joint has a collateral ligament on each side for joint stability and to keep the finger from bending in directions it's not supposed to. That's why these are the most commonly sprained finger ligaments.

A finger sprain can happen in any number of ways—it's pretty simple to do, you just bend it in a way it doesn't appreciate—but if you play a team sport with a ball, you're a prime candidate.

FIX IT

- **Check your rotation.** Bend all of your fingers toward your palm at the third knuckle (the base of your fingers), as if your fingers are taking a bow. If the injured finger crosses over one of its neighbors, you have what's called rotational deformity and you need to see a doctor immediately to see how extensive your injury is.

- **Take a break.** If you injure your finger during a game, hit the sidelines for a bit until you can determine how badly you're hurt. If you've got a lot of pain, swelling, and joint instability, you're out; see "When to Call a Doctor." If your pain improves and you have a full range of motion and normal hand strength, you can get back in the game, but you should...

- **Buddy tape it.** Do this whether you're going back in the game or to see a doctor. It's an easy way to give your injured finger support and protect it from accidental banging or bending.

For a simple sprain, tape the injured finger to the finger next to it, one strip above and one below the injured joint. A strip of foam padding between the two fingers can add extra protection.

- **Employ dynamic rest.** Avoid using that finger as much as possible. Use the time off to jack up your running, swimming, and lower-body workouts not just to keep fit, but also to get in even better shape.

- **Ice it.** Applying ice to the area for 15 minutes 4 to 6 times a day for the first 2 days can help relieve swelling. Wet and freeze a washcloth to use for the icing; once it thaws a bit, you can wrap your whole finger in it. Submerging your finger or hand in cold water also works well.

- **Try an NSAID.** An antiinflammatory like ibuprofen or naproxen can help with swelling and inflammation.

PREVENT IT

- **Prepare.** That's shorthand meaning get in the best shape you can, use proper form, and keep your eyes, ears, and brain in the game at all times. The fact is, sprained fingers are common and sometimes things just happen.

But if you're in top shape and fully aware of what's happening in the game at all times, you might catch that basketball instead of bending your finger back. Carelessness can be an athlete's biggest enemy.

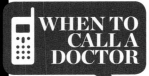

WHEN TO CALL A DOCTOR

A simple sprain is painful, but not necessarily a big deal. However, if you have extreme pain, swelling, and joint weakness or instability, see a sports doctor ASAP. Also see a doctor if what you think is a "simple sprain" doesn't improve within a couple of days or the swelling and pain get worse. X-rays and MRIs will show fractures and connective tissue tears.

As mentioned, buddy taping is a good idea for mild sprains and an effective stopgap measure until you can get a more severe sprain to a doctor. But these more severe cases will benefit from a splint. Do not splint your finger on your own and assume everything will be peachy. There are different ways to splint different injuries, and you don't want to get it wrong. Leave it to your doctor.

DO YOU NEED SURGERY?

It depends on various factors like the severity of your injury and which joint was injured. Certain nasty tears and full ruptures of connective tissues could require reconstruction. You won't know until you consult with a doctor.

FOREARMS, WRISTS & HANDS

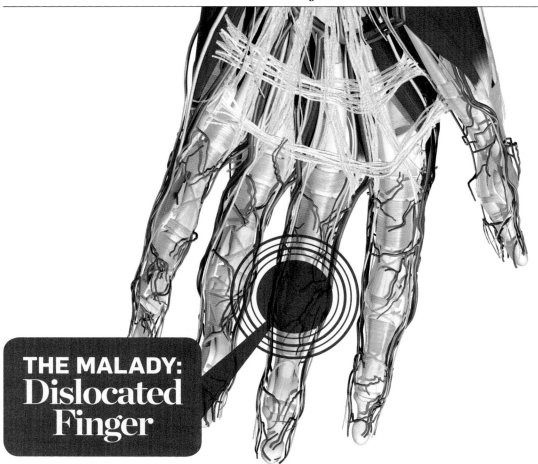

THE MALADY:
Dislocated Finger

THE SYMPTOMS

Extreme pain, swelling, and finger deformity after an impact on the finger. Your finger bone will literally look as though it's out of its joint—because it is.

WHAT'S GOING ON IN THERE?

A dislocation happens when your finger takes some sort of impact or is twisted and a finger bone (called a phalanx) is forced out of its joint. The most common causes are taking a ball off the end of your finger, snagging your finger in someone's jersey or pad, and falling awkwardly.

The most commonly dislocated finger joint by far is the proximal interphalangeal joint (the second knuckle), but the distal interphalangeal joint (the one near the fingernail) and the metacarpophalangeal joint (the base of the finger) can also take hits. Each of these joints is reinforced by two collateral ligaments (one per side) and the volar plate, a ligament-cartilage attachment under the joint. They do their best to keep things in line, but if the force is too great, they can give way—and be damaged. (Thumb dislocations are rare.)

It's also possible to have a partial dislocation, which is called a subluxation. This usually heals on its own with buddy taping to the adjacent finger and application of the self-care measures in "Fix It."

FIX IT

- **Don't "self-reduce."** The medical term for realigning or "popping" a dislocated bone back into its joint is reduction. Time is a factor here because the longer you wait to reduce the joint, the more time it has to swell and the muscles have to spasm, which could make reduction more difficult. You or a buddy or a coach may be tempted to reduce a dislocated finger on the spot after it happens. Even with the time factor, I don't recommend this. The fact is, neither you nor your well-meaning friend is a trained physician. I recommend going to the ER pronto and letting a pro do the work (see "When to Call a Doctor"). Yes, the dislocation is very painful and will hurt all the way to the hospital, but you don't want to risk long-term damage to the joint because someone thinks it's easy (or cool) to pop a bone back in.

NOTE: If your finger pops out and quickly pops back in by itself, I still recommend making a doctor visit for imaging tests to see if the joint is damaged.

POST-REDUCTION:

- **Employ dynamic rest.** Avoid using that finger as much as possible. Use the time off to jack up your running, swimming, and lower-body workouts not just to keep fit, but also to get in even better shape.

- **Ice it.** Applying ice to the area for 15 minutes 4 to 6 times a day for the first 2 days can help relieve swelling. Wet and freeze a washcloth to use for the icing; once it thaws a bit, you can wrap your whole finger in it. Submerging your finger or hand in cold water also works well.

- **Try an NSAID.** An antiinflammatory like ibuprofen or naproxen can help with swelling and inflammation.

PREVENT IT

- **Prepare.** That's shorthand meaning get in the best shape you can, use proper form, and keep your eyes, ears, and brain in the game at all times. Sometimes a dislocated finger just happens. But if you're in top shape and fully aware of what's happening in the game at all times, you might catch that football instead of bending your finger back or land with more strength and athleticism. Carelessness and lack of preparation can be an athlete's biggest enemy.

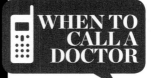

WHEN TO CALL A DOCTOR

If you dislocate your finger, go to the ER. Doctors are trained to handle dislocations and will use the proper techniques to reduce it. Also, a doctor in an ER can give you a local anesthetic to ease the pain caused by the reduction itself.

Even if the finger "self-reduces," or pops out and then goes right back in, you should still see a doctor to rule out other injuries.

Once the dislocation is properly reduced, the doctor will splint or buddy tape your finger to allow healing. An x-ray and MRI can confirm a fracture and soft tissue damage. **IMPORTANT:** If the skin around the injury is broken in any way, get medical attention immediately. Also hit the ER if you have numbness in the finger, or if it's cold, pale, or blue. Nerve and vascular injuries are serious.

DO YOU NEED SURGERY?

It's possible, depending on the extent of the damage to the joint. Torn ligaments and other joint injuries can go hand in hand with a dislocation. If you do need surgery, you're most likely looking at a recovery period of several months, depending on the injury. Your doctor will let you know the full story after an exam and tests.

FOREARMS, WRISTS & HANDS

HEAD

The head is where sports really happen—you see, you react, your brain tells your body to move. When folks talk about sports injuries of the human head, the first thing they say is concussion. Yes, that's one of the most serious sports injuries for your noggin—you'll find all the info you need on concussions here—but there are others that can take you out of the action just as quickly and easily. Read on for simple ways to keep your head where it belongs—in the game.

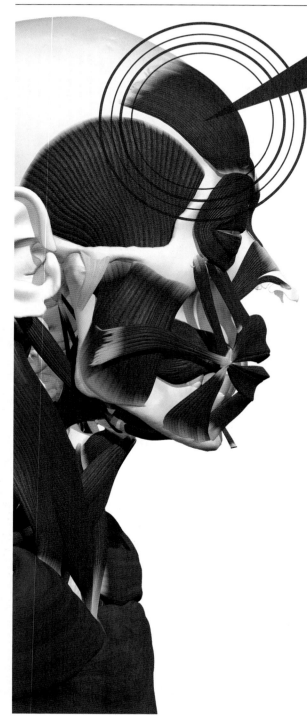

THE MALADY:
Concussion

THE SYMPTOMS

Immediately after a blow to the head, any number of the following: headache, loss of memory, loss of consciousness, confusion, dizziness, visual disruptions like double vision or seeing stars, ringing in the ears, pupil dilation, nausea or vomiting, slurred speech, and sluggishness. Later on, concentration problems, irritability, and sensitivity to light and noise. Understand that if you didn't get hit very hard, some of the symptoms might be subtle.

WHAT'S GOING ON IN THERE?

In medical terms, a concussion is a mild traumatic brain injury, but in reality there's nothing mild about it. It's serious. Government stats estimate that there are more than 300,000 sports-related concussions every year, but those are just the cases reported from ER visits. The actual number could be triple that, many of them occurring in youths participating in organized sports.

When you get whacked in the head, the force makes nerves twist and stretch and your brain hits the inside of your skull. Researchers theorize that these aggravated nerve cells release a neurotransmitter called glutamate, which binds to brain cells and allows potassium to escape and calcium and sodium to enter the cells.

The calcium slows down energy production in your brain cells and constricts blood vessels. This is why you feel groggy and lethargic. If the impact is hard enough, cellular energy production can be halted and you lose consciousness.

In response to all of this, your cells try to draw potassium back in, releasing the sodium to make room for it. This forces the cells to operate beyond their capacity, so they're unable to store information. This is why you can lose memory of the incident.

Over the next 10 days, the calcium inside your brain cells dissipates as the cells recover. During this time, your brain is in a state of metabolic depression, so you can't activate it fully. This makes you susceptible to headaches, memory loss, dizziness, and grogginess. You could have trouble concentrating.

If you get hit on the head again during this time, you could end up with permanent brain damage (see "Concussion Red Flag: Second Impact Syndrome," below).

Remember, once you've had a concussion, you're three to five times more susceptible to future concussions when you take a hit. For example, it's estimated that nearly one-quarter of NFL players have had three or more concussions in their careers.

FIX IT

- **Get out of the game.** Even the mildest concussion is a brain injury. Avoid strenuous activity while any concussion symptoms are present and allow your brain time to heal. For the average concussion, it takes 2 weeks for symptoms to go away and the brain to return to operating at full capacity. Don't mess with this healing time. See "When to Call a Doctor."

- **Try acetaminophen.** To treat pain during the healing period, try acet-

aminophen. Avoid NSAIDs like ibuprofen, naproxen, and aspirin because they can promote bleeding.

- **Rest your brain.** Avoid tasks requiring close concentration while giving your brain time to heal. That means no video games, texting, or computer work, and minimize TV watching.

- **Get clearance.** Once you're symptom free after a concussion, see a doctor for evaluation and clearance before you return to your sport.

CONCUSSION RED FLAG: SECOND IMPACT SYNDROME

There's been a paradigm shift on concussions in the past 5 to 10 years. As doctors, we understand now that they are far more serious than was previously thought. We hope that this recognition of their seriousness will trickle down to coaches and parents, because the days of an athlete getting his or her "bell rung" and getting right back in the game are over. Why? One of the reasons is what's known as second impact syndrome.

After you get a concussion, you have a big window of vulnerability while you're healing. If you take a second hit before you have fully recovered from the first one, you risk major brain injury or, if the injury is severe enough, death. That's why the first injury must be completely healed before you return to activity. Only a doctor can give you that clearance (not a coach, parent, teammate, or friend).

Cont'd on page 206

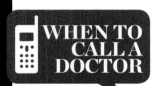

WHEN TO CALL A DOCTOR

As soon as possible after a head blow, even if it's just as a precaution. However, four specific things warrant an immediate trip to the ER: first, any dizziness and/or a lingering headache. Second, tingling arms and/or legs; this can signal bleeding in the brain (see "Is It a Concussion? Or Something Worse?" on page 206). Third, memory loss. If you hit your head hard enough to lose even a few seconds' worth of memory, you need to go to the ER to get checked out. And fourth, loss of consciousness. Again, any blow to the skull hard enough to knock you out for even 1 second is serious. If you take a hit and black out or can't remember it, assume the worst.

A doctor can order a CT scan or MRI to check your brain. And don't be fooled by a "clean" scan. A CT scan can't pick up cellular changes in your brain, though it will show bleeding and swelling. If you have a good CT scan but still have concussion symptoms, give yourself time to heal.

DO YOU NEED SURGERY?
Doubtful, but it's possible if you have a serious head injury with internal bleeding or other injuries.

HEAD

PREVENT IT

It's so easy to say, "Don't get knocked on the noggin," but things do happen when you're playing all-out. This collection of information and advice will both help keep you prepared on the playing field and give you a course of action if you or someone around you takes a shot to the skull. The "Fix It" section on the previous page tells you what to do after a concussion. This section contains all the things you need to know before it happens.

IS IT A CONCUSSION? OR SOMETHING WORSE?

To add even more weight to the head-injury discussion, when you take a hit to the skull, the injury may be even worse than a concussion. If the blow breaks blood vessels inside your head, bleeding can result in a mass of blood called a hematoma (another word for a bruise). They're called different things based on where they occur in relationship to the dura, a protective layer that lies between the inner side of your skull and your brain, and they need to be distinguished from concussions—and one another.

• **Subdural hematoma.** Subdural means below the dura, so the bleeding happens between the dura and your brain. This is a venous bleed, meaning that veins have been lacerated. The symptoms: After a head hit, you have a headache on one side of the head that gets progressively worse over the first 6 to 12 hours after the hit. You sometimes also experience visual changes. Get to an ER immediately.

• **Epidural hematoma.** Epidural means above the dura, so the bleeding happens between your skull and the dura. This is an arterial bleed, meaning that an artery has been lacerated. The symptoms: At first, you may seem fine. But as the bleeding occurs and increases the pressure inside the skull, you can have a severe headache, dizziness, and vomiting, and one pupil may be larger than the other. You can also have sudden weakness or tingling in your arms and/or legs. Later, more dangerous symptoms develop, including lethargy, shallow breathing, and loss of consciousness. A recent high-profile case: In 2009, actress Natasha Richardson died from an epidural hematoma after a fall while skiing. It's very simple: An epidural hematoma is a medical emergency.

USE YOUR BRAIN (DON'T BRUISE IT)

The commonsense precautions are obvious: Wear proper headgear for your sport, and in high-contact games like football and hockey, never involve your head in the contact (as you do when you make a helmet-first tackle). Heading a soccer ball won't give you a concussion, but if two players try to head the ball simultaneously, they could head each other.

WEAR A MOUTH GUARD.

Research shows that mouth guards can lower your chances of concussion if you take hit.

PRESEASON NEUROCOGNITIVE TESTING:
A MUST FOR ALL ATHLETES

One way to help quickly diagnose and evaluate the severity of a concussion—and also to help determine when an athlete can return to action—is using computerized neurocognitive testing (one of the most widely used testing software packages is ImPACT).

Before an athletic season starts, each player's brain function is evaluated so coaches, trainers, and doctors have a baseline—a set of data that's considered that player's normal state. Then, if the player suffers a head injury, doctors can quickly test his or her brain function and compare it to the baseline data to see how severe the injury is.

Two of the keys to properly treating a concussion are figuring out how bad it is and when it has healed. This type of testing is critical because some athletes may report feeling fine and even appear to be fine after a period of healing, but testing can reveal that they still aren't ready for action. That can help prevent second impact syndrome and a potentially devastating brain injury.

PREPARE

That's shorthand meaning get in the best shape you can, use proper form, and keep your eyes, ears, and brain in the game at all times. Even if you do all of that, however, sometimes a head hit just happens. But if you're in top shape and fully aware of what's happening in the game at all times, you might be able to avoid the hit altogether, or at least have another body part take the hit instead. Carelessness and lack of preparation can be an athlete's biggest enemy.

KIDS AND CONCUSSIONS

IMPORTANT: Youth sports coaches and parents have to understand something about kids and injuries: With almost all sports injuries, kids generally heal faster than adults—except for concussions. Children heal more slowly than adults with the same grade of concussion, so their windows of vulnerability for second impact syndrome are much longer. Only a doctor can clear a child to return to sports after a concussion. Also, parents should consider whether allowing the child to return to that sport is worth the risk of him or her getting a second (or third, or fourth...) concussion. Remember: Kids have long lives ahead of them. Is the risk of having another concussion or a serious brain injury worth it?

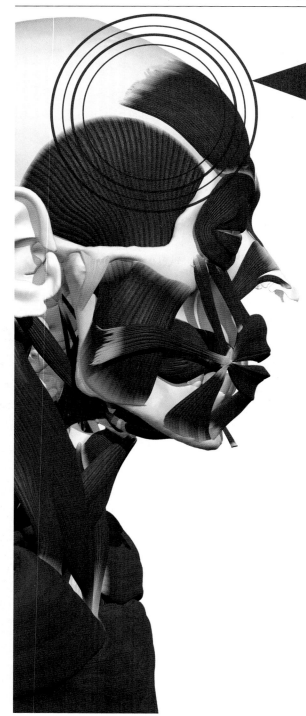

THE MALADY: Exercise-Induced Headache

THE SYMPTOMS

A sudden, intense, throbbing headache, usually on both sides of your head, during or after a workout or game. You may also have dizziness, vomiting, blurred vision, or neck rigidity if it's more serious.

WHAT'S GOING ON IN THERE?

There are two kinds of exercise headaches, primary and secondary. One is painful but ultimately harmless. The other can be scary.

No one is sure what causes primary exercise-induced headaches, which makes them frustrating. They most commonly come on after running, weight lifting, or another hard, strenuous activity. Hot weather and training at a high altitude may contribute, and poor hydration could factor in as well. Determining the true cause of these headaches is sketchy because they seem so individual, but dilated blood vessels in and around your brain could contribute. This type of headache comes and goes and is treated like most headaches (see "Fix It" on page 211).

The secondary type of exercise-induced headache is caused by some underlying health problem, but even those vary widely. Bleeding in the membrane surrounding the brain, a problem with the blood vessels in the brain, a tumor, or even a sinus infection could be the cause.

How can you tell the difference between the two types?

Primaries give you a throbbing and even nasty headache, but that's all. Secondaries deliver more serious symptoms along with the head pain: nausea, vomiting, dizziness, loss of consciousness, double vision, or neck rigidity.

Your risk of developing a primary headache rises if you train in hot weather or at a high altitude. If you're prone to having migraines, you have a higher risk of getting exercise headaches, though they aren't the same thing. Exercise headaches come on fast, like a thunderclap, and don't last as long as migraines.

FIX IT

• **Go over-the-counter.** A common pain reliever like acetaminophen or ibuprofen can help with the pain, though some exercise headaches are brief and may be gone before the med kicks in. Take it only if you really need it.

• **Hydrate.** At the first sign of pain, down a cup or two of water. This alleviated headaches in 65 percent of sufferers within 30 minutes, according to a study in the journal *Headache*. If you've been exercising, chances are you're at least a little dehydrated.

• **Chill it.** Putting a cold washcloth on your forehead or the back of your neck for 10 to 15 minutes may bring some relief. The thinking here is that the chill may constrict dilated blood vessels.

• **Try acupressure or massage.** Two key pressure points for reducing pain with acupressure: First, the web between your forefinger and thumb. Pinch the area and apply pressure in a circular motion (switch hands when you finish). Second, under the skull's bottom edge on the back of the head, about halfway between the bony bumps just behind the ears and the middle of the skull; use your thumbs to apply pressure there in a circular motion. Work either area for 5 minutes, several times a day as needed.

• **Eat a pencil.** Well, not eat, exactly. Put a pen or pencil between your teeth, but don't bite. Leave it there for 5 minutes. This relaxes your jaw muscles, which could be tensed up.

PREVENT IT

• **Try to predict when they'll hit.** Some exercise headaches are predictable, occurring either under certain conditions—hot weather and high altitude are common triggers—or with a specific activity. You can either avoid these conditions or use medication prophylactically by taking a pain reliever an hour before your activity.

• **Warm up.** Doing a proper warmup before a hard workout can help as well. And by proper I don't mean 5 minutes on a treadmill or a set of 10 bench presses with an empty barbell. A proper warmup leaves you sweaty. A good 10-minute set of activation exercises will prepare your muscles for the work to come: Try forward and backward lunges with trunk rotation, side lunges, cariocas (sideways running with crossover steps), pogo hops, arm windmills, and inchworms (begin in the top pushup position, then walk your feet toward your hands as your butt rises in the air; at the top, walk your hands back out until you return to the pushup position). See the Iron Strength workout section on page 264 for details on a proper warmup.

See the Iron Strength workout section on page 264 for details on a proper warmup.

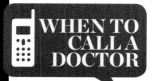

WHEN TO CALL A DOCTOR

If you experience a sudden, intense headache for the first time during or after a hard workout, see a doctor, especially if the pain is ongoing or worsens at night. Even if your headache lasts for only a few minutes or hours, it's probably benign, but it's best that your doctor hears about it and examines you.

Head to an ER immediately if you have secondary headache symptoms like nausea, vomiting, vision disturbances, or neck rigidity. This could be a serious problem in or around your brain. Your doctor will want to do a CT scan or MRI to see what's going on in your head. A prescription anti-inflammatory medication and perhaps a blood pressure medication could help. If your headaches are predictable, you can use the meds preventively.

DO YOU NEED SURGERY?

Not unless you have a serious brain abnormality that's causing the symptoms. The vast majority of exercise-induced headaches are benign.

HEAD

THE MALADY:
Migraine

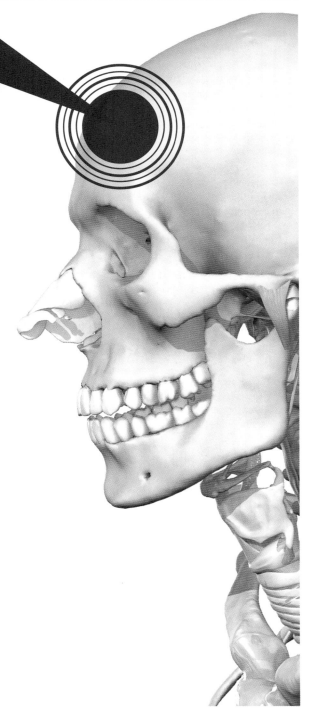

THE SYMPTOMS

Mild to severe head pain, usually on one side. It can be accompanied by nausea and/or sensitivity to noise and light. Migraines generally come on gradually and can last for hours or even days.

WHAT'S GOING ON IN THERE?

More than 28 million people in the United States get migraines. It's a complex disease that is still shrouded in mystery because the headaches can be so varied. Are they genetic? Yes. Are they environmental? Yes—they can arise from either or both sources. We know that the brain's serotonin level drops during migraines, which spurs the production of neuropeptides that travel to the outer layer of the brain. This can trigger pain.

The most frustrating thing about coping with and preventing migraines is trying to pinpoint your personal triggers and symptoms, because they seem to vary for everyone.

Common triggers: alcohol, changing hormone levels, poor sleeping habits, dehydration, stress, chemicals in certain foods (chocolate, wine, cheese, the nitrates in processed meats, and monosodium glutamate—MSG—are prime culprits), perfume, weather changes, seasonal changes, altitude changes, bright lights, loud noises, and low blood sugar.

Common signals that one is coming: Some people experience subtle changes one or two days before an attack, such as constipation, diarrhea, depression, stiff neck, irritability or hyperactivity, or food cravings. Other migraines are preceded by sensory disruptions such as seeing swirling lights (called auras) or blind spots and possibly having tingling in your arms or legs.

FIX IT

- **Stop exercising.** If you feel a migraine coming on during a workout, stop. Working out during a migraine is a bad idea, because having dilated blood vessels is part of the problem and you could make it worse. Many people get migraines so bad that exercise is out of the question anyway.

- **Catch it early.** As soon as you feel a migraine signal, take whatever remedy it is that you normally use. It may help lessen the severity of the attack.

- **Hydrate.** At the first sign of a migraine, down several cups of water. Dehydration can worsen headache pain (it's also a cause of migraines).

- **Try some caffeine.** A cup of coffee may help. Caffeine is in many over-the-counter migraine medications because it helps constrict dilated blood vessels around your temples. It can also increase the efficacy of pain meds.

- **Pick a pill.** An over-the-counter med like acetaminophen, ibuprofen, or naproxen may help. A migraine-specific med that combines acetaminophen, aspirin, and caffeine can also help. You need to experiment to see which one is most effective for you. See "When to Call a Doctor" for information on prescription meds you can try.

- **Find your cave.** Some migraine suffers get hit so badly that they have to lie down in a dark room until the misery subsides. If this is you, go for it. The faster you relieve the symptoms, the faster you can get back to your game.

PREVENT IT

- **Stay hydrated.** Dehydration can help trigger a migraine, so be sure to drink ample fluids throughout the day, especially after exercise. Also, alcohol can dehydrate you, so . . .

- **Avoid alcohol.** Alcohol is at the top of the list of the most common food triggers of migraines. It's a vasodilator, meaning that it expands blood vessels and can trigger a migraine. Red wine (more so than white), beer, champagne, and eggnog are most frequently mentioned as triggers. Dark-colored spirits like scotch, rye, bourbon, brandy, sherry, and cognac seem more likely to trigger headaches than light-colored drinks like gin, vodka, and white wine.

- **Keep a headache diary.** Every time you have a migraine, write down some stats: time of onset, intensity and duration, what you ate that day, what medications you took, and any factors that may have triggered the headache. If you start to see common patterns, you'll be able to avoid some of the triggers.

- **Sleep.** Poor-quality or insufficient sleep contributes to migraines. Strive for your 7 to 8 hours a night.

- **Experiment with alternatives.** A variety of alternative migraine treatments have been shown to help, though they are not sure things. The following supplements and treatments should be on your radar: acupuncture, biofeedback, the herbs feverfew and butterbur, vitamin B_2 (riboflavin), magnesium, and coenzyme Q10. Every patient is different and gets different results, but if your migraines are bad, search for what works.

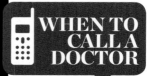

WHEN TO CALL A DOCTOR

If your migraines are mild enough to endure with over-the-counter meds and home remedies, a doctor visit isn't necessary. But if you have severe attacks, see your doctor for an exam and to talk about prescription remedies. Before you go, however, keep a headache diary so you have a written record of triggers, headache intensity and duration, and other factors that can help your doctor evaluate you.

One of the most common migraine meds is a triptan. It helps with the pain and nausea, and also tempers the sensitivity to light and sound. Ergots are another variety of medication that contains caffeine; they're cheaper than the triptans but less effective.

The FDA has also approved Botox injection as a migraine treatment. It works for some folks, but injections have to be done every 12 weeks.

Also, various cardiovascular meds like beta-blockers and some anti-depressants have been shown to help prevent migraines, though they aren't long-term solutions. Your doctor may have you try them and, if your migraines stop, taper you off the medication to see if the migraines return.

DO YOU NEED SURGERY?
No.

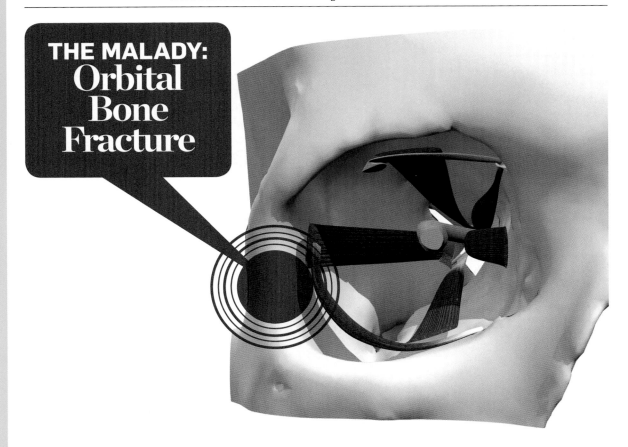

THE MALADY:
Orbital Bone Fracture

THE SYMPTOMS

Intense pain after an impact to the eye and the bones around the eye. You can also have vision problems and eye movement problems.

WHAT'S GOING ON IN THERE?

You call it your eye socket, but the proper name for it is the orbit. Seven bones make up the orbit (thus, all of them are orbital bones), and when you run your finger along the rim of your eye socket, you're feeling the bones that can be involved in an orbital fracture. But that's just the beginning.

Severe orbital fractures can include what's called a blowout fracture, in which the inside of the eye orbit—most commonly the floor, or bottom—cracks open. This includes a serious eye injury about a third of the time. Associated injuries include corneal abrasion, lens dislocation, eye alignment and movement problems, and other issues (as if the fracture weren't enough by itself).

So what causes an orbital fracture? An impact. Martial arts, boxing, and ball games are some of the most common causes because a hard impact from a fist (even one in a boxing glove), a baseball, or a softball can crack bone. Oh, and don't underestimate a hockey puck's destructive talents.

This is a traumatic injury, obviously, and other issues can go along with it, such as loss of consciousness and concussion, depending on the force of the impact.

FIX IT

- **Head to the ER.** Don't mess with eye injuries. Even if you can see just fine, swelling that could be caused by a blowout fracture can cause problems later. You do not want to risk your eyesight because you think you'll be all right. Also, if you took a good shot, you may have a concussion.

- **Ice it.** Applying ice can help with swelling after you've been seen by a doctor and gone home. Don't simply ice your eye after an impact and think that will take care of it. Eye trauma needs medical attention before anything else.

- **Try an NSAID.** Taking ibuprofen is usually recommended for orbital fractures that don't require hospital admission (see "When to Call a Doctor").

PREVENT IT

- **Keep your head in the game.** It's easy to say that, but because injuries sometimes just happen, it's best to make sure you're well prepared for any competition: That will lessen the chance that you'll take a shot to the eye that might break bone. If you're in a hand-to-hand combat sport like boxing or martial arts, proper conditioning and preparation mean your opponent will have less of a chance of getting through your defenses. In baseball or softball, the advice is simpler: Keep your eye on the ball (but not literally).

- **Wear your gear.** If your sport requires headgear, don't be stupid and leave it in the car.

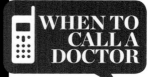

WHEN TO CALL A DOCTOR

ASAP. All eye injuries are serious, but taking a hit to the eye can be flat-out scary. Even if your eyesight doesn't seem to be affected, head to the ER to get checked out.

A blowout fracture sounds gruesome, but the fact is, if you have one with no other apparent eye injury (about two-thirds of cases), you may not even be admitted to the hospital. The injury resolves itself once the swelling goes down. As the orbit heals in the ensuing weeks, if you have any changes such as increasing pain, problems with visual acuity, or seeing flashing lights, get back to the ER pronto. If healing proceeds without a problem, you'll just have to make a follow-up visit with the doctor for the final okay to get back in the game.

DO YOU NEED SURGERY?

It's possible, but only for very serious injuries. The procedure depends on the specific complication. Serious eye injuries with blowout fractures are generally referred to an eye surgeon or an otolaryngological (ears, nose, and throat) surgeon.

HEAD

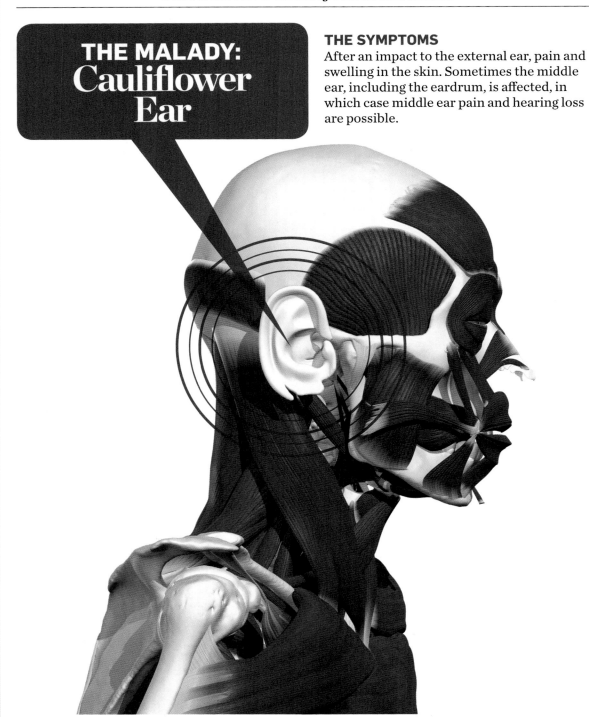

THE MALADY:
Cauliflower Ear

THE SYMPTOMS

After an impact to the external ear, pain and swelling in the skin. Sometimes the middle ear, including the eardrum, is affected, in which case middle ear pain and hearing loss are possible.

WHAT'S GOING ON IN THERE?

The external ear, called the pinna, is basically cartilage and skin. When it's traumatized—by a direct hit, pulling, or folding over—bleeding under the skin (a hematoma) can cause swelling and pain.

The real problem comes if the cartilage in the pinna and the skin surrounding it are somehow pulled apart. That skin is the cartilage's only source of blood, which means that the skin is what's keeping the cartilage alive. A hematoma beneath the skin, or the impact itself, can pull the skin away from the cartilage or otherwise disrupt the skin-cartilage connection. Once that happens, the cartilage begins to die.

When the cartilage is necrotic (dead tissue), it shrivels up and turns white. The skin around it shrivels as well, and you now have a permanent deformity known as cauliflower ear (because that's what it looks like).

The athletes most at risk for this type of injury (and the subsequent cauliflower ear) are wrestlers, mixed martial artists, rugby players, and boxers.

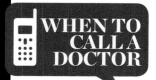

WHEN TO CALL A DOCTOR

Serious pain and swelling are indications of a hematoma, which is a big cause of cauliflower ear. If you want to avoid having a deformed ear, you need to have that hematoma drained. That will allow the skin and cartilage to heal up and keep that cartilage supplied with nutrients transported by the blood. Draining it is a simple procedure, but you need to let a pro do it under sterile conditions.

If you have hearing issues to go along with your injury, get to an ER to see what kind of damage has been done. Don't let it go, folks.

DO YOU NEED SURGERY?

No (unless you count draining the hematoma as a surgical procedure). But if you let the injury go and develop cauliflower ear, you may want to have plastic surgery to fix it.

FIX IT

- **Ice it.** For mild trauma to the external ear, applying ice should be enough.

- **Don't drain it yourself.** If your ear is swollen from a big hematoma, it needs to be drained so the skin can maintain contact with the cartilage. You may see videos on the Web showing you how to do this with an insulin needle. I don't recommend this. It's too easy to hurt yourself or get an infection. If your hematoma needs to be drained, let a pro do it under sterile conditions.

- **Try an NSAID.** Use ibuprofen to help with the pain and inflammation.

PREVENT IT

- **Wear your headgear.** Wearing protective headgear that covers your ears is the single best preventive measure for an external ear injury. In sports like mixed martial arts and wrestling, there's certainly a tough-guy mentality. And that's fine. But why risk your dashing good looks (not to mention your hearing) when you don't have to?

THE MALADY:
Broken Nose

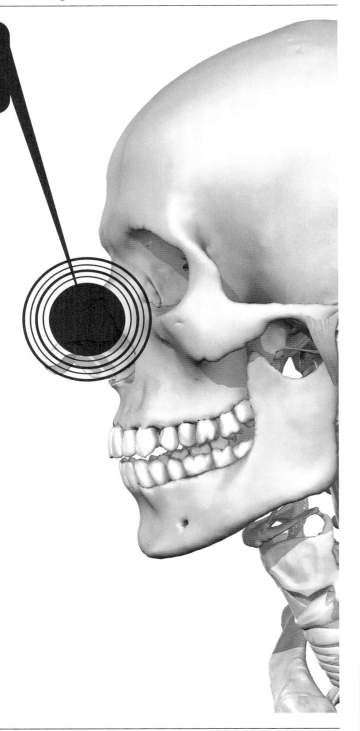

THE SYMPTOMS

After an impact to the nose, pain, swelling, and bruising of the nose and under the eyes. Your nose could look "out of joint" and you could be having trouble breathing through it. The nose might bleed, but not necessarily. Note that symptoms sometimes don't show up immediately, but rather days later.

WHAT'S GOING ON IN THERE?

Your nose is essentially a breathing structure of bone and cartilage that keeps your nasal airways open (that also allows you to smell and filters the air that comes through it). If you take a hard hit to the front of the nose or across the bridge of the nose, the bone and cartilage could fracture, sometimes in multiple places. It's incredibly painful, disorients you, makes your eyes tear, and can be scary to look at if you have bleeding and deformity.

Virtually any sport puts you at risk for a broken nose (okay, golf not so much), including team sports like football, basketball, hockey, and soccer. And one-on-one impact sports are also common nose breakers: martial arts, boxing, wrestling, and, when the gloves come off, hockey. You can even break your nose going over a bike's handlebars or lifting weights without a spotter.

FIX IT

- **For a minor nasal fracture,** there isn't much you can do except treat your pain and swelling. As these symptoms subside, the nose should heal on its own.

- **Don't swallow the blood.** If your nose is bleeding, lean forward so the blood drains and doesn't run down the back of your throat, which can add nausea and vomiting to your problems.

- **Ice it.** Apply ice immediately after the injury, as well as for 15 minutes several times a day to help reduce the swelling and bruising. Be careful not to put too much pressure on the nose.

- **Try an NSAID.** Over-the-counter ibuprofen or another pain reliever like naproxen or acetaminophen can help with the pain.

- **Keep your head up.** When you're lying down, keep your head elevated so the swelling (and throbbing) doesn't get any worse.

PREVENT IT

- **Wear your headgear.** Using whatever protective gear it is that your sport requires (helmets and face masks for football and hockey) is the single best preventive measure for a broken nose. In sports having no head protection gear, the best prevention is good training and paying attention. And never leading with your head.

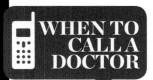

WHEN TO CALL A DOCTOR

Head to an ER if you have any of the following problems after the impact: bleeding that won't stop, a crooked or deformed nose, or a hard time breathing through your nose. X-rays aren't usually needed; the doctor can generally diagnose a broken nose with a physical evaluation.

Most broken noses can be "set" manually by a process called closed reduction. The doctor gives you a local anesthetic and, using tools and hands, sets the nose.

Also head to the ER if you have any secondary symptoms that signal a head or neck injury, such as a headache, nausea, vomiting, neck pain, or loss of consciousness.

DO YOU NEED SURGERY?

It's very rarely needed for a broken nose itself unless the patient has waited more than 14 days after the injury to be seen, in which case surgery is necessary to set and shape the nose. If the injury causes a deviated septum that inhibits your breathing, surgery is the only way to correct it. Another rare complication is bleeding in the nasal cartilage, called a septal hematoma. This big clot can block one or both nostrils and must be drained.

HEAD

PART TWO

THE MOST ANNOYING SPORTS MALADIES EVER—CURED!

Athletes face a lot of issues that have nothing to do with an "injury." I put that word in quotation marks because the maladies in this section aren't exactly breakdowns in bones, muscles, or connective tissues, but any athlete will tell you that they are indeed painful, irritating, and, in severe cases, debilitating. Luckily, there are terrific remedies for all of them. Get ready to feel a whole lot better.

Abrasion (brush burn, road rash)

You can scrape up your skin a hundred ways, but here I'm talking about taking off a big patch of epidermis and dermis (the first two of the three layers of skin, which means, yes, it hurts like crazy). Examples include when a cyclist crashes and gets road rash and when a fast-pitch softball player slides into third and scrapes off a big patch of his or her calf. It's not an especially deep injury, but it can bleed and is definitely painful.

If the abrasion is large—say, twice the size of your palm—see a doctor. Also see a doctor if it is on your face, hands, feet, or genitals. Otherwise, see if it will respond to home treatment with these tactics.

CLEAN IT. Clean the area with a mild soap and water. Abrasions like these are loaded with dirt from whatever surface it was that you dragged yourself across. Scrub gently—you don't want to cause any more damage. If you can't scrub it because it hurts too much, try pouring soapy water over it. Use tweezers to remove any gravel. Oh, and take an NSAID like ibuprofen or naproxen to help with the throbbing, because this will hurt.

DRESS IT. Apply a layer of triple-antibiotic ointment (like Neosporin) to the entire area. It's also helpful to apply a layer of petroleum jelly on top of that to prevent the bandage from sticking to the flesh. Cover it with a sterile gauze pad and tape. Change the dressing once a day. It will be gooey and ooze, which is nasty but normal. Big abrasions usually heal from the deeper layers of the skin outward, and also from the edges toward the center. If the bandage sticks to the wound, don't try to pull it loose. Soak it in the bathtub for about 20 minutes and it should come off easily.

WATCH IT. If you see redness and swelling and the wound feels hot or secretes pus, it could be infected. See a doctor.

Anemia (menstrual)
[WOMEN]

I see many female patients who complain of fatigue and weakness. Those symptoms don't point to any specific malady, especially in women whose sleep quality and diet are good. But for these athletes, many times iron-deficiency anemia is the problem.

Anemia is a condition in which you have a low number of red blood cells, meaning that there aren't enough to carry all the oxygen your active body needs. When this happens, the symptoms include fatigue, light-headedness, decreased endurance, and a feeling that you're just not as fit as you should be given your training.

There are other definitive physical signs: A rapid heartbeat because the heart has to move more blood to deliver oxygen and a lighter shade of red under the fingernails and in the rims of the eyelids are both among the first signs of a decreased number of red blood cells.

Iron-deficiency anemia is common in female athletes for two reasons. The first is because of the monthly menstrual cycle, which of course causes blood loss. The second results from hard training, especially endurance training, in which the repeated microtrauma literally sucks the life out of your blood, possibly because, according to one theory, repeated footstrikes destroy red blood cells, affecting the cell count as the miles pile up. A bonus reason could be diet: Some women don't take in enough iron.

If you suspect that you have iron-deficiency anemia, see your doctor, who can confirm the diagnosis with a blood test. If that is indeed your problem, you can rectify it in a few months with these simple solutions.

TRY IRON SUPPLEMENTS. Women need roughly 15 milligrams of iron a day, and supplements will help build up your body's iron stores.

REVAMP YOUR DIET. Iron is in many foods, but the body absorbs only 1 milligram of iron for every 10 to 20 milligrams of it consumed. Vitamin C enhances the absorption of iron, so eating citrus fruits or taking C supplements can help you absorb iron more effectively.

What to eat? Oysters are the best source of iron, but easier sources are meat (especially red meat), fish, leafy green vegetables (especially spinach), and nuts (all things you should be eating anyway).

Athlete's foot

Athlete's foot is the most common form of tinea, a fungal infection of the nails, skin, or hair. The fungus lives on the skin and breeds best in warm, moist conditions. If you go barefoot and pick it up in a locker room, pool, or bathroom, your sweaty sneakers let it thrive. The fungus triggers redness, swelling, cracking, burning, scaling, and intense itching between your toes. A nasty case can take a few weeks to cure, and if you don't take the proper steps, it'll come back. So here are some ways to strike back.

SOOTHE THE SORES. Use compresses to cool the inflammation, ease the pain, lessen the itching, and dry the sores. Dissolve 1 packet of Domeboro powder or 2 tablespoons of Burow's solution (both available over-the-counter at pharmacies) in 1 pint of cold water. Soak a washcloth in the liquid and apply it as a compress for 15 to 20 minutes 3 or 4 times a day.

MEDICATE YOUR FOOT. Over-the-counter antifungal medications can help, but try a gel as opposed to a cream or lotion because the gels also contain a drying agent. Apply it 2 or

3 times a day up until 2 weeks after the problem seems to have cleared up.

SCRUB AWAY DEAD SKIN. When the acute phase of the attack has died down, remove any dead skin. It houses living fungi that can reinfect you. In the shower, work the entire foot lightly but vigorously with a bristle scrub brush.

CHANGE YOUR SHOES. Having two pairs of athletic shoes and alternating between them is a good idea, because it takes shoes a good 24 hours to dry out thoroughly. Also, dust the insides of your shoes with antifungal powder or spray. Another way to kill fungus spores: Spray a disinfectant (like Lysol) on a rag and wipe the insides of your shoes whenever you take them off.

DRY YOUR TOES. Allow your feet to dry for 5 to 10 minutes after coming out of the shower and before putting your shoes on. You can speed the process with a hair dryer; wiggle your toes to dry between them.

COVER UP IN PUBLIC PLACES. Wear slippers or shower shoes in areas where other people go barefoot. If you're prone to fungal infections, you can pick them up almost anyplace that's damp.

Black eye

Black eye is something of a misnomer. Very dark blue eye or rainbow-of-colors eye would be better. Whether you took an elbow in a soccer game or a left hook in hockey, the skin around your eye is so thin that blood shows up as dark blue. Over the week it takes to heal, the blood is reabsorbed back into the body, in the process presenting a kaleidoscope of colors that signifies healing. Here are some ways to soothe the pain and swelling that don't involve raw steak.

PACK IT IN ICE, THEN HEAT. A cold pack will keep the swelling down and, by constricting the blood vessels, decrease the internal bleeding. Apply ice (a bag of frozen peas works great, too) for 15 minutes 4 to 6 times a day for the first 2 days. Then switch to warm compresses on the same schedule.

TRY VITAMINS C AND K. Taking vitamin K is an old Chinese remedy for a black eye. It helps the blood clot so it doesn't spread across your face. Vitamin C can help prevent the wild discoloration.

REDUCE SWELLING WITH TEA. Using a wet black tea bag as a topical compress can help reduce swelling. The chemical epigallocatechin gallate in the tea acts as an antiinflammatory. The caffeine is a natural diuretic, which can help reduce swelling.

SEE HOW YOU SEE. A black eye shouldn't be taken lightly since it can involve serious internal eye injuries, including a detached retina and internal hemorrhages, that may not be evident at first. If you have difficulty seeing, you need medical attention immediately. If you have pain in the eye, sensitivity to light, blurred or double vision, or see specks floating in your field of vision, see a doctor.

Blisters

Blisters are your body's way of saying it's had enough. Be it too much friction or too much ambition, a blister—much like a muscle cramp or side stitch—is designed to slow you down and make you prepare better for physical activity. A blister forms because you've ruptured cell tissue and released plasma (the fluid in a blister), and the ballooned outside skin is your body's way of preventing infection.

TO POP OR NOT TO POP. If you pop a blister, you risk infection. If you don't, you have to protect it. I recommend popping blisters that are big enough to inhibit your sports activity. If you pop it, use a needle sterilized in alcohol. Wash the blister several times a day and cover it with some antibiotic ointment and a waterproof bandage. If you don't pop it, cut a piece of moleskin in a doughnut shape and place it over the blister, with the blister in the open center. The moleskin will absorb the friction of activity, and as long as the skin is clean and dry, it will adhere. Moleskin and other "second skin" products should allow you to get back to your regular activities.

BEWARE STRANGE COLORS. If your blister is painful, oozing pus, and red around the edges, you may have an infection. See a doctor.

LET IT BREATHE. Air and water are good for healing, so at night remove the dressing, soak the blister in some water for 10 minutes, and then let it air out for the rest of the night.

KILL ANY ITCH. If the blister itches or burns, apply a little of the hemorrhoid cream Preparation H. It works.

WEAR FASHIONS THAT FIT. Properly fitted shoes and socks won't give you blisters. If you feel a part of your foot rubbing, back off and address the problem. A thick waterproof bandage can help protect the area, and in a pinch, so will a piece of duct tape applied directly over the blister.

PREVENT THEM. Anything that reduces friction in the area will prevent blisters. Runners, buy and try double-layer socks. Putting petroleum jelly between your toes can also help.

Bonking (hypoglycemia)

Athletes, especially endurance athletes, speak of bonking as a horrible fate. And it is. You only need to experience exercise-induced hypoglycemia once to know you don't ever want it again. Your body—and especially your brain—runs on glucose, and having low blood sugar means your body is out of fuel. It's that "bonk" of hitting the wall, often after about 2 hours of exercise. I've had it many times during training and races. It starts as a headache and can also include nausea, fatigue, and a slowed pace. Once you attack hypoglycemia, it usually takes about a half hour or more to cure—more than enough time to spoil any race or event. Severe cases can make you feel horrible for days.

WHEN YOU BONK, INGEST CARBS. Sports drinks and gels are usually what's readily available, but a sectioned orange is a pure sugar injection for your system.

THE KEY IS PREVENTION. During long exercise sessions, your body needs fuel, period. Gels and drinks are the easiest ways to keep your blood sugar from dropping. Pre-race nutrition is important as well: Those pre-marathon spaghetti dinners are offered for a reason.

Bonking, part 2 (hyponatremia)

When I was in the running stage of my first Ironman in Lake Placid back in 2000, a strange and scary feeling set in at mile 14. It came over my whole body like a wave: The pain of pounding out steps lessened. And then my entire drive evaporated. I no longer cared about the race. My awareness of where I was diminished and soon I felt myself not caring about anything. By mile 15, I wanted to sit by the side of the road and take a nap.

Just at that point, I saw a strange sight: an old man with a jar of salt. What the...? A jar of salt? Why? I didn't know why, and yet my brain guided me right to him. I opened my hand, took an entire handful of salt, and devoured it right in front of him. Almost immediately, I felt better. The turnaround was amazingly fast: My mind cleared, the world was in focus again. Even the water that had been sloshing around in my stomach stopped sloshing. Onward I went. When I passed the old man again on my way back, I took another salt hit for the road. During the last miles of the race, I was upright and smiling. I know one thing: Without that old man and the jar of salt, I wouldn't have finished the race.

So what happened to me? As a doctor, I was amazed at both the speed of the onset and the speed of the cure. It was hyponatremia—a loss of sodium in the blood. My symptoms were classic.

Hyponatremia is common during endurance events, especially those lasting more than 4 or 5 hours. Much as with in my experience, the symptoms are often not apparent as they're happening to you. When athletes sweat in hot and humid conditions, they lose both water and electrolytes like sodium and potassium. The pace this happens at is known as your sweat rate.

Sweat rate is influenced by a number of factors, including the athlete's fitness level, the "bulb index" (a combination of the temperature and humidity on that particular day), and plain old body chemistry, which makes some people sweat more than others. The better your physical fitness, the higher your sweat rate. Heavy sweaters can lose 2 to 3 liters of fluid every hour. These folks look as if they're covered in chalk at the end of a long race—it's all the dried salt. (I talk about sweat rate in more detail in "General Guidelines for Sports Nutrition," page 303).

The symptoms of hyponatremia are different from those of hypoglycemia. The main difference is the changes in mental status that are the hallmarks of hyponatremia: confusion and an inability to focus on where you are. Muscle cramping and swelling of the fingers and toes can also occur.

There are laboratories that can test athletes to calculate their sweat rates, but as you might imagine, they aren't readily available to the average athlete. One of the best ways to prevent hyponatremia is to down sodium in electrolyte drinks and gels instead of water during the race, especially during the second half of your event. As for how much, everyone is different, so go by how you feel. If you've had hyponatremia before, you know exactly what I'm talking about. And if anyone sees an old man in Lake Placid holding a jar of salt, please thank him for me.

Bruises

Every athlete has bruises. But there are ways to treat them and help them disappear faster.

ICE IT, THEN HEAT IT. Apply ice or a cold pack for 15 minutes several times a day during the first 2 days. After that, use heat to help dilate the blood vessels and improve circulation in the area, which will help the body remove the blood in the bruise. Elevating the bruise above the level of your heart at any time can also help.

KNOW YOUR MEDICINE'S SIDE EFFECTS. Aspirin, NSAIDs, antidepressants, and asthma medications can thin the blood and make you bruise easily. Alcohol or drug abusers tend to bruise easily as well.

UP YOUR VITAMIN C. If you bruise easily, you could be vitamin C deficient. C helps build protective collagen around blood vessels in the skin. Take a supplement or up your intake of citrus fruits, leafy green vegetables, and bell peppers.

USE VITAMIN K. Vitamin K helps erase bruising by helping blood to clot. Rub some vitamin K cream (available at your local drugstore) on a bruise a few times a day to help it clear faster.

TRY ARNICA. Arnica (available at most drug and health food stores) is a plant-based supplement and homeopathic remedy that has been shown to prevent and minimize bruising. A topical gel, it acts as an antiinflammatory and also helps dilate capillaries under the skin, which allows blood to move out of the injured area.

Chafing (common)

What starts off innocently as your skin rubbing on something else—be it more skin, your jogging shorts, or your bra—can quickly become more sinister. A little friction can make skin become red, hot, and inflamed, and in severe cases, it may even cause bleeding. Try these strategies to deal with it.

KEEP IT CLEAN. If your chafing is bad enough that the area's bleeding or on the verge of bleeding, clean it with hydrogen peroxide, then apply some antibiotic ointment and cover it with sterile gauze and athletic tape or bandages.

WEAR TIGHTS. Athletic tights and spandex cycling shorts stretch and cause no friction against the skin.

ROLL ON RELIEF. Most sports stores carry sticks of roll-on lubricant that you can rub on before an activity that may lead to raw skin.

Chafing of the nipples

For male distance runners, nipple chafing is a very real, very painful side effect of running with a shirt on. (Women tend not to get nipple chafing because sports bras protect them, but those bras can chafe just as badly where the elastic meets the skin.) You see pictures after every marathon of men crossing the finish line with two red streaks down the fronts of their shirts. And if you think it's no big deal, well, your first shower after the race will teach you a new definition of the word *sting*. Here's what to do.

If your nipples are chafing during a race or long run: If you can, take off your shirt. That eliminates the friction. If that's not an option, you can hold your shirt out, away from your nipples, as you run. Not very convenient, but it works.

If your nipples have already chafed: Treat them like what they are, open wounds. Clean them with hydrogen peroxide (yup, stings like crazy!), then apply some antibiotic ointment and cover them with sterile gauze and athletic tape or bandages.

If you want to prevent this from ever happening: You have several options. Putting a waterproof bandage across each nipple can work. Sweat may make them come loose, however. Also, NipGuards, small, round adhesive pads that cover your nipples, work pretty well and are available at running stores. Pack extras in case sweat works them loose.

Chapped lips

Chapped lips give new meaning to the expression crack a smile. Athletes training in dry, cold weather or even in intense sunshine can develop chapped lips. The skin on the lips is very thin, so there's nothing to protect them from the elements.

UP THE MOISTURE FACTOR. You could be dehydrated. Make sure you're drinking enough fluids that your urine runs clear.

MIND YOUR NUTRITION. Nutritional deficiencies, especially in the B-complex vitamins and iron, can play a role in scaling of the lips. A multivitamin should give you what you need. Taking an omega-3 supplement (or eating more fatty fish like salmon) is also a good idea, because chapped lips can be caused by a lack of unsaturated fatty acids in the epithelial tissue.

SHOP FOR THE RIGHT LIP BALM. A waxy lip balm can cover your lips and help prevent chapping, but if they're already chapped, forget it. You need moisture. Petroleum jelly is very effective. Also look for lip balms that have only natural ingredients like olive oil, almond oil, beeswax, and shea butter.

AND IN A PINCH… If you're outside and have nothing else handy, rub your finger alongside your nose, then rub it on your lips. Your finger will pick up a little of the natural oil on your skin, which is the kind of oil the lips are looking for anyway.

Chipped or knocked-out tooth

A chipped or broken tooth is definitely a job for your dentist. If an entire tooth gets knocked out with the root intact, see your dentist ASAP for reimplantation. Don't try to clean the tooth—the root is delicate and easily damaged. The best way to transport a tooth is to put it either in its natural environment—your mouth, maybe between your cheek and gum—or in a glass of salt water or milk.

Common head cold

The conventional wisdom when you have a cold bug is that if it's above the neck (in your head only), you should train. If it's below the neck (in your lungs), don't. The fact is, even if you have a mild head cold, you don't want it to turn into something worse that makes you cough up green junk for 2 weeks. Here are some ideas.

SEE IF VITAMIN C WORKS FOR YOU. C might cut back on the coughing, sneezing, and other symptoms, but scientific studies have produced mixed results. One summary of

30 studies that was published in 2000 found "a consistently beneficial but generally modest therapeutic effect on duration of cold symptoms." So it can't cure a cold, but it may help reduce your symptoms.

TRY ZINC. Sucking on zinc lozenges can cut colds short, from an average of 8 days down to an average of 4, say researchers from the Cleveland Clinic. Study subjects sucked on 4 to 8 lozenges a day, each containing 13.3 milligrams of zinc. It doesn't necessarily work for everyone, but give it a try. Don't take zinc at the same time as vitamin C, because the two bind together and make the zinc less effective—leave at least 1 hour between taking them. Also, watch your zinc intake. More than 40 milligrams a day can cause nausea, dizziness, or vomiting.

USE A SALINE RINSE. A nasal saline rinse (available at any pharmacy) goes a long way in keeping your sinuses clear, not only allowing you to breathe, but also helping to make sure that phlegm doesn't pool in your sinuses and promote a sinus infection.

DON'T SPREAD YOUR GERMS. If you are going to work out with a head cold, please do society a favor and do it solo. Spreading the love at the gym is just mean.

Erectile dysfunction caused by nerve compression [MEN]

Erectile dysfunction is generally a reason to see your doctor because it can be a harbinger of heart disease. That is, if you're not getting good blood circulation in the smaller vessels of the penis, it could mean you'll have bigger blockage issues in larger blood vessels later on. But here I'm talking about a form of erectile dysfunction that is usually seen in cyclists and triathletes. If you have ED and don't ride a bike for long periods, see a doctor. However, if you experience sexual performance issues or numbness in the region and train hard on a bicycle, read this.

I've seen patients and have trained with men who have experienced numbness and erectile dysfunction after long rides, and the symptoms worsen with the more time you spend in the saddle. The problem is compression of the pudendal nerve, which runs just beneath the ischial tuberosity, otherwise known as the sit bones. (Women can also have this problem, but they experience numbness.)

Athletes can alleviate the ED by getting a better-fitting bike saddle. What qualities should you look for in a good seat? Comfort, comfort, and comfort. Some other good preventive ideas: Stand up in the pedals every once in a while, and change the pressure points on your crotch by shifting forward and backward in the saddle during a long ride.

This generally fixes the "problem." If your ED continues, see a doctor.

Foot odor

Your feet have more sweat glands per square inch of skin than any other part of your body—an average of 250,000 of them. So you can imagine what's going on after a good workout. Your feet being encased in shoes and socks allows the bacteria proliferating on your skin to produce an evil substance called isovaleric acid that makes your feet reek. The American Podiatric Medicine Association says that 25 percent of us have foot odor issues. I think the percentage among athletes is much higher. Here are some ideas to make life better for everyone around you.

WASH, DRY, AND POWDER. Wash your feet thoroughly, especially between the toes, every day. Dry them well and apply a foot odor powder or cornstarch. And don't forget to apply the powder inside your shoes as well.

TRY ANTIPERSPIRANT. Putting regular antiperspirant on your feet can reduce the sweating. Try a roll-on or solid, however, instead of a spray. A lot of spray is lost to the air.

USE TWO PAIRS OF SHOES. Alternating days on the same make and model of shoe allows each pair time to dry out. You can also try running the insoles through the washing machine (but not the dryer, which can destroy their shock-absorbing abilities; let 'em air-dry).

UP YOUR ZINC INTAKE. Foot odor is one of many symptoms of zinc deficiency. Replenish your zinc level with oysters, nuts, peas, eggs, whole grains, and pumpkin seeds.

Groin hit [MEN]

A hit to the testicles brings ungodly pain and even nausea, but it's usually a transient thing. The testicle is a delicate network of tubules that make up a man's sperm factory, but testes are spongy and pretty decent shock absorbers by design. If you take a direct hit and have significant ongoing pain and swelling, you'll want to have it checked to see if you've got testicular torsion, where the testicle twists on itself, or, more rarely, testicular rupture. Both are as nasty as they sound.

Groin hit [WOMEN]

The male groin hit gets all the press, but ask any woman in a contact sport like martial arts if a groin hit hurts. In most cases, you're talking about a bruise that will simply heal. But if you're hit hard enough, you could have an internal injury—there's a lot of reproductive machinery in that region—or you could have a pelvis fracture. If you experience continued pain and/or bleeding, see a doctor immediately.

Heat exhaustion

A lot of athletes exercise in hot weather and sometimes in extreme heat. Signs of heat exhaustion often begin suddenly. The combination of heat, heavy perspiration, and inadequate fluid intake takes away your body's ability to cool itself and your internal temperature starts to rise, sometimes as high as 104°F. The symptoms resemble the onset of shock: You feel weak, dizzy, nauseated, or worried. You could have a headache and/or a fast heartbeat.

Don't confuse heat exhaustion and heatstroke. The latter is the potentially deadly condition, and you get it by ignoring the signs of the former. No one goes directly from feeling fine to the brink of death no matter how hot it is, so give yourself 30 minutes to respond positively to the following self-care measures. If your symptoms don't improve by then, go to the ER immediately. When you go from having weakness and confusion to having difficulty walking or loss of consciousness, you've crossed over from heat exhaustion to heatstroke.

Here's what to do for heat exhaustion and how to prevent it.

GET OUT OF THE HEAT—FAST. The obvious answer, but people often ignore it. You need shade or air-conditioning. And after you feel better, know that returning to the sun even hours later can spur a relapse. Be careful.

DRINK COOL FLUIDS. Drinking cold water and sports drinks not only works well for fast hydration, but also will help lower your internal temperature.

GET WET. Cold water on the skin is a big help. Cold water on the skin in front of a fan is even better. Spray it on, drizzle it over your head and neck, or wipe yourself down with cold, wet towels.

CHECK YOUR WEIGHT. If you train in hot weather, weigh yourself before and after a workout to see how much water weight you've lost. Then replenish. The next day, weigh yourself again before the workout—and every day thereafter. If your weight doesn't return to your original number or drops further, you may be slowly dehydrating yourself. Make sure you drink enough fluids that your urine runs clear.

KEEP YOUR SHIRT ON. You pick up more radiant heat exposure with your shirt off. Once you perspire, a shirt can act as a cooling device when the wind blows on the wet material.

STAY AWAY FROM ALCOHOL. A good summer workout, or even a long round of golf in the sun, may make you feel that it's time for a beer afterward. Watch it. Alcohol dehydrates you and can make even mild heat exhaustion worse. Hydrate first, celebrate later.

WAIT A WEEK. If you do get heat exhaustion, try to stay out of extreme heat for the next week. You're especially vulnerable to a relapse during that time. Train indoors.

WAIT A WEEK, PART 2. If you train in normal temperatures and know you have a big athletic event coming up in hot weather, give your body time to acclimate to it. Train in that weather for at least a week beforehand.

MIND YOUR MEDS. Certain medications, such as diuretics, blood pressure medicines, allergy meds, cough and cold medicines, laxatives, and benzodiazepines, can decrease the body's ability to regulate its temperature, increasing your risk. If you have to be on any of those, consider exercising in air-conditioning.

Hemorrhoids

Hemorrhoids are among the most common health ailments. More than half of us will develop them, usually after age 30, according to the American Society of Colon and Rectal Surgeons. A hemorrhoid is a swollen vein in or around the anus. There are several causes, including pregnancy and childbirth, poor diet, lifting heavy things, pushing during bowel movements, and sitting on hard surfaces. Heredity is also a factor. Whatever the cause, the tissue supporting the vessels stretches. The vessels then dilate, their walls become thin, and they bleed. If the stretching and

pressure continue, the weakened vessels bulge. The symptoms are pain, itching in the anal area, bleeding during a bowel movement, and a protrusion in the anal area.

Many athletes suffer through hemorrhoids (some of you may recall Baseball Hall of Famer George Brett dealing with hemorrhoids during the 1980 World Series). Cyclists have it especially tough. Still, most hemorrhoids improve dramatically with simple measures.

ADD FIBER TO YOUR DIET. The American Gastroenterological Association suggests that drinking water and eating enough fiber are the two biggest ways to ease hemorrhoid flare-ups. This softens the stools and makes them easier to pass, reducing pressure on the hemorrhoids. Easy fiber sources include fruits and vegetables, beans, whole grains, and high-fiber cereals. A typical adult needs 25 to 30 grams of fiber daily.

GO WHEN YOU GOTTA GO. When the urge hits, head to the bathroom immediately. Don't wait for a more convenient time. The stool can back up, which can result in increased pressure and straining later.

LIMIT YOUR TOILET TIME. An awful lot of folks read on the toilet. Not a good idea if you have hemorrhoids. Prolonged toilet sitting causes blood to pool and enlarge the vessels.

CLEAN YOURSELF TENDERLY. Regular toilet paper can feel like sandpaper on hemorrhoids. Dampen toilet paper before each wipe. Premoistened alcohol-free wipes also work well.

USE MEDICATION. Yes, hemorrhoid creams and suppositories reduce pain and swelling. But more isn't necessarily better; use them as directed.

WORK WONDERS WITH WITCH HAZEL. A bit of witch hazel (found at your pharmacy) applied to the anus with a cotton ball is a terrific remedy. It causes the blood vessels to shrink and contract. Chill the bottle of witch hazel in the fridge—it feels even better when applied cold.

EAT BERRIES. The flavonoids found in blueberries and blackberries can help reduce the thinning of veins. In a study of 120 people with frequent hemorrhoid flare-ups, those who received a twice-daily supplement of 500 milligrams of flavonoids had fewer and less severe hemorrhoid attacks than those who didn't. Another study, published in the *British Journal of Surgery*, looked at the effect of flavonoids on 100 patients facing surgery to fix their hemorrhoids. After 3 days of treatment, bleeding stopped in 80 percent of the patients. Continued treatment prevented a relapse in nearly two-thirds of the patients.

   A NOTE ABOUT ANAL BLEEDING: Hemorrhoids can bleed after a bowel movement and blood in the toilet or on toilet paper can be a disturbing sight. But bleeding in the gastrointestinal tract works like this: The higher up the bleeding, the darker it is when it comes out. That's why bleeding farther up the line, which signals more serious health issues, appears as a tarry, dark stool. Bright red blood that shows up only occasionally usually signals hemorrhoids. If you have chronic bleeding or dark stools, see a doctor.

Nosebleed

Whether you took a ball, a fist, or even a head (soccer!) to the nose, nosebleeds are painful and ugly. Vast amounts of blood circulate through capillaries in the nose, so bleeding can be copious when blood vessels there break. Nosebleeds can also occur if you're training indoors in winter, when dry heat irritates your mucous membranes. Here are some strategies for stemming the red tide.

BLOW OUT THE CLOT. Before you try to stop your nosebleed, give your nose one good, vigorous blow. That should remove any clots that are keeping blood vessels open. A clot can act like a wedge in a door. Blood vessels have elastic fibers, and if you can get any clots out, the elastic fibers can contract around the tiny opening, helping to stop the bloodflow.

USE COTTON. A cotton ball or a portion of one is a good nasal plug. It will soak up blood, and if you want to be even more aggressive, put some nasal decongestant spray, like Afrin, on the cotton before you stick it up your nose. This can help shrink blood vessels so a scab can form.

PINCH. Once the cotton is in place, pinch the soft part of your nose shut. Using a cold washcloth to do this with isn't a bad idea, either. Apply continuous pressure for 10 minutes, then remove the cotton. If the bleeding doesn't stop, pinch again for another 5 to 7 minutes. Most nosebleeds will have stopped by then.

DON'T LEAN BACK. Leaning your head back when you have a nosebleed can cause blood to run down the back of your throat. This tastes horrible, of course, but it can also start a coughing fit. Even worse, if enough blood goes down your throat, it can irritate your stomach and cause vomiting.

KEEP COOL. Putting another cold washcloth on the back of your neck is a good idea, too. This can help constrict blood vessels and slow the flow.

DON'T PICK. It takes 7 to 10 days to heal the blood vessel rupture that caused the nosebleed. Bleeding stops after a clot forms and the clot becomes a scab. If you pick your nose during this process, you'll open the scab and have another nosebleed. So hands (or, rather, fingers) off.

STOP SMOKING. If you happen to smoke, among the other 2,001 bad things it does to you is that smoking dries out the nasal cavities, making you more prone to nosebleeds.

Poked eye

Playing any close-quarters, full-contact sport can get you poked in the eye. Most times, you'll be just fine after a few minutes. But here are some things to do and look out for to make sure you see well for the rest of your life.

DON'T TOUCH OR RUB THE EYE. You'll just irritate it even more or cause more damage.

ANALYZE THE PAIN. Does it hurt to move your eye from side to side? Up and down? In either case, see a doctor to make sure you don't have a serious injury.

WATCH FOR VISION PROBLEMS. If you have any disruptions in your vision, head to an ER ASAP. Common eye-poke complications are a scratched cornea (which feels like you have sandpaper in your eye when you blink), bleeding in the eyeball, and a detached retina. Only a doctor can diagnose and treat these problems.

USE YOUR BRAIN, AND YOUR GEAR. It's commonsense advice that bears repeating: If your sport requires protective headgear that covers your eyes...use it.

Saddle sores

Cyclists can develop abrasions on their rumps from excessive friction and long rides. Saddle sores start out as a rubbing abrasion or "hot spot." This is when you should treat it. Don't wait. Full-blown sores are excruciating and dangerous because of the infection risk. Here are some tips for preventing them on the long hauls.

WEAR THE RIGHT SHORTS. Wearing well-fitting cycling shorts is a commonsense step. Try different brands and ask other riders what works for them.

CHECK YOUR BIKE FIT. A bike properly fitted to your body—including the seat that suits you best—won't outlaw saddle sores, but it can help reduce the risk. Generally, the higher the saddle is for your body, the more friction. See your local bike shop for a checkup.

USE PETROLEUM JELLY (OR CHAMOIS CREAM). Apply a layer of petroleum jelly to the vulnerable area before each ride. It's a simple lubricant that helps reduce a lot of friction. You'll also find some commercial lubricants at your cycling shop. See what works best for you.

GET OFF YOUR BUTT. Standing in the pedals periodically during a ride removes the offending friction. And you can stand pretty much whenever you want: going uphill, downhill, on a straightaway.

USE WHAT THE COWS USE. A lot of riders like Bag Balm for treating hot spots and also as a preventive lubricant. The stuff was developed to sooth the friction sores on cows' udders caused by milking. If it's good for the udders, it'll do you just fine.

SEE A DOCTOR. If you develop a full-blown saddle sore, especially if it appears to be infected, see your doctor for a potential antibiotic prescription. And let it heal before you get back on your bike.

Stinger

A stinger (or burner) is a classic football injury, though it can happen in any sport. A concentrated string of nerves called the brachial plexus comes out of the spinal cord into the shoulder, neck, and upper arm. When this nerve group is stretched or compressed, the result is a wicked stinging pain in the neck and shoulder and sometimes down the arm into the fingers, along with possible tingling and weakness. Tackling and blocking are prime causes.

In general, the pain subsides after a few minutes, but in some cases it may last for hours. If symptoms subside and you have normal strength, neck motion, and reflexes, you can return to action. If symptoms remain after the game, however, see a doctor to ensure that the injury isn't more serious, such as nerve damage or a fracture. Also see a doctor if stingers are a chronic problem for you, because this can signal the presence of other issues, such as spinal stenosis (narrowing of the spinal canal).

Sunburn

An interesting thought struck me as I was speaking to a group of triathletes recently. They were fit, intense, and motivated. But, man, the ones who had been doing it for a while looked a bit weather-beaten. Bottom line: No matter what your sport, if you spend a lot of time in the sun, you must take care of your skin.

Dermatologists I've spoken with tell me that the number of people coming into their offices with sundamaged skin and sun-related cancers has grown tremendously in the past 10 years. Genetics play a part, of course, since your skin pigmentation and where your family originally hails from are factors. People with fair complexions, blue or green eyes, freckles, and light-colored hair get sunburned the fastest. But even more significant in skin cancer risk is having a history of deep sunburn. Repeated, deep, painful sun damage has been strongly linked to precancerous skin lesions.

If you train outdoors, you must slather on a waterproof sunblock with no less than SPF 30 and reapply it regularly, especially if you're sweating a lot. Athletes overlook this crucial detail all the time, especially if they get deep into a workout or match and

stop thinking about the sun.

And if you have a new or funny-looking mole or patch on your skin? Speak to your doctor or see a dermatologist. All forms of skin cancer are easier to treat when they're caught early.

All that said, sunburns still happen to the best of us, even if we're smart enough to know better: Forty-two percent of people polled recently admitted to getting at least one sunburn per year, according to the Skin Cancer Foundation. Here's how to manage a bad burn.

APPLY COLD COMPRESSES. Following a burn, the skin is inflamed. Cool it down by applying ice-water soaks, which can be soothing and help the burn heal faster. Soak some washcloths in a bucket of ice water, wring one out, and lay it over the burned skin. You'll feel the washcloth get warm after several minutes. Replace it with another cold cloth. Do this for 15 minutes several times a day.

SOOTHE THE RED WITH WHITE. If your sunburn is mild (meaning that you have no blisters), apply distilled white vinegar to the burn. The acetic acid in the vinegar acts as a topical antiinflammatory. For extra cooling power, chill it before application.

SEEK HYDROCORTISONE RELIEF. Try a topical lotion, spray, or ointment containing 1 percent hydrocortisone, such as Cortaid or

Cortizone-10. Hydrocortisone is an antiinflammatory.

SAY GOOD-BYE WITH ALOE. Apply refrigerated pure aloe vera gel (available in pump bottles at most pharmacies) to the burn. Aloe can speed wound healing and is also a terrific moisturizer.

TRY SOME TEA. If your eyelids are burned, apply tea bags soaked in cold water to decrease swelling and relieve pain. Tea has tannic acid, which can ease sunburn pain.

Swimmer's ear

All it takes to come down with a stubborn bout of swimmer's ear is an ear and lots of moisture. Swimmer's ear begins as an itchy ear. Left untreated, it can turn into a full-blown infection, which is excruciating. Try these strategies to stop it before it starts.

GO OVER-THE-COUNTER. Most drugstores carry eardrops that help dry up swimmer's ear. If ear itchiness is your only symptom, this might be enough to ward off an infection. Use drops each time your ear gets wet.

LEAVE YOUR EARWAX ALONE. Earwax serves several purposes, including harboring friendly bacteria. Cooperate with your body's natural defenses by not swabbing the wax out. Wax coats the ear canal and protects it from moisture. Rubbing a cotton swab in your ear is a surefire recipe for swimmer's ear.

TRY DROPS. Several fluids are good for killing germs and drying your ears, especially if you spend a lot of time in the water. Tilt your head to the side, pull your ear up and back to open up the canal, and use an eyedropper to apply drops of one of the following: rubbing alcohol; a solution of equal parts rubbing alcohol and white vinegar; or, for preventive protection before swimming, mineral oil, baby oil, or lanolin. Once you put the drops in, turn your head to the other side and let them drain out naturally.

PLUG 'EM UP. Wax or silicone earplugs found at any drugstore can keep the water out whenever you swim or shower.

Yeast infection
[WOMEN]

As many as three out of four women will have at least one diagnosis of vaginal yeast infection during their lifetimes. Yeast infections are one of the most common causes of vaginitis, which is inflammation of the vagina. Athletic women in particular are prone to yeast infections because of all that time they spend raising their body temperatures; sweating; and wearing shorts, bathing suits, and other clothing that can trap moisture. Under normal circumstances, the vagina is a self-cleaning organ. The vulva and vagina produce an average of 1 to 2 grams (about ¼ to ½ teaspoon) of vaginal discharge every 8 hours, and its consistency varies. This is normal and healthy. However, if the discharge smells bad or is accompanied by burning, itching, or other discomfort, see your doctor. There are several ways to prevent a yeast infection.

MIND YOUR PH. Wash with water and a perfume-free, pH-balanced soap like Dove.

ALLOW SOME AIRFLOW DOWN THERE. You want the moisture to evaporate. Always wear cotton underwear during the day and go pantyless at night.

EAT YOGURT DAILY. Inside your vagina, the bacterium *Lactobacillus* helps keep nastier bacteria in check. It also crowds out yeast spores, another normal inhabitant of the vagina, which can otherwise grow into an itchy infection. A daily cup of yogurt that contains *Lactobacillus acidophilus* can help keep its vaginal population high.

AVOID TAKING ANTIBIOTICS UNNECESSARILY. They kill off the good bacteria along with the bad.

PART THREE

HOW TO WIN

AT EVERYTHING

Sport-specific secrets for staying injury free and on top of all the games you play

All athletes have a bit of mad scientist inside them. Whether you love one sport or play multiple sports with equal zeal, you're always tinkering, experimenting, searching for the little things that can give you an edge. Maybe it's about conditioning, or performance, or avoiding injury, but I'll bet you're on the lookout for cool, proven ideas you can take to your next training session or game. Well, I aim to please.

I want to see you both excel and remain healthy, so here's an entire chapter devoted to just those kinds of ideas. I start you off with a section of general, non-sport-specific tips that apply to all athletes, then I move into the sport-specific info. Give 'em a try, play mad scientist, and enjoy the ride.

Smart Ideas for Every Athlete

LEARN TO JUGGLE.

Sound goofy? Think about it. Juggling is all about hand-eye coordination. And better hand-eye coordination means faster, smoother reactions and fewer rushed, jerky, wrenching motions that can cause both errors and injuries. Put simply, juggling can help make you a better all-around athlete.

BUY SOME DENTAL INSURANCE.

Athletes who wear custom-fitted mouth guards reduce their risk of dental injuries by 82 percent, according to a study from the University of North Carolina at Chapel Hill. "What does this have to do with improving my performance?" you may ask. A well-protected athlete concentrates on the game, not on what might happen if he or she takes a bone-rattling hit or an elbow to the jaw. Lay out the money for a custom-fitted guard and it'll last for years. So will your smile.

RESPECT THE HEAT.

Humid environments—i.e., anywhere south of Maine and east of Colorado—take their toll on training performance and can make conditions like asthma even worse. If you train outdoors, train early. The temperature will be lower, and so will the humidity and ozone levels that can mess with your lungs. And while we're on the subject...

CHECK THE OZONE LEVEL.

When you hear the words *ozone alert day*, move your workout indoors. A study in the the *Lancet* medical journal found that those who exercise in high-ozone conditions are three times more likely to develop asthma than those who skip overheated workouts on those days.

CHECK YOUR WATER LOSS.

A simple loss of body water can decrease your performance, though you may not feel it. Weigh yourself before and after a long workout in hot weather. If you've lost more than 2 percent of your body weight by the time you're finished, you're dehydrated and could be at risk for heatstroke (you'll find more detailed hydration info in the nutrition section). Endurance athletes, invest in a water pack so you can easily sip throughout your workout. And water's not enough for exercise lasting more than an hour—your body also loses salt in sweat, so you need a sports drink containing carbohydrates and electrolytes.

LOWER YOUR CORE TEMPERATURE.

If you play any sport in hot weather, staying cool is crucial. Here are two tricks.

• **Drown your hands.** During a break from the action, submerge both hands in a bucket of ice water for as long as you can stand it. There are a lot of blood vessels in your hands and fingers, so you're cooling a lot of blood via that surface area. The blood circulates throughout your body, helping to bring your internal temperature down.

• **Make some Florida water.** An old-school heat remedy from the Deep South, Florida water is used in youth and adult sports from football to baseball to tennis. You mix a small amount of spirits of ammonia (not, I repeat, not regular household ammonia) with a few gallons of ice water and soak some small towels in the solution. The spirits of ammonia, which you can find at your pharmacy, opens your pores and cools you faster than regular ice water can.

Try this recipe: Fill a bucket or small cooler halfway with ice, then fill it the rest of the way with water and 1 ½ ounces of spirits of ammonia for every gallon of water. Soak small towels or washcloths in the mixture. During game breaks, wring out a washcloth and wipe yourself down. Do not drink Florida water or stick the washcloth in your mouth. Nasty.

CRUSH PRE-PERFORMANCE ANXIETY.

Back in 2005, I raced in the Ironman World Championship triathlon in Hawaii for the first time. I felt prepared, but as the race approached, I felt increasingly excited, nervous,

PLAY THROUGH THE PAIN? OR BAIL ON A COMPETITION?

So there I sat, a week out from an Ironman race in Lake Placid. I had to decide: Do I go forward with the race? Or do I bail and trash months of training and preparation? The joy of race day is offset by a lot of sacrifice to get there. My brothers were competing in this race as well (and I hate losing to them!) and our parents were coming in.

Herein lies the rub: My stupid left foot, specifically the ridiculous plantar fascia, was telling me not to run. Living through this debilitating heel pain was enough to elicit a string of words unsuitable for a family publication. Of course, I tried all the treatments and even had some ideas for race day. But here and now, a week before, I didn't think I could run.

So ask yourself: When do you pull the plug on a big sporting event? Is it worth starting and perhaps hurting yourself even more? The questions are simple. The answers are more complicated.

Having dealt with these issues with my patients for some time, here's the algorithm that seems to make the most sense. First of all, is there a risk for a more serious or severe injury? If so, the answer is immediate: Don't do it.

If there is little risk of further injury, what will the experience be like? Agonizing? Fun? A mix? Will the pain be so great that you can't perform the way you normally would? My general rule here is that if pain limits an athlete's ability to perform normally, it's best to stop. Why? Because injuries from improper form can take months to heal and create even worse problems than the one you're dealing with now.

Another good strategy: Consult with your doctor, not your coach. Your coach wants you in the game, but your doctor will be straight with you about your risks. Consider all of these factors when deciding whether to "play with the pain."

Me? I agonized over my decision for the next week. And then I finished that Ironman in just under 12 hours.

and agitated. Questions raced in my brain: Will I bonk? Will I stumble across the finish line? Will a shark see me as a tasty treat? Will the famed winds of Kona knock me off my bike?

Anxiety is an irrational fear that delivers a physical reaction: rapid breathing, increased heart rate, and sweating. The anxiety you feel before a big game or race is anticipatory anxiety. If all your energy is spent worrying, anticipating, and getting nervous, the body doesn't work very well. Bloodflow is diverted, sleep quality declines, and helpful energy is wasted in the days and hours leading up to the event. A little bit of anxiety is good—it keeps the mind sharp and the muscles ready. But too much for too long is a big negative.

I've spoken with sports psychologists about this, and in the days leading up to a big race—like that big triathlon I mentioned—I use positive visualization and get good results. I visualize everything going right, breaking down each step in my mind, rehearsing how it will work. This boosts my confidence and alleviates self-doubt. Before a triathlon, I envision a smooth swim with tropical fish. I see myself cruising along on the bike with the wind at my back. I see myself running with a strong stride, pain free and smiling.

Are these images true? No way! However, they do allow me to focus and quell my anticipatory anxiety. Running the event in your head allows for a positive mind-set, but it also allows you to focus on the task in a detailed way before you do it. You no longer have time to think about the things that make you nervous.

PRACTICE HARDER AND SMARTER.

It's simple: If you do everything you need to do to prepare for an event, you'll perform better because you'll be more relaxed and confident in your skills and conditioning. Science backs this up: Performance anxiety can narrow your peripheral vision by as much as 3 degrees and slow your reaction time by 119 milliseconds, according to the *Journal of Sports Sciences*. Any athlete knows what a difference those tiny numbers can make.

DROP THE TOBACCO.

A study of army recruits found that smokers were nearly 50 percent more likely than clean-lunged privates to suffer fractures, sprains, and other injuries. Smoking may interfere with wound healing and muscle repair. And it's counterproductive to conditioning.

UNWIND THE ANKLE TAPE.

It loosens after 10 minutes of play, according to the *American Journal of Sports Medicine*. Researchers found that those who wore ankle braces after an injury returned to full participation 2 days sooner than those who were taped. But wearing an ankle brace doesn't give you a free pass on being smart about your injury. Keep it braced for at least 6 months, advises the National

Center for Injury Prevention and Control. Most foot and ankle injuries are caused by incomplete healing of prior injuries.

GIVE UNSEXY MUSCLES THEIR DUE.

Men work their chest and biceps, women want a great butt and legs. These are the vanity muscles, and we forget that the shoulder, for example, is a balanced joint that needs strong muscles on the front and back. Strong quads give you great-looking legs, but if your hamstrings are neglected, you're headed for an injury. Whatever exercise you do, be sure to perform an equal number of reps for the opposing movement. For example, for every set of chest presses you do, perform a set of seated rows as well.

STRAP IN YOUR BOYS. [MEN]

A recent study in the *Clinical Journal of Sport Medicine* found that 47 percent of male high-school and college athletes involved in contact sports do not wear any kind of genital protection. The good news? These Darwin Award winners will be less likely to breed.

BUY THE RIGHT SPORTS BRA. [WOMEN]

A well-fitted sports bra can make the difference between a pleasant training session and discomfort, chafing, and an all-around miserable experience. Here are some tips for finding the right fit.

• Look for sports bras that encapsulate each breast in a separate chamber; they reduce bounce and support better than simple shelf bras.

• Try to find sports bras that come in cup and band sizes rather than just small, medium, and large; they usually fit more precisely.

• Look for strategically placed seams and stitching, which help cushion the breast. Or go seamless. Companies like Isis, Asics, and Champion make seamless sports bras.

• Pick high-performance fabrics (like CoolMax and Double Dry) that wick away sweat to minimize chafing.

• Own a variety of sports bras, and when in doubt, choose a higher-impact bra for a lower-impact sport—never the other way around.

• Get fitted by an expert. You can find bra fitters at most department stores and lingerie shops.

• Before buying, jump, swing your arms, and move around. If a bra pokes, rubs, slips, doesn't support you, constricts your breathing, or bulges, put it back. Also, it should fit on the first hook; as it loses elasticity over time, you'll need room to tighten it.

• Rotate your bras and wash them regularly so you can get at least a year's use out of each one.

CROSS-TRAIN WITH A BRAIN.

If you want to last longer at your chosen sport, cross-training can help keep you from overtraining or overusing the same muscles.

But cross-train with your brain and try out different sports that complement the muscles and movements you already do. Natural pairings: skiing and soccer, swimming and martial arts, running and cycling, tennis and hoops.

TRAIN YOUR BRAIN TO HEAL YOUR ANKLE.

Training sensory receptors in your ankles can help prevent recurrent injury, according to research from the Netherlands. Try a wobble board to get better at something known as proprioception: the subconscious bond between your nerves and the muscles that do your brain's bidding. Try standing on a wobble board for 5 minutes a day—say, while you're watching *SportsCenter*. When that becomes easy, balance with your eyes closed (and listen to sports on Sirius).

KEEP A COOL HEAD FOR A SOUND BODY.

You've seen them before, the hot-tempered, ultracompetitive players who bring a good dose of rage to the game. Hey, maybe that's you. Nothing wrong with wanting to win. But when you bring all your anger and stress to the field, you not only take away others' enjoyment, you jack up your own injury risk. Researchers found that athletes with high levels of stress off the field are five times more likely to experience injuries than even-keeled people. Think about it: Mixing anger and a need to win could make you do some-

ON LONG RUNS AND BIKE RIDES, BEWARE "MAN'S BEST FRIEND"

If you train for long periods, especially on rural roads or in farming regions, either on a bike or on foot, chances are you'll encounter a surly dog at some point. Even a nip can break the skin or rip your shorts, so it's best not to let Fido get that close to you. Some solutions:

If you're on a bike, squirt him with your water bottle. In the face. Never let him get in front of you. Running him over could cause a crash that hurts you worse than him. (And then he has a roadside meal!)

If you meet the dog on a regular route, start carrying biscuits. You might make a friend.

If he's behind you and closing in, turn around and jog backward. It's never a good idea to turn your back on a barking dog—he'll think your derriere is fair game. If you face him, however, or take a step toward him, a lot of "all bark" dogs will back off.

If a dog flat-out attacks you, use whatever you've got to fight with and scream to wake the dead. The situation is no joke, and you need help from whoever's in earshot. Like the dog's owner, for example, who now has just as serious a problem with you as you do with his or her dog.

thing stupid that could hurt yourself or another athlete.

PROTECT YOUR KNEES.

No one really likes kneepads, but boy, do they make a difference. In a recent University of Iowa study, researchers examined young amateur athletes involved in contact sports—basketball, volleyball, and wrestling—and found that wearing kneepads reduced the rate of lower-extremity injuries by 67 percent. That's big. It's the same principle I mentioned about mouth guards—a protected athlete isn't just a healthy athlete, but also a confident athlete.

IF YOU CAN'T RUN WITH THE BIG DOGS, DON'T.

This is a major issue. Sometimes people want to prove how good they are and get into situations they shouldn't. So be smart: Choose a league or race appropriate to your skill level. Injuries tend to happen when things get out of control, but even if you don't get hurt, you'll definitely frustrate yourself and/or your teammates with your inability to compete at the same level.

Now, that said, here's an idea. Compete at the lower level, but practice and train with the more-advanced players. That will reduce your injury risk and frustration level, but your skill level will jump. And maybe you'll eventually dominate the lower level enough that you'll be ready for that next level naturally.

Smart ideas for every
Runner

BUY RUNNING SHOES AFTER WORK.

Shop at night, when your feet are swollen after a day of pounding. That approximates how big your feet will be after the first 3 miles of your run. Also, try to find a running shoe store that offers video analysis of your stride, which can help you find the right shoe.

EXERCISE OFF-ROAD.

Unstable surfaces train stable ankles.

DON'T RUN IN WET SHOES.

Soggy midsoles have 40 to 50 percent less shock-absorbing capability than dry sneaks. But don't toss your shoes in the dryer; heat can degrade cushioning and support components.

TO STRENGTHEN MUSCLE, LENGTHEN IT.

Muscles that are strengthened as they lengthen can absorb more force, and this means less potential for tendon trouble. Try some eccentric training, meaning you go slower on the lowering part of a lift. Here's a good move for runners: In a calf raise, lift for 2 seconds, then spend 10 seconds lowering the weight. The tissue is lengthening as it's contracting, and that trains it for force absorption and greater strength.

HOW TO MANAGE YOUR, AHEM, MORE EMBARRASSING BODILY FUNCTIONS DURING A RACE.

I'll never forget this quote. I was standing in line with 300 of my closest friends in 2008 at the EagleMan triathlon. It was 6 in the morning and pre-race jitters were rampant. And I heard this from a fellow racer a few places back: "Dear Lord, please let everything work for me in the porto-potty."

Any endurance athlete knows exactly what he was talking about. The truth is that bad bathroom prep can ruin a race. Racers have succumbed to any number of gastrointestinal emergencies—none of them pretty.

Good bathroom prep depends on a phenomenon called gastrointestinal transit time. Some foods, such as fiber-heavy and carb-heavy foods, move quickly through the GI tract, often completing the trip in 12 hours or less. And some, fat-laden foods in particular, can take up to 36 hours to pass.

In planning your pre-race bathroom strategy, make sure that on the day before, and particularly in the last meal before the race, your diet is heavy in foods that won't cause problems the next morning. That means that pre-race meals should be consumed about 10 to 12 hours before the start time. And avoid fatty foods.

And beware caffeine. It jacks up the muscular contraction in the intestines, moving things along faster. If you want caffeine, have it 2 hours before the race, never right before the gun.

Naturally, even the best-laid plans fail. For that reason, many racers carry toilet paper during a race. It's also a good idea during your training weeks, especially on long runs. If there are such things as better and worse reasons for a bad race, poor bathroom prep has to be among the very worst. Good luck out there.

EVEN OUT UNEVEN SURFACES.

Road running is necessary for a lot of runners, and you might have noticed that most roads are designed with a crown, meaning the center of the road is higher than the sides. This allows rain to run off to the roadside. But running on a crowned surface means that one foot will always be striking at a higher level than the other. This uneven surface could cause a muscle imbalance if you don't compensate for the other leg. And that's easy: If you run one way on a road like that, run back in the opposite direction for the same distance, staying on the same side so your other leg gets equal time.

Smart ideas for every Cycler

TRY PRE-RACE CAFFEINE.

In a University of Georgia study, cyclists who downed caffeine before a 30-minute ride had significantly less thigh pain than those who took a placebo. For longer rides, however, avoid caffeine in large amounts (5 to 7 cups of coffee a day), which can dehydrate you. Caffeine can also stimulate your digestive system. You know what that means.

"PULL" ON THE PEDALS.

When pedaling, don't press down with the balls of your feet, because that's tough on your knees. Rather, press with your heel, then pull back and up with your calves in a circular motion. This generates power and speed.

RAMP UP CYCLING FITNESS.

Here are three ways to change up your rides.

1. Once a week, go for distance. Work up to 2 hours or more, depending on the length of the race you're training for.

2. Every other week, do 20 to 30 minutes of "tempo riding" at an increased pace. Begin and end these sessions with at least 10 minutes of easy riding.

3. Every other week, or even every 3rd week, do some speed. After 15 minutes of easy cycling, push hard for a minute, then go easy for a minute. Repeat 10 to 20 times, finishing with 15 minutes of easy riding.

Smart ideas for every Swimmer

HIT THE POOL EARLY.

Inhaling organic material, such as particles of hair, skin, or urine (even on a microscopic level), can cause breathing problems. Schedule your lap sessions early: Fewer people in the pool means less splashing and less of their debris left behind in the water.

DRILL FOR BETTER FORM.

In each of these four drills, swim short repeats (25 meters or so) slowly and easily, and try to feel what's described in each drill. Between repeats, take three to five deep, slow breaths until you feel ready to swim again without fatigue.

DRILL 1: Hide your head

Why: Good head-spine alignment is essential to smooth swimming.
How: Lead with the top of your head, not your forehead. Feel water flowing over the back of your head. Look at the pool bottom directly under you, not in front of you.

DRILL 2: Swim downhill

Why: Balance—feeling completely supported by the water—is the essential skill for efficient swimming.
How: "Lean" on your chest until your hips and legs feel light. Your hips and legs should actually be slightly higher in the water than your head and torso.

DRILL 3: Lengthen your body

Why: A longer body line reduces drag, making swimming easier.
How: Extend a "weightless" arm slowly. Slip your arm into the water as if you're sliding it into a jacket sleeve. Keep extending it until you feel your shoulder touch your jaw.

DRILL 4: Flow like water

Why: Making waves and creating turbulence takes energy, all of it supplied by you.
How: Pierce the water; slip through the smallest possible hole. Swim as quietly as possible. Try not to make waves or disturb the water.

Smart ideas for every
Triathlete

KEEP IT SIMPLE.

To keep your training schedule as simple as possible, plan to do two runs, two swims, and two bike sessions each week, with 1 day of rest. This is how your week might look.
• Monday: Swim
• Tuesday: Cycle
• Wednesday: Run
• Thursday: Off
• Friday: Swim
• Saturday: Cycle
• Sunday: Run

FOR THE SWIMMING STAGE…
Don't go too slow. Triathlon coaches warn against simply logging laps at a slow pace. The problem with it is that before long your form deteriorates and you adopt poor habits. Go with interval training instead, such as 5 bursts of 25 meters each with rests between repeats.
Increase overall strength. With swimming, you increase muscle mass in your upper body while giving your legs a break. This is crucial because it actually helps your running improve.
Improve fitness without the injury risk. You should never run hard 2 days in a row, but you can swim hard the day after a hard run, because you're working completely

different muscles. Therefore, you'll be boosting fitness capacity without increasing your injury risk.

FOR THE CYCLING STAGE...

Remember that cycling is not running. In terms of training effect, running 1 mile equals cycling about 3 miles, but cycling can take considerably more time. For example, a 5-mile run may take you 45 minutes. An equivalent bike ride of 15 miles could take you at least an hour, depending on terrain and other conditions. Plan your schedule accordingly.

Push smarter, not harder. A common cycling mistake that novice triathletes make is mashing big gears—that is, using higher gears in the hope that it will get them in cycling shape faster. But this can lead to knee injuries and stalled progress. Instead, do what cyclists call "spinning": Stay in the lower gears at a cadence of at least 90 revolutions per minute.

FOR THE RUNNING STAGE...

To maintain your running speed and endurance, concentrate on these three running workouts.

• Every Sunday, do a long run at an easy training pace. If you're training for an Ironman, work up to 20 miles for your long run.

• Every other Wednesday, do a 15- to 20-minute tempo run slightly slower than 10-K-race pace.

• On the Wednesdays you're not doing tempo, do 800- to 1,600-meter repeats at about 5-K-race pace, with plenty of rest between the repeats.

FIND A TRIATHLON.

If you're new to triathloning, you should probably look for short-distance "sprint" triathlons, especially those with pool swims as opposed to open-water swims. Sprint triathlons usually include a ¼-mile swim, a 15-mile bike ride, and a 5-K run. For a large listing of triathlons, go to usatriathlon.org, or check *Triathlete* magazine's Web site at triathletemag.com. Both sites have national race calendars.

Smart ideas for every
Baseball & Softball Player

STOP AND START TO FIGHT MUSCLE STRAINS.

Sprint-based sports like baseball and softball churn out a lot of lower-body muscle strains (especially in "beer leagues" where training may not be the biggest priority). The fix: stop-and-start drills.

Run 40 yards at about 70 percent of your maximum effort, slow to a jog for 10 yards, then pick it up again for another 40 yards. Repeat 4 or 5 times. You'll be conditioned to sprint to first base, slow down, and charge for second.

LOOSEN YOUR SHOULDERS.

An injured rotator cuff can shut down a shoulder. Add external- and internal-rotation stretching to protect your rotator cuffs.

External. Stand with your right arm straight out to the side and parallel to the floor. Bend your elbow so your arm forms a right angle and your forearm points straight up, palm facing forward. Keeping your elbow in place, move your hand back until you feel slight tension in your shoulder. Hold for 30 seconds. Repeat on the left side.

Internal. Do as directed above, but point your forearm straight down toward the floor at the start, palm facing behind you. Hold for 30 seconds, then repeat on the other side.

AVOID THE GUY SLIDING INTO SECOND.

When you see a guy get flipped, it's usually because he went outside the bag to make the throw. If you can't jump and throw, use the bag to protect yourself by standing directly behind it. You may not be able to throw to turn a double play, but at least the runner won't get a piece of you.

SLIDE SAFELY INTO THIRD.

Aim up and over the side of the bag. Slide over it so your foot or hand does not catch on it. If your slide comes to a sudden stop, your joints take most of the impact.

Smart ideas for every
Soccer Player

AIM HIGH AND TIGHT.

In a recent study, Hong Kong researchers found that goalkeepers rarely stand in the center of the goal. They favor one side, hoping to bait the opposition into kicking toward the open side, which in turn enables them to anticipate the shot. Eliminate this advantage by aiming your shots at the corner above the goalkeeper's head. Top corner shots can't be stopped. A soccer ball's sweet spot: bottom right (if you're right-foot dominant). Strike it with the top of your big toe.

KEEP YOUR FEET MOVING.

Try this classic drill to blast your lungs and legs simultaneously. Place a soccer ball a foot in front of you. Jumping quickly, alternate touching your big toes on top of the ball without kicking it forward. Do this for 40 seconds, rest for 60 seconds, and repeat twice more. For an added challenge, circle the ball as you work.

KICK IT OLD-SCHOOL.

For a great conditioning and sports workout (that also helps your soccer game), trade a 30-minute jog for 10 minutes of intermittent sprints while dribbling a soccer ball from foot to foot. Simply sprint with the ball for 20 seconds, rest for 60 seconds, and repeat 7 times.

Smart ideas for every Basketball Player

BEWARE EYEBALL BUSTERS.

Interesting stat: Basketball is responsible for the most eye injuries, according to the University of Michigan Kellogg Eye Center. No, basketball goggles don't look all that flattering, but then neither do black eyes or bloody eyeballs.

WARM UP ALL OVER THE PLACE.

Think about the wild gyrations you perform during one turnover from offense to defense in basketball. If your groin, back, and leg muscles aren't ready, you'll pull up in pain. Before the game, run backward, forward, sideways, and in quick combos of all directions.

MASTER THE HIP CHECK.

To dominate on the glass, place your backside or elbow firmly against your opponent's hip as soon as the ball hits the rim. You'll be able to rebound and score easy put-back points. It's simple and fundamental, but effective.

STAY IN MOTION.

Break to the basket after every pass you throw. Don't get the ball? Immediately switch to an L cut. Here's how: Once you're under the goal, lock your defender behind you with a hip check (above). Then run to the free-throw line. As soon as your foot touches the line, break horizontally toward the closest wing, your body facing the ball. You'll be wide open to receive a pass. From there...

PRACTICE TO DECEIVE.

A good head fake is the most important but least used move in pickup basketball. Pump the ball as if you're about to shoot. Then, as you bring the ball back down, throw a strong head fake to the left, and drive right. The first move gets your defender in the air and the second gets him or her moving in the wrong direction, leaving you an open path to the hoop.

DON'T OVEREXTEND YOURSELF ON BLOCKS AND DUNKS.

Stiff arms are more easily injured. Keep a 15-degree bend in your elbow when going for a block or a dunk. Overextending your arm makes you prone to injury.

PROTECT YOUR FEET.

Add arch supports to your basketball shoes, even if you don't have flat feet. It'll cut down on pressure on the outer edge of your foot—a common site for stress fractures. Over-the-counter insoles in general work great, and they'll save you a hundred bucks over custom inserts.

Smart ideas for every

Jumping-Sport Athlete

CUSHION YOUR LANDING.

The huge majority of ACL injuries occur when players are pivoting or landing awkwardly after a jump. Hitting the ground with your knees bent instead of nearly straight greatly reduces the risk, according to a report published in the *Journal of the American Academy of Orthopaedic Surgeons*.

ELIMINATE THE HEEL-STRIKE.

When you land after a jump, make sure it's toes first, then heel. If you land either flat-footed or on your heels, you'll be putting a lot of stress on your Achilles tendons, which may cause your knees to hyperextend.

Smart ideas for every

Skier & Snowboarder

KNOW HOW TO FALL.

Learning to snowboard is a snap—for your wrists. When you fall, let your butt and back share the impact with your forearms. And wear wrist guards; they may not look sexy, but neither will a cast and sling.

TRAIN YOUR BRAIN TO STAY UPRIGHT.

Here's another good reason to invest in a wobble board: It helps you work on maintaining your sense of balance and keeping your center of gravity low for snowboarding, skateboarding, and surfing. It also requires you to move your ankles in a fashion that's similar to what you'll be doing during your ride.

REMEMBER COLD-WEATHER HYDRATION.

Skiing is just like running track. The difference: You're wearing a lot more clothes. Your body loses moisture during all activity, even in cold weather; if you can see your breath, you're venting moisture. Store a water bladder under your parka so it won't freeze.

MASTER THE SNOWBOARD ACCELERATOR.

Gravity's your gas on a snowboard, but there are right and wrong ways to accelerate off the line. Consider your front leg to be first gear, your back leg overdrive. As you start from a standstill, lean on the front leg to start moving (rock back and forth if you're rooted in place), then ease into a balanced position once you get going. Leaning on your back leg too much is like punching the gas in a funny car: Your front end will lift off the ground, and you'll lose control of where you're headed.

AND ITS BRAKES.

Slowing down without sitting down is one of the toughest skills to nail. Apply pressure to whatever edge of the board is uphill, dragging yourself against the slope like a knife shaving butter. Your knees should be slightly bent, with your body angled slightly uphill to maintain your center of gravity. The same technique will help you regulate speed between turns.

Smart ideas for every Golfer

SHOW UP EARLY.

Most amateurs show up late and rush to the first tee, take a practice swing, and play. How can you not hook it into the pro shop with that approach? Show up early enough to stretch and hit a bucket of balls. By gradually warming up for that first strike, you'll guard against incorrect body rotation on your takeaway—the primary cause of golf-related back injuries (and lost balls).

USE A LIGHT GRIP.

Most wrist and elbow injuries occur because people are not gripping the club lightly enough. Gripping a golf club should feel like holding a bird. To get the feel, swing two clubs at once—it can't be done with a tight grip.

IF YOU CAN, FORGET THE GOLF CART.

Walking the course will keep your back and hips loose between shots, helping to prevent muscle strains.

STRETCH YOUR SWING MUSCLES.

If you refuse to give up the golf cart (or the course requires it), use it as a stretching tool: Stand about a foot away from the cart and facing it. With your knees slightly bent, reach out and grab the handle on the side. Keeping your arms fully extended, sit back so your buttocks and hips extend away from the cart. You should feel a stretch in the lower part of your back. Hold for 10 seconds. Repeat 2 times at every hole.

LOOSEN UP BEFORE EACH SWING.

Try this before each golf shot: Grasp a club in both hands like a handlebar, hold it parallel to the ground, and lift it overhead. Bend forward at the waist to make your shoulders as parallel to the ground as possible. With your arms extended, raise the club as far as you can overhead and behind you.

Smart ideas for every

Tennis & Racquetball Player

SWING WITH YOUR LEGS.

People forget to use their legs when they're hitting their serve or other strokes. For example, when you toss the ball up for a serve, you stress your lower back if you don't use your legs. Bend your knees and push up and through the serve with your legs. You'll gather power from the strongest part of your body.

PLAY ON CLAY OR GRASS.

Natural surfaces are naturally kinder to your body. Plus, soft surfaces absorb less heat, reducing heatstroke risk.

PLAY TENNIS IN TENNIS SHOES.

Sounds silly, but a lot of people play tennis in running shoes. Unlike running shoes, however, which have an angled bottom to promote linear movement, tennis-shoe soles are flat, for optimal side-to-side motion.

PART FOUR

IRON STRENGTH WORKOUTS

Build every muscle, achieve tip-top conditioning, and prevent injuries with these simple (but intense!) workouts

I treat patients for a living, but I also teach fitness classes on the weekends. It's some of the most fun I have because it hits the two areas that I'm concerned most about as a doctor and an athlete: injury prevention and better performance. I sure want the benefits as much as I want to give those benefits to the folks who train with me. What follows is a sampling of the kinds of workouts I lead—bootcamp-style using body weight or a light set of dumbbells.

I'll be honest: The workouts are brutal. When I run a class, we go for about an hour, and go hard. You'll adjust the length and intensity of your workouts based on your fitness level; you'll see how easy it is to adapt them to your specific needs in a moment. The exercises are designed to hit every muscle in your body, increase dynamic flexibility, boost explosive power, and allow you to go harder for longer in your chosen sport.

For the dumbbells, I recommend hexagonal style, as we use the dumbbells as a base for some of the exercises, and you don't want a dumbbell to roll out from under you. For women, 8 to 10 pounds is fine. For men, 12 to 15 pounds.

The best part about these workouts is you can do them just about anywhere. Outside in a park or your backyard, indoors at the gym or in your bedroom (one workout is specifically designed for outdoors). You have no excuses about location, equipment, or facilities here, my friends. So smile and let's have some fun ...

The Best Injury-Prevention Workout You're Not Doing
FOAM-ROLL EXERCISES

Foam rolling is in many ways like a deep massage—but you give it to yourself. By rolling the hard foam over your thighs, calves, and back, you'll loosen tough connective tissue (like the fascia, which stretches over many of your muscles and can tighten up) and decrease the stiffness of your muscles. The result? Better flexibility and mobility, and muscles that can function properly. I recommend foam rolling before any workout, but in reality, you can do it anytime. The easiest time is to pull out the foam roller while you're watching TV.

If you've never foam-rolled before, be prepared. It's uncomfortable and can even be painful when you start. Don't worry—the more painful it is, the more that muscle needs foam rolling. The good news is that the more you do it, the less discomfort you'll feel. For each muscle that you work, slowly move the roller back and forth over it for 30 seconds. If you hit a really tender spot, pause on it for 5 to 10 seconds.

Definitely focus on the muscles that need rolling the most. You'll know which ones they are just by trying it. You'll find 36-inch foam rollers at most sports or fitness shops, but in a pinch you can also use a basketball, tennis ball, or even a length of PVC pipe.

1 HAMSTRINGS ROLL

Place a foam roller under your right knee, with your leg straight. Cross your left leg over your right ankle. Put your hands flat on the floor for support. Keep your back naturally arched.

Roll your body forward until the roller reaches your glutes. Then roll back and forth. Repeat with the roller under your left knee.

NOTE: If rolling one leg is too difficult, perform the movement with both legs on the roller.

2 GLUTES ROLL

Sit on a foam roller with it positioned on the back of your right thigh, just below your glutes. Cross your right leg over the front of your left thigh. Put your hands flat on the floor for support.

Roll your body forward until the roller reaches your lower back. Then roll back and forth. Repeat with the roller under your left glute.

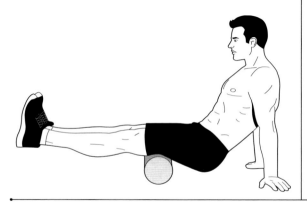

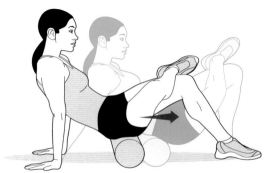

3 ILIOTIBIAL-BAND ROLL

Lie on your right side and place your right hip on a foam roller. Put your hands on the floor for support. Cross your left leg over your right and place your left foot flat on the floor.

Roll your body forward until the roller reaches your knee. Then roll back and forth. Lie on your left side and repeat with the roller under your left hip. If this becomes too easy over time, place your right leg on top of your left instead of bracing it on the floor).

IMPORTANT NOTE: Your iliotibial band—commonly called the IT band—is a tough strip of connective tissue that runs down the side of your thigh, starting on your hip bone and connecting just below your knee. When you start foam rolling, you'll probably find that this tissue is one of the most sensitive areas that you can roll over, perhaps due to the high tension of the band. Remember, pain means you need to roll it. Make this a priority, because over time, if your IT band is too tight, it could cause knee pain.

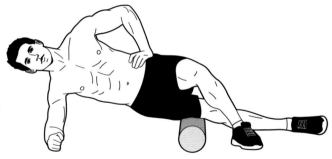

4 CALF ROLL

Place a foam roller under your right ankle, with your right leg straight. Cross your left leg over your right ankle. Put your hands flat on the floor for support and keep your back naturally arched.

Roll your body forward until the roller reaches the back of your right knee. Then roll back and forth. Repeat with the roller under your left calf. (If this is too hard, perform the movement with both legs on the roller.)

5 QUADRICEPS-AND-HIP-FLEXORS ROLL

Lie facedown on the floor with a foam roller positioned above your right knee. Cross your left leg over your right ankle and place your elbows on the floor for support.

Roll your body backward until the roller reaches the top of your right thigh. Then roll back and forth. Repeat with the roller under your left thigh. (If that's too hard, perform the movement with both thighs on the roller, as shown.)

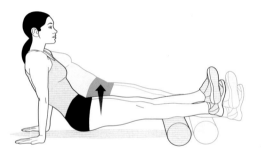

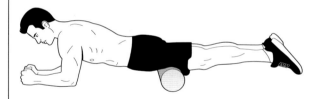

6 GROIN ROLL

Lie facedown on the floor. Place a foam roller parallel to your body. Put your elbows on the floor for support. Position your right thigh nearly perpendicular to your body, with the inner portion of your thigh, just above the level of your knee, resting on top of the roller.

Roll your body toward the right until the roller reaches your pelvis. Then roll back and forth. Repeat with the roller under your left thigh.

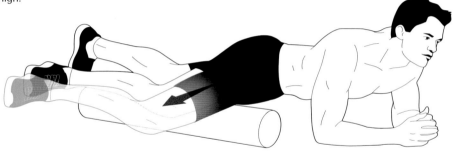

7 UPPER-BACK ROLL

Lie faceup with a foam roller under your mid-back, at the bottom of your shoulder blades. Clasp your hands behind your head and pull your elbows toward each other. Raise your hips off the floor slightly.

Slowly lower your back downward, so that your upper back bends over the foam roller. Raise back to the start and roll forward a couple of inches—so that the roller sits higher under your upper back—and repeat. Roll forward one more time and do it again. That's 1 rep.

8 LOWER-BACK ROLL

Lie faceup with a foam roller under your mid-back. Put your hands flat on the floor for support. Your knees should be bent, with your feet flat on the floor. Raise your hips off the floor slightly. Roll back and forth over your lower back.

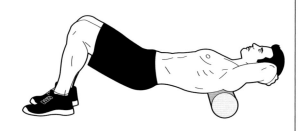

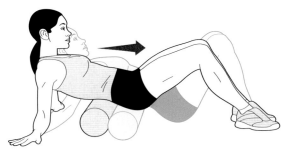

9 SHOULDER-BLADES ROLL

Lie faceup with a foam roller under your upper back, at the tops of your shoulder blades. Cross your arms over your chest. Your knees should be bent with your feet flat on the floor.

Raise your hips so they're slightly elevated off the floor. Roll back and forth over your shoulder blades and your mid- and upper back.

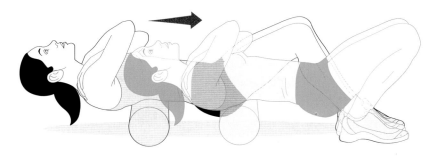

Stretching: The Truth

What do you consider a "warm-up" before a workout? Chances are, it's far less than you need. See, a lot of people short-change themselves on the warm-up. They'll do 5 minutes on a treadmill or do a set of bench presses with an empty barbell. Maybe they'll add in some perfunctory stretches.

That's not warming up. A proper warm-up leaves your body prepared for a hard workout, so if you do it right, you'll be sweating when you finish and your muscles will be ready for action. In a way, it's like throwing a power switch in your body. If you activate your muscles before a workout, they'll be more prepared for performance and less inclined to break down because of too much stress, too soon.

So what is a "proper" warm-up? First, let's talk about the most common activity done during a warm-up: stretching.

CAN STRETCHING PREVENT INJURY?

It depends on what kind of stretching you do. There are two major types of stretching: static and dynamic. You're probably more familiar with the former. A static stretch for your hamstrings is what you think it is—a movement in which you lean forward until you feel a slight discomfort in the target muscle, then stretch the muscle by holding that position for a few seconds.

Although it's often prescribed as an injury-prevention measure, static stretching before a workout might be the worst of all strategies. It forces the target muscle to relax, which temporarily makes it weaker. As a result, a strength imbalance can occur between opposing muscle groups. For example, stretching your hamstrings causes them to become significantly weaker than your quadriceps. And that may make you more susceptible to muscle strains in the short term.

Static stretching also reduces bloodflow to your muscles and decreases the activity of your central nervous system—meaning it inhibits your brain's ability to communicate with your muscles, which limits your capacity to generate force. The bottom line: Never perform static stretching before you work out or play sports.

Now, before you abandon static stretching for good, realize that it does have value. Improving your "passive" flexibility through static stretches is beneficial for all the movement you have to do during your day-to-day life—bending, kneeling, squatting, etc. All you have to know is the right stretch for the right time.

YOUR GUIDE FOR EFFECTIVE STATIC STRETCHING

Stretch twice a day, every day. Do it any less frequently and you won't maintain your gains in flexibility—which is why most flexibility plans don't work. Twice a day may seem like a lot, but each "session" will require as little as 4 minutes of your time. Also, there's no need to "warm" your muscles before stretching; that's a myth. So you can stretch at work, while you're watching TV, or while you're grilling burgers.

Keep in mind that duration matters. You can increase passive flexibility with a static stretch that's held for as little as 5 seconds, but you get optimal gains by holding it between 15 and 30 seconds, the point of diminishing returns.

Finally, do just one stretch for each tight muscle (hamstring, calf, quad, etc). Most of the improvements in flexibility are made on the first stretch, so repeating the same movement provides little benefit.

DYNAMIC STRETCHING

A dynamic stretch is the opposite of a static stretch. In this version, you quickly move a muscle in and out of a stretched position. Example: A body-weight lunge is a dynamic stretch for your quadriceps and hips.

Here's why the difference matters: Improvements in flexibility are specific to your body position and speed of movement. So if you do only static stretching—as most guys are advised—you'll primarily boost your flexibility in that exact posture while moving at a slow speed. That's great if you're a contortionist, but it has limited carryover to the flexibility you need in sports and weight training, which require your muscles to stretch at fast speeds in various body positions. That's why dynamic stretching is a necessary component of any program: It improves your "active" flexibility, the kind you need in every sport.

Dynamic stretching also stimulates your central nervous system, and increases bloodflow, as well as strength and power production. So it's the ideal warm-up for any activity. And when you regularly perform both dynamic and static stretches, some of the flexibility improvements from one will transfer to the other.

A Proper Warmup

This warmup is simple.
Do 10 reps of each of these exercises
with no rest between sets.

1 JUMPING JACKS

Stand with your feet together and your hands at your sides. Simultaneously raise your arms above your head and jump up just enough to spread your feet out wide. Without pause, quickly reverse the movement and repeat.

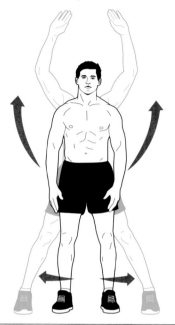

2 WALKING HIGH KNEES

Stand tall with your feet shoulder-width apart. Without changing your posture, raise your right knee as high as you can and step forward. Repeat with your left leg. Continue to alternate back and forth.

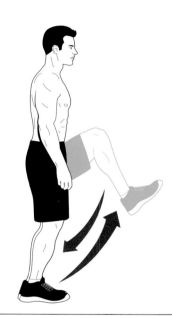

3 WALKING HIGH KICKS

Stand tall with your arms hanging at your sides. Keeping your knee straight, kick your left leg up—reaching with your right arm out to meet it—as you simultaneously take a step forward (just imagine that you're a Russian soldier).

As soon as your left foot touches the floor, repeat the movement with your right leg and left arm. Alternate back and forth.

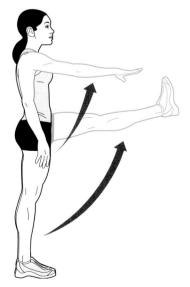

4 SQUAT THRUSTS (DUMBBELLS OPTIONAL)

Stand with your feet shoulder-width apart and your arms at your sides. Push your hips back, bend your knees, and lower your body as deep as you can into a squat.

As you squat down, place your hands on the floor in front of you, shifting your weight onto them. Kick your legs backward, so that you're now in a pushup position.

Quickly bring your legs back to the squat position. Stand up quickly and repeat the movement.

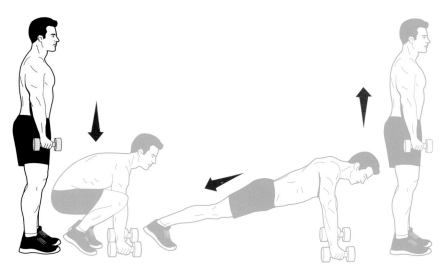

5 LUNGE WITH SIDE BEND

Stand tall with your arms hanging at your sides. Step forward with your right leg and lower your body until your right knee is bent at least 90 degrees.

As you lunge, reach over your head with your left arm as you bend your torso to your right. Reach for the floor with your right hand. Return to the starting position.

Complete the prescribed number of reps, then lunge with your left leg and bend to your left for the same number of reps.

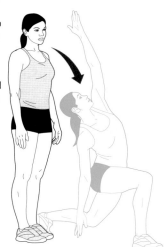

6 REVERSE LUNGE WITH REACH BACK

Stand tall with your arms hanging at your side. Brace your core and hold it that way. Lunge back with your right leg, lowering your body until your left knee is bent at least 90 degrees.

As you lunge, reach back over your shoulders and to the left. Reverse the movement back to the starting position.

Complete the prescribed number of reps with your left leg, then step back with your left leg and reach over your right shoulder for the same number of reps. Keep your torso upright for the entire movement.

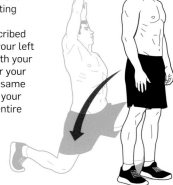

7 LOW SIDE-TO-SIDE LUNGE (DUMBBELLS OPTIONAL)

Stand with your feet set about twice shoulder-length apart, your feet facing straight ahead. Clasp your hands in front of your chest.

Shift your weight over to your right leg as you push your hips backward and lower your body by dropping your hips and bending your knees. Your lower right leg should remain nearly perpendicular to the floor. Your left foot should remain flat on the floor.

Without raising yourself back up to a standing position, reverse the movement to the left. Alternate back and forth.

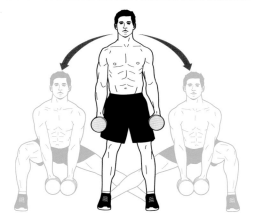

8 INVERTED HAMSTRING

Stand on your left leg, your knee bent slightly. Raise your right foot slightly off the floor. Without changing the bend in your left knee, bend at your hips and lower your torso until it's parallel to the floor.

As you bend over, raise your arms straight out from your sides until they're in line with your torso, your palms facing down. Your right leg should stay in line with your body as you lower your torso.

Return to the start. Complete the prescribed number of repetitions on your left leg, then do the same number on your right.

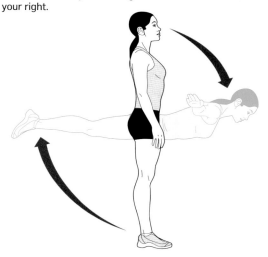

9 INCHWORM

Stand tall with your legs straight and bend over and touch the floor. Keeping your legs straight, walk your hands forward (if you can't reach the floor with your legs straight, bend your knees just enough so you can; as your flexibility improves, try to straighten them a little more). Keeping your core braced, walk your hands out as far as you can without allowing your hips to sag.

Then take tiny steps to walk your feet back to your hands. That's 1 repetition. Do 5 forward, and then 5 more in reverse.

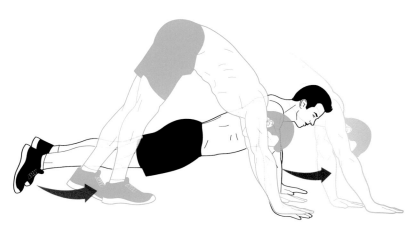

The Iron Strength Workout

This is a high-volume, high-intensity workout. You can tweak the timing and reps to your level of fitness, as well as add in rest. Listen to your body and don't hurt yourself. You can also make the workout more challenging by shortening the rest and/or doing more than one circuit of all the exercises. Again, let your fitness level be your guide here.

For the standard workout, do each exercise for 40 seconds, then rest for 20 seconds. Move on to the next exercise. Once through the entire circuit, rest for 2 minutes and repeat. And again, adjust the timing and intensity as you need to.

FIRST: A PROPER WARM-UP (SEE PAGE 264)

1 BODYWEIGHT JUMP SQUATS

Place your fingers on the back of your head and pull your elbows back so that they're in line with your body. Perform a bodyweight squat until your thighs are parallel to the floor, then explosively jump as high as you can (imagine you're pushing the floor away from you as you leap). When you land, immediately squat and jump again. Hold dumbbells at your side to make it more challenging.

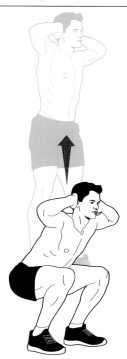

2 SPLIT JUMP (WITH OR WITHOUT DUMBBELLS)

Stand in a staggered stance, your right foot in front of your left. Lower your body as far as you can. Quickly switch directions and jump with enough force to propel both feet off the floor. While in the air, scissor-kick your legs so you land with the opposite leg forward. Repeat, alternating back and forth with each repetition.

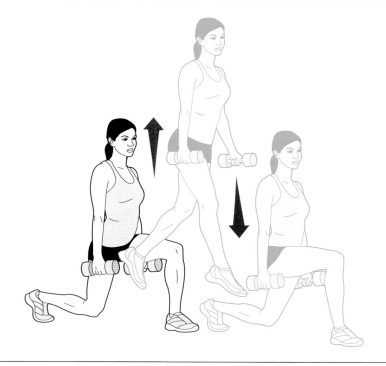

3 SINGLE-ARM DUMBBELL SWING

Hold a dumbbell at arm's length in front of your waist. Without rounding your lower back, bend at your hips and knees and swing the dumbbell between your legs. Keeping your arm straight, thrust your hips forward and swing the dumbbell to shoulder level as you rise to a standing position. Swing the weight back and forth. Halfway through your time, switch arms.

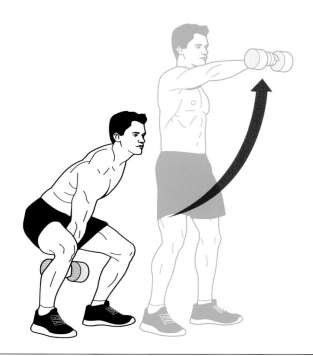

4 PISTOL SQUAT (WITH OPTIONAL PLYO)

Stand holding your arms straight out in front of your body at shoulder level, parallel to the floor. Raise your right leg off the floor and hold it there. Keeping your right leg straight, push your hips back and lower your body as far as you can without breaking form. As you do this, raise your right leg so that it doesn't touch the floor, and keep your torso as upright as possible. Pause, then push your body back to the starting position. Halfway through the prescribed time, switch legs.

For a bigger challenge, as you rise out of the squat, add in a jump off your plant leg.

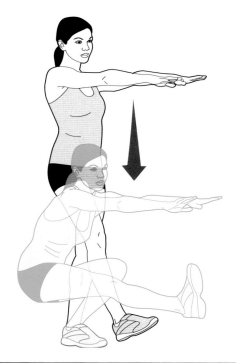

5 DUMBBELL ROWS FROM PLANK

Get into pushup position gripping dumbbells in your hands as a base. Do a single-arm row, pulling the dumbbell toward your chest. Halfway through your prescribed time, switch arms.

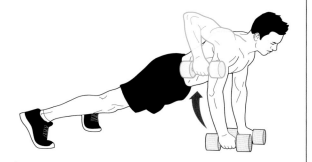

6 PUSHUPS

Get into pushup position gripping hexagonal dumbbells in your hands as a base. Keeping your body straight from your head to your ankles, lower your body until your chest nearly touches the floor. Pause at the bottom and then push yourself back to the starting position as quickly as possible.

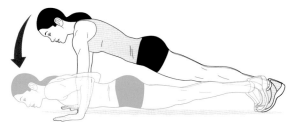

7 WRIST-TO-KNEE CRUNCH

Lie faceup with your hips and knees bent 90 degrees so that your lower legs are parallel to the floor. Place your fingers on the sides of your head. Lift your shoulders off the floor as if doing a crunch. Twist your upper body to the right while bringing up your right knee to touch your left wrist. Simultaneously straighten your left leg. Return to the starting position and repeat to the other side.

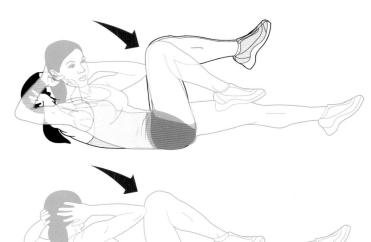

8 MOUNTAIN CLIMBERS

Get in pushup position with your arms straight. Use the ground or a bench as your base. This is the starting position. Lift your right foot and raise your knee as close to your chest as you can. Touch the ground with your right foot and then return to the starting position and repeat with your left leg. Go as fast as possible.

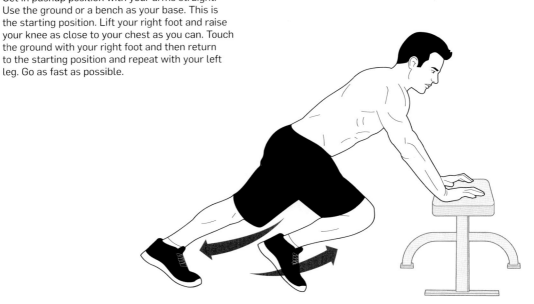

9 DUMBBELL PUSH PRESS

Stand holding a pair of dumbbells just outside your shoulders, with your arms bent and palms facing each other. Stand with your feet shoulder-width apart and knees slightly bent. Dip your knees and explosively push up with your legs as you press the weights straight over your shoulders. Lower the dumbbells back to the starting position and repeat.

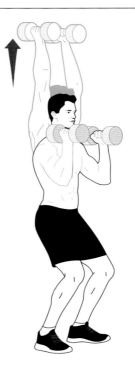

10 BURPEES (DUMBBELLS OPTIONAL)

Stand with your feet shoulder-width apart and arms at your sides. Lower your body into as deep a squat as you can. Now kick your legs backward so that you're in pushup position. Do a pushup, then quickly bring your legs back into the squat position. Stand up quickly and jump. That's 1 rep.

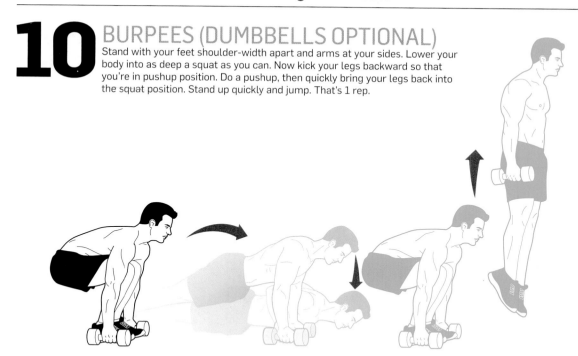

11 PLANKS

Get into pushup position, but bend your elbows and rest your weight on your forearms. Your body should form a straight line from your shoulders to your ankles. Brace your core and hold.

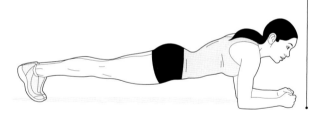

12 SIDE PLANK

Lie on your side and use your forearm to support your body. Raise your hips until your body forms a straight line from shoulder to ankles. Hold and repeat for the other side.

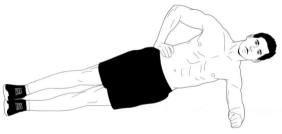

The Iron Strength Workout 2
DUMBBELL FUN

This is a variation on the first workout that involves more dumbbell work. Tweak the timing and reps to your level of fitness, as well as add in rest if you need it. Listen to your body and don't hurt yourself. You can also make the workout more challenging by shortening the rest and/or doing more than one circuit of all the exercises. Again, let your fitness level be your guide here.

For the standard workout, do each exercise for 40 seconds, then rest for 20 seconds. Move on to the next exercise. Once through the entire circuit, rest for 2 minutes and repeat. Adjust the timing and intensity as you need to.

FIRST: A PROPER WARM-UP (SEE PAGE 264)

1 SINGLE-ARM DUMBBELL SNATCH

Grab a dumbbell with an overhand grip. With your feet slightly wider than shoulder-width apart, bend at your hips and knees to squat down until the weight is centered between your feet, your arms straight. Your lower back should be slightly arched.

In a single movement, bend your arm, raise your elbow as high as you can, and try to throw the dumbbell at the ceiling (without letting go of it). Keep the dumbbell as close to your body as possible at all times. You should be thrusting the dumbbell upward so forcefully that you rise up on your toes. Allow your forearm to rotate up and back from the momentum of the lift, until your arm is straight and your palm is facing forward. Pull your body under the weight.

That's 1 rep. Halfway through the prescribed time, switch arms.

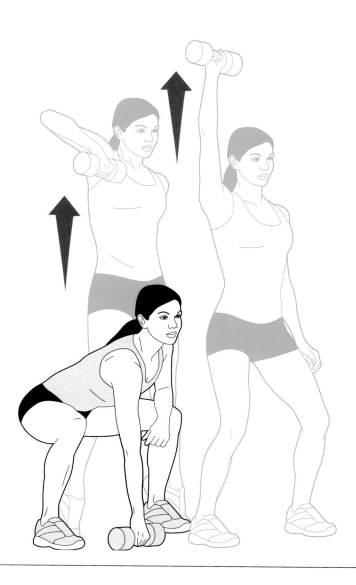

2 V-UP

Lie faceup on the floor with your legs straight and your arms straight above the top of your head, in line with your body. In one movement, simultaneously lift your torso and legs as if you're trying to touch your toes. Keep your head in line with your body; don't crane your neck. Your legs should be straight and your torso and legs should form a V. Lower your body back to the starting position.

3 DUMBBELL SPLIT SQUAT

Hold a pair of dumbbells at arm's length next to your sides, your palms facing each other. Stand in a staggered stance, your right foot in front of your left, with your feet set 2 to 3 feet apart. Slowly lower your body as far as you can. Pause, then push yourself back up to starting position as quickly as you can. Keep your torso upright and brace your core for the entire movement. Halfway through the prescribed time, switch feet.

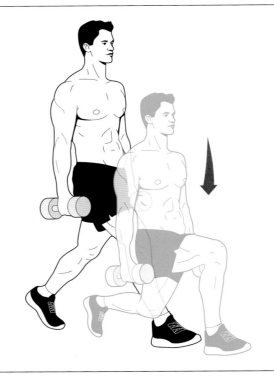

4 SINGLE-LEG DUMBBELL DEADLIFT

Grab a pair of dumbbells and stand on your left foot. Lift your right foot behind you and bend your knees so your right lower leg is parallel to the floor. Bend forward at your hips and slowly lower your body as far as you can, or until your right lower leg almost touches the floor. Pause, then push your body back to the starting position. Halfway through the prescribed time, switch legs.

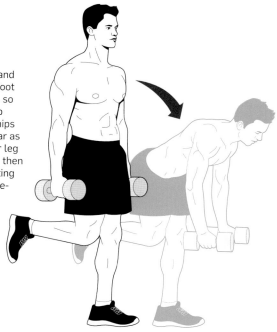

5 DUMBBELL CHOP

Grab a dumbbell and hold it with both hands above your right shoulder. Stand with your feet shoulder-width apart. Brace your core and rotate your torso to your right. While keeping your arms straight, swing the dumbbell down and to the outside of your left knee by rotating to the left and bending at your hips. Reverse the movement to return to the start. Halfway through the prescribed time, switch sides.

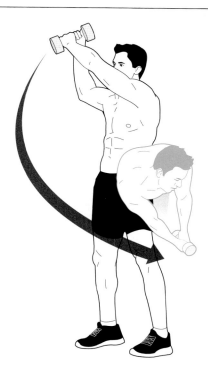

6 SIDE LUNGE AND PRESS

Grab a pair of dumbbells and stand with your feet hip-width apart. Press the dumbbells over your head so that your arms are straight. Brace your core, then step to the left and lower your body into a side lunge as you lower the left dumbbell to your shoulder. Keep your torso as upright as possible. Reverse the movement and push yourself back to the start. Halfway through the prescribed time, switch to the other side.

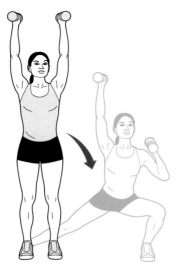

7 T-PUSHUP

Place a pair of hexagonal dumbbells at the spot where you position your hands. Grasp the dumbbells' handles and set yourself in pushup position with your feet hip-width apart. The dumbbells should be slightly wider than shoulder-width apart. Lower your body to the floor. As you push yourself back up, in one fluid motion, rotate the right side of your body upward as you bend your right arm and pull the right dumbbells to your torso. Then straighten your arm so that the dumbbell is above your right shoulder (your arms should form a T with your body). As you rotate your body, pivot on your toes and then lower your heels to the floor. Lower the dumbbell back down and repeat, this time performing the move to your left.

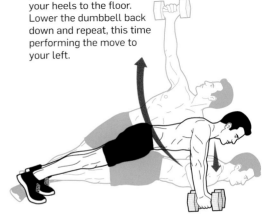

8 WIDE-STANCE PLANK WITH OPPOSITE ARM AND LEG LIFT

Start to get in the pushup position, but bend your elbows and rest your weight on your forearms instead of on your hands. Your body should form a straight line from your shoulders to your ankles. Move your feet out wider than your shoulders.

Brace your core by contracting your abs as if you're about to be punched in the gut. Now raise your left foot and right arm off the floor and hold. Halfway through the prescribed time, switch to the other arm and leg.

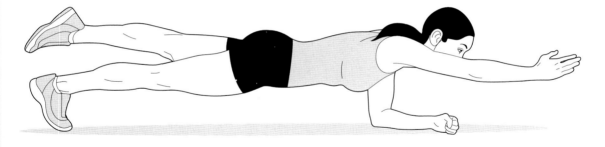

9 ROWS FROM PLANK.

Get into pushup position gripping dumbbells in your hands as a base.

While bracing your core, do a single-arm row, pulling the dumbbell toward your chest. Alternate arms for the prescribed time.

10 PRONE COBRA

Lie facedown on the floor with your legs straight and your arms next to your sides, palms down.

Contract your glutes and the muscles of your lower back, and raise your head, chest, arms, and legs off the floor.

Simultaneously rotate your arms so that your thumbs point toward the ceiling. At this time, your hips should be the only parts of your body touching the floor. Hold this position for the prescribed time. (Note: If you can't hold it for the entire time, hold for 5 to 10 seconds, rest for 5, and repeat as many times as needed. If the exercise is too easy, you can hold light dumbbells in your hands while you do it.)

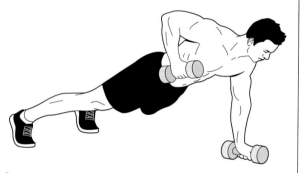

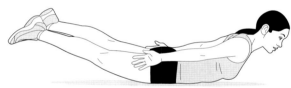

11 SINGLE-LEG SIDE PLANK

Lie on your side and use your forearm to support your body. Raise your hips until your body forms a straight line from shoulder to ankles. Then raise your top leg as high as you can and hold it that way for the duration of the exercise. Halfway through the prescribed time, switch sides.

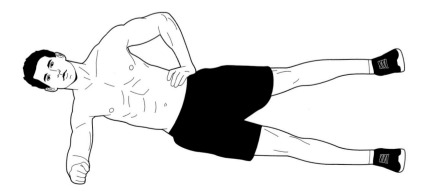

The Iron Strength Workout 3
THE GREAT OUTDOORS

This is a variation on the first workout that takes the action outside and involves interval (a.k.a. sprint) work, a great way to change up your routine, enjoy good weather, and get some fresh air. Tweak the timing and reps to your level of fitness, as well as add in rest if you need it. Listen to your body and don't hurt yourself. You can also make the workout more challenging by shortening the rest and/or doing more than one circuit of all the exercises. Again, let your fitness level be your guide here.

For the standard workout, do each exercise for 40 seconds, then rest for 20 seconds. Then move on to the next exercise. Once through the entire circuit, rest for 2 minutes and repeat. Adjust the timing and intensity as you need to.

FIRST: A PROPER WARM-UP (SEE PAGE 264)

1 WALKING LUNGE (DUMBBELLS OPTIONAL)

Perform a lunge, but instead of pushing your body backward to the starting position, raise up and bring your back foot forward so that you move forward (as if you're walking) a step with every rep. Alternate the leg you step forward with each time.

Halfway through your prescribed time, perform backward walking lunges to return to your starting point.

For a bigger challenge, hold dumbbells at your side.

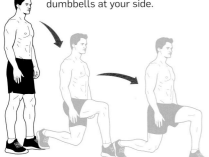

2 PUSHUPS

Get into pushup position using your hands as a base (you can also grip hexagonal dumbbells as your base). Keeping your body straight from your head to your ankles, lower your body until your chest nearly touches the ground. Pause at the bottom and then push yourself back to the starting position as quickly as possible.

You can also try pushup variations: Decline pushups with your feet on a bench; wide-hand or close-hand pushups; and staggered-hand pushups with one hand placed several inches forward.

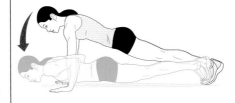

SPRINT

Run at full speed. Halfway through the prescribed time, turn around and return to your starting point.

3 SUICIDES (SHUTTLE RUN)

Sprint 5 paces, touch the ground, then return to your starting point and touch the ground. Without stopping, now sprint 10 paces, touch the ground, then return to your starting point and touch the ground. Halfway through the prescribed time, start working back down the distance ladder (15 paces, 10 paces, 5 paces, etc).

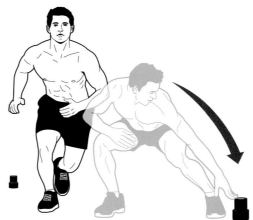

FOR THE SPRINTS:

Several variations are suggested here, but invent your own based on what outdoor terrain is available to you. Do you have access to stairs or steep hills? Use them. Do directional change drills (those little orange cones you can buy at the sporting goods store are great for this). Heck, if you have a nice line of trees, run a slalom between them. The point is, sprinting is great exercise, but adding in variations surprises your body and your muscles, which helps you improve not just your cardiovascular fitness, but your balance and ability to change direction explosively.

4 BODYWEIGHT JUMP SQUATS

Place your fingers on the back of your head and pull your elbows back so that they're in line with your body. Perform a bodyweight squat until your thighs are parallel to the floor, then explosively jump as high as you can (imagine you're pushing the floor away from you as you leap). When you land, immediately squat and jump again. Hold dumbbells at your side to make it more challenging.

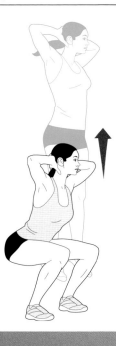

SPRINT
Run at full speed. Halfway through the prescribed time, turn around and return to your starting point.

5 WRIST-TO-KNEE CRUNCH

Lie faceup with your hips and knees bent 90 degrees so that your lower legs are parallel to the floor. Place your fingers on the sides of your head. Lift your shoulders off the floor as if doing a crunch. Twist your upper body to the right while bringing up your right knee to touch your left wrist. Simultaneously straighten your left leg. Return to the starting position and repeat to the other side.

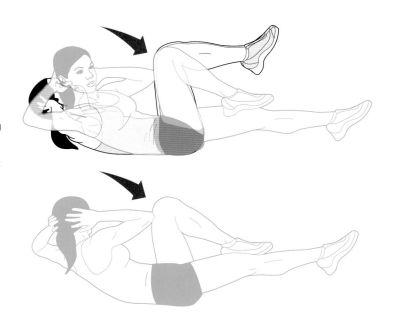

6 BURPEES (DUMBBELLS OPTIONAL)

Stand with your feet shoulder-width apart and arms at your sides. Lower your body into as deep a squat as you can. Now kick your legs backward so that you're in pushup position. Do a pushup, then quickly bring your legs back into the squat position. Stand up quickly and jump. That's 1 rep.

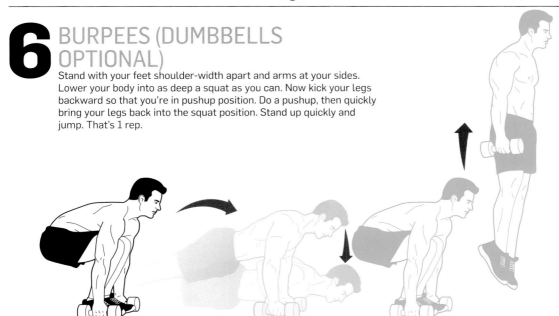

FIGURE-8 SPRINT

Run full speed in a figure-8 pattern. The tighter the figure 8, the more challenging it will be. Halfway through the prescribed time, run in the opposite direction.

7 PLANKS

Get into pushup position, but bend your elbows and rest your weight on your forearms. Your body should form a straight line from your shoulders to your ankles. Brace your core and hold.

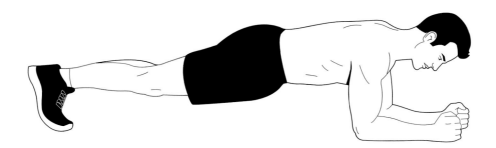

FREESTYLE SPRINT

Run at full speed using any surrounding features to make it more challenging (and fun!): hills, tree slalom, suicides, etc.

The Iron Strength Workout 4
THE CORE BLASTER

This is an intense core workout. Tweak the timing and reps to your level of fitness, as well as add in rest if you need it. Listen to your body and don't hurt yourself. You can also make the workout more challenging by shortening the rest and/or doing more than one circuit of all the exercises. Again, let your fitness level be your guide here.

For the standard workout, do each exercise for 40 seconds, then rest for 20 seconds. Move on to the next exercise. Once through the entire circuit, rest for 2 minutes and repeat. Adjust the timing and intensity as you need to.

FIRST: A PROPER WARM-UP (SEE PAGE 264)

1 CAT CAMEL

Position yourself on your hands and knees. Gently arch your lower back—don't push—then lower your head between your shoulders and raise your upper back toward the ceiling, rounding your spine. That's 1 repetition. Move back and forth slowly, without pushing at either end of the movement.

NOTE: The cat camel may look funny, but slowly flexing and extending your spine in small ranges of motion is a great way to prepare your core for any activity.

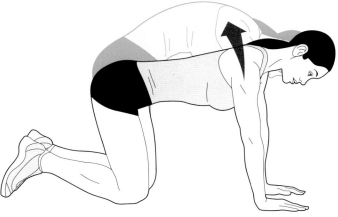

2 REVERSE CRUNCH

Lie faceup on the floor with your palms facing down. While holding your feet together, bend your hips and knees at 90 degrees. Raise your hips off the floor and crunch them inward—your knees should move toward your chest (imagine that you are emptying a bucket of water that's resting on your pelvis). Your hips and lower back should raise up off the floor. Pause, then slowly lower your legs until your heels nearly touch the floor.

3 MOUNTAIN CLIMBERS

Get in pushup position with your arms straight (use the ground or a bench as your base). This is the starting position. Lift your right foot and raise your knee as close to your chest as you can. Touch the ground with your right foot and then return to the starting position and repeat with your left leg. Go as fast as possible.

4 ROLLING SIDE PLANK

Start by performing a side plank with your right side down. Hold for 1 or 2 seconds, then roll your body over onto both elbows—into a traditional plank—and hold for 1 or 2 seconds. Next, roll all the way up onto your left elbow so that you're performing a side plank facing the opposite direction. Hold for another second or two. That's 1 repetition. Make sure to move your whole body as a single unit each time you roll.

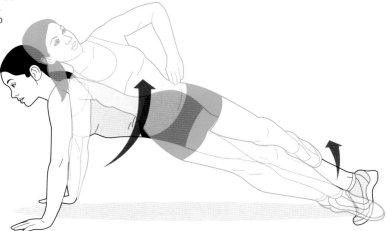

5 CORE STABILIZATION

Sit on the floor with your knees bent. Hold a weight plate straight out in front of your chest. Your feet should be flat on the floor. Lean back so your torso is at a 45-degree angle to the floor, and brace your core.

Without moving your torso (your belly button should point straight ahead at all times), rotate your arms to the left as far as you can. Pause for 3 seconds. Rotate your arms to the right as far as you can. Pause again, then continue to alternate back and forth.

NOTE: If you don't have a weight plate, you can substitute a light dumbbell, a basketball, a rock, or if you have no object (or need the exercise to be easier), simply clasp your hands together in front of you.

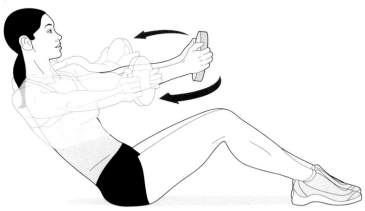

6 WRIST-TO-KNEE CRUNCH

Lie faceup with your hips and knees bent 90 degrees so that your lower legs are parallel to the floor. Place your fingers on the sides of your head. Lift your shoulders off the floor as if doing a crunch. Twist your upper body to the right while bringing up your right knee to touch your left wrist. Simultaneously straighten your left leg. Return to the starting position and repeat to the other side.

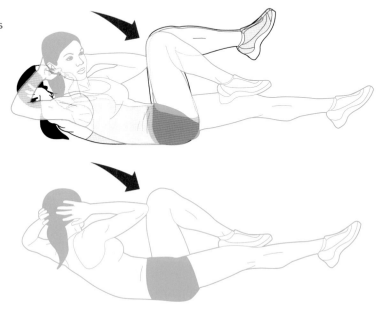

The Iron Strength Workout 5
ANYWHERE, ANYTIME

This is a variation on the first workout, based completely on body weight, which makes it a perfect workout for road warriors or anyone who doesn't have easy access to a gym. Tweak the timing and reps to your level of fitness, as well as add in rest if you need it. Listen to your body and don't hurt yourself. You can also make the workout more challenging by shortening the rest and/or doing more than one circuit of all the exercises. Again, let your fitness level be your guide here.

For the standard workout, do each exercise for 40 seconds, then rest for 20 seconds. Move on to the next exercise.

There are two ways you can approach this workout. It's divided into 3 circuits, so you can pick one circuit and cycle through it 3 times (resting 2 minutes between circuits). Or, you can go through all 3 circuits one time (resting 2 minutes between circuits). Adjust the timing, number of circuits, and intensity as you need to.

FIRST: A PROPER WARM-UP (SEE PAGE 264)

CIRCUIT 1

1 BODYWEIGHT BULGARIAN SPLIT SQUAT

Stand in a staggered stance, your left foot in front of your right 2 to 3 feet apart. Place just the instep of your back foot on a bench or chair. Pull your shoulders back and brace your core. Lower your body as deeply as you can, keeping your back foot on the bench. Keep your shoulders back and chest up through the movement. Pause, then return to starting position. Halfway through the prescribed time, switch to the other foot.

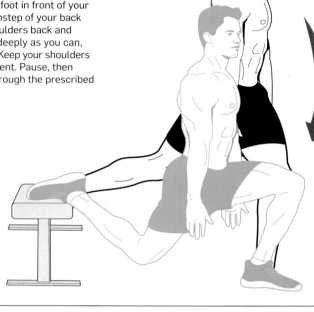

2 PUSHUPS

Get into pushup position using your hands as a base (you can also grip hexagonal dumbbells as your base). Keeping your body straight from your head to your ankles, lower your body until your chest nearly touches the ground. Pause at the bottom and then push yourself back to the starting position as quickly as possible.

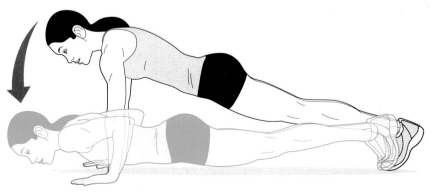

3 HIP RAISE

Lie faceup on the floor with your knees bent and your feet flat on the floor. Place your arms out to your sides at 45-degree angles, your palms facing up. Raise your hips so your body forms a straight line from your shoulders to your knees. Squeeze your glutes as you raise your hips. Make sure you're pushing with your heels. To make it easier, you can position your feet so that your toes rise off the floor. Pause for 5 seconds in the up position, then lower your body back to the starting position.

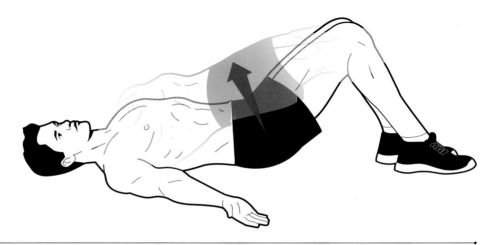

4 SIDE PLANK

Lie on your side and use your forearm to support your body. Raise your hips until your body forms a straight line from shoulder to ankles. Hold and repeat for the other side.

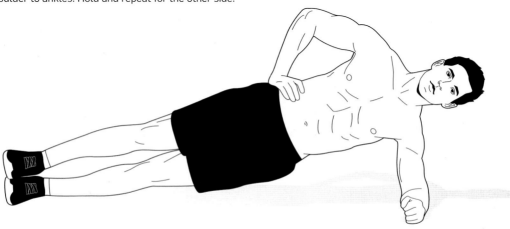

FLOOR Y-T-I RAISES

NOTE: Do one full set of each letter.

5 Y RAISE

Lie facedown on the floor. Allow your arms to rest on the floor, completely straight and at a 30-degree angle to your body, your palms facing each other (thumbs up). Your body should resemble the letter Y. Raise your arms as high as you can, pause, then slowly lower back to the starting position.

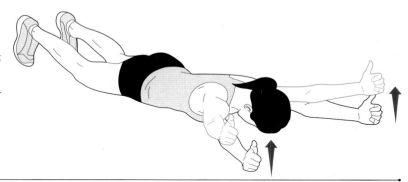

6 T RAISE

Lie facedown on the floor. Move your arms so they're out to your sides—perpendicular to your body with the thumb sides of your hands pointing up—and raise them as high as you can. Pause, then slowly lower back to the starting position.

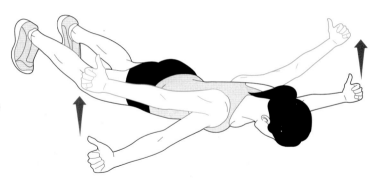

7 I RAISE

Lie facedown on the floor. Position your arms straight above your shoulders so your body forms a straight line from your feet to your fingertips. Your palms should be facing each other, thumbs pointing up. Raise your arms as high as you can, pause, then slowly lower back to the starting position.

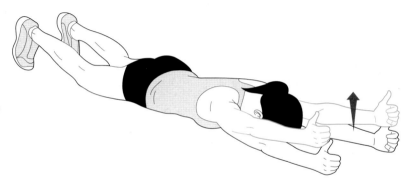

CIRCUIT 2

1 ISO-EXPLOSIVE BODYWEIGHT JUMP SQUATS

Place your fingers on the back of your head and pull your elbows back so that they're in line with your body. Perform a bodyweight squat until your thighs are parallel to the floor, then explosively jump as high as you can (imagine you're pushing the floor away from you as you leap). When you land, immediately squat and jump again. Hold dumbbells at your side to make it more challenging.

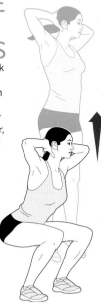

2 ISO-EXPLOSIVE PUSHUP

Assume the pushup position. Bend your elbows and lower your body until your chest nearly touches the floor. Pause 5 seconds in the down position. Then press yourself up so forcefully that your hands leave the floor.
NOTE: This 5-second pause technique eliminates all the elasticity in your muscles, which allows you to activate a maximum number of fast-twitch muscle fibers. These are the fibers with the greatest potential for size and strength gains.

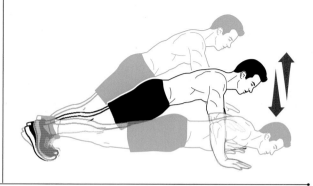

3 SINGLE-LEG HIP RAISE

Lie faceup on the floor with your left knee bent and your right leg straight. Raise your right leg until it's in line with your left thigh. Place your arms out to your sides at 45-degree angles to your torso, palms facing up. Push your hips upward, keeping your right leg elevated and in line with your left thigh. Be sure to push up from your heel (you can raise your toes to help). Your body should form a straight line from your shoulders to your knees. Pause, then slowly lower your body and leg back to the starting position. Halfway through the prescribed time, switch legs.

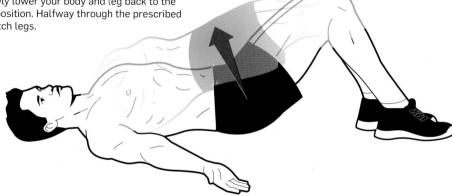

4 INVERTED SHOULDER PRESS

Assume a pushup position, but place your feet on a bench or chair and push your hips up so that your torso is nearly perpendicular to the floor. Your hands should be slightly wider than your shoulders, and your arms should be straight.

Without changing your body posture, lower your body until your head nearly touches the floor. Pause, then return to the starting position by pushing your body back up until your arms are straight.

NOTE: While the inverted shoulder press is technically a pushup, the tweak to your form shifts more of the workload to your shoulders and triceps, reducing the demand on your chest.

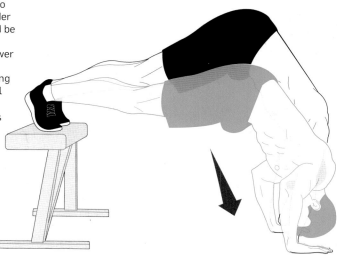

5 PRONE COBRA

Lie facedown on the floor with your legs straight and your arms next to your sides, palms down.

Contract your glutes and the muscles of your lower back, and raise your head, chest, arms, and legs off the floor.

Simultaneously rotate your arms so that your thumbs point toward the ceiling. At this time, your hips should be the only parts of your body touching the floor. Hold this position for the prescribed time. (Note: If you can't hold it for the entire time, hold for 5 to 10 seconds, rest for 5, and repeat as many times as needed. If the exercise is too easy, you can hold light dumbbells in your hands while you do it.)

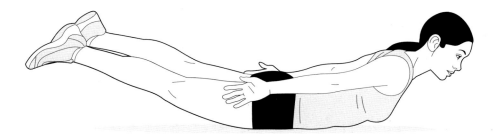

CIRCUIT 3

1 JUMPING JACKS

Stand with your feet together and your hands at your sides. Simultaneously raise your arms above your head and jump up just enough to spread your feet out wide. Without pause, quickly reverse the movement and repeat.

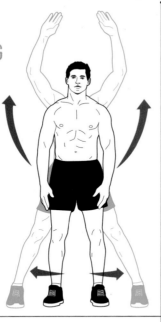

2 PRISONER SQUAT

Stand as tall as you can with your feet spread shoulder-width apart. Place your fingers on the back of your head (as if you have just been arrested). Pull your elbows and shoulders back, and stick out your chest. Lower your body as far as you can by pushing your hips back and bending your knees. Pause, then slowly push yourself back to the starting position.

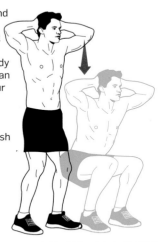

3 CLOSE-HANDS PUSHUP

Assume standard pushup position, but place your hands directly under your shoulders (placing your hands closer together works your triceps harder). Keeping your body straight from your head to your ankles, lower your body until your chest nearly touches the ground. Pause at the bottom and then push yourself back to the starting position as quickly as possible.
NOTE: Keep your elbows tucked close to your sides as you lower your body.

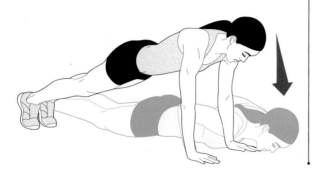

4 WALKING LUNGE

Perform a lunge, but instead of pushing your body backward to the starting position, raise up and bring your back foot forward so that you move forward (as if you're walking) a step with every rep. Alternate the leg you step forward with each time.

Halfway through your prescribed time, perform backward walking lunges to return to your starting point.

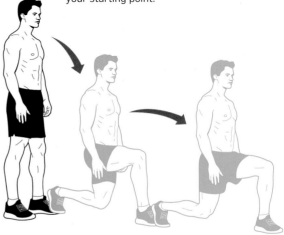

5 MOUNTAIN CLIMBERS

Get in pushup position with your arms straight. Use the ground or a bench as your base. This is the starting position. Lift your right foot and raise your knee as close to your chest as you can. Touch the ground with your right foot and then return to the starting position and repeat with your left leg. Go as fast as possible.

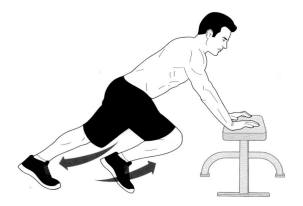

6 INVERTED HAMSTRING

Stand on your left leg, your knee bent slightly. Raise your right foot slightly off the floor. Without changing the bend in your left knee, bend at your hips and lower your torso until it's parallel to the floor.

As you bend over, raise your arms straight out from your sides until they're in line with your torso, your palms facing down. Your right leg should stay in line with your body as you lower your torso. Return to the start. Switch legs halfway through the allotted time.

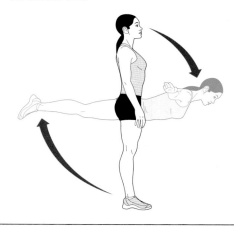

7 JUDO PUSHUP

Begin in standard pushup position, but move your feet forward and raise your hips so your body almost forms an upside-down V. Keeping your hips elevated, lower your body until your chin nearly touches the floor. Lower your hips until they almost touch the floor as you simultaneously raise your head and shoulders toward the ceiling. Reverse the movement back to the starting position and repeat.

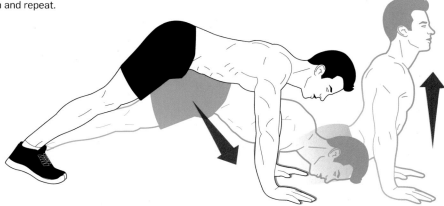

PART FIVE

THE ATHLETE'S GUIDE TO GREAT EATING

A meal-by-meal breakdown of everything you need to fuel training, boost performance, and prevent injury

Y ou've heard it 100 times before because it's 100 percent true: The smarter you eat, the better your body feels and performs. Maybe you've heard it put other ways. "Food is fuel"; "Eat clean"; and even the crusty old classic, "You are what you eat."

There's wisdom in all of that. But these rules of thumb don't tell the whole story . . .

Why?

Those rules don't delineate the actual problem for active people: After reading the injury section of this book, you might have come to the conclusion that all sports injuries come from too much, too little, or simply misguided exercise. But almost all health problems have a nutritional component as well, such as inadequate hydration and vitamin deficiencies. And too many athletes rely on fast fixes—meal replacement bars, energy drinks, and vitamins—instead of just plain eating right.

Eating right means eating whole foods. When NFL teams report to training camp every summer, the team nutritionists don't serve them protein bars, omega-3 pills, and energy drinks at mealtime. They serve them meat, fish, vegetables, pasta, fruits, and milk. Sure, there are sports drinks on the field, but off the field, these guys eat real food to fuel their workouts. And that's just one example.

Another complicating factor for active folks like you: the tons and tons of advice that's out there about what to eat and when. A lot of it is good advice, like you should eat five to six small meals a day to keep yourself fueled. That's smart eating. But there can be so much noise, so much static, that it's easy to get confused or, worse, to overthink eating. And once it becomes a chore, a pain the butt, something that sucks up too much brain time, you lose your discipline.

We can do better. My goal here is to make eating right as simple as possible. And you can do that by following one simple rule: Eat foods that have a purpose.

An athlete needs foods that have specific purposes in his or her body. Examples:

- It provides energy.
- It hydrates.
- It helps maintain muscle.
- It helps repair muscle.

- It helps prevent muscle cramping.
- It replaces what you lose in sweat (like sodium and potassium).

    If a food has no purpose, don't eat it. Simple.

    In a way, you can think of this as selfish eating. Look at the food in front of you and ask, "What's in it for me?" If the answer is, "Nothing," don't eat it. When it comes to food, it pays to be self-centered.

    Your hand moves toward the potato chips: "What's in it for me?"

    You want something sweet and you see a soda. Or an apple. "What's in it for me?"

    You already know the answers, and that's what makes this so simple. You're reminding yourself to question not just the quality of the food, but also your nutritional cravings before you eat something. If you crave soda, you crave sugar, so have the sweet apple and watch the craving disappear. And the apple has something in it for you: If there's a more portable, convenient, satisfying, and nutritious snack than an apple, I don't know what it is.

    You know what else "What's in it for me" makes you think about? All those hours you've spent training to become good at your sport. All that sweat equity. That's yours. You have a right to be selfish about that, to want to protect it rather than sabotage it.

    Think about how easy "What's in it for me" makes your life. If you ask

A WORD ABOUT SUPPLEMENTS

My philosophy? Always eat whole foods. If you do that, you shouldn't need supplements. But I certainly know that many athletes out there use them every day. Whey protein isolate, for example, is an effortless way to raise your protein intake when you're trying to build muscle. And other supplements can give your health a boost: omega-3 fatty acids, for one. But you can also get that from eating fish. And that's the point: A supplement is just that, something that "supplements" an intelligent diet. Supplements should never be a substitute for an intelligent diet. And I know a lot of people out there down vitamins and other pills without thinking very much about how they match up with the rest of the food they're eating that day. If you're looking for vitamins and minerals, and you think about it in a logical way, why would you ever need more than a standard multivitamin that gives you a day's worth of all those things?

    I suggest using the same approach to supplements that you use for food. Before you take it, ask yourself, "What's in it for me?"

that one simple question at every meal, everything in your diet falls into line. It eliminates lousy food. It eliminates reckless and mindless eating. It reinforces discipline, the hardest part of healthy eating.

What to Eat— and When

I've given you a food philosophy. Now you need a specific plan. Susan M. Kleiner, PhD, RD, is one of the world's foremost authorities on nutrition, especially sports nutrition. She's helped establish the eating plans for NFL teams, and her consulting company, High Performance Nutrition, has helped clients use cutting-edge nutrition concepts to achieve a broad range of goals. One of her books, *The Powerfood Nutrition Plan,* is one of the best resources out there for learning how to eat to fuel high performance.

Kleiner has outlined two specific eating plans, as well as given you 1 week of menus for each. One is for building strength. The other is for expanding endurance. Read on and she'll tell you how and when to use each, and what the plans will

ANOTHER REASON TO LIKE VEGETABLES

Alkaline foods are good for your body—and don't worry, that's not nearly as exotic as it sounds. Foods have either an acidic or alkaline effect on the body as they're digested. An acidic profile is terrible for your bones (a tooth dropped into a can of cola dissolves). But boosting the blood's alkaline level helps wounds heal faster. It will also make your blood less acidic, which cuts inflammation. What are the best highly alkaline foods? That's easy: vegetables. Any food that's naturally vibrant in color, especially those that are green, is good.

do for you. If you want to get serious about eating for sports, here's your guide.

YOUR STEP-BY-STEP EATING PLAN

By Susan M. Kleiner, PhD, RD

If you're a competitive person, nutrition can be your secret weapon—and you need to take it seriously. What I've found is that athletes need their nutrition plans to be as regimented as their training and recuperation. You can't think of it haphazardly, like, "Oh, yeah, I know I'm supposed to eat a little more protein, so I'll throw some of that in." People at the top of their game know exactly what they need to eat, and they plan their menus accordingly. They shop for the right foods and, when necessary, they take the time to prepare their meals. When they leave home, they make sure they have what they need in their backpacks or carrying cases, whether it's turkey jerky, fruits, nuts, a peanut-butter-and-jelly sandwich, or a ready-to-drink protein shake. That way, they have access to the right foods at the right times.

The successful athletes I've worked with never go anywhere

ANOTHER REASON TO LIKE PROTEIN

Protein provides the raw material needed to repair all of our daily tissue damage—not just muscles after a workout (which it also does, of course). Example: Our bodies replace each red blood cell every 90 days or so. That's a lot of repair work, and protein helps fuel it.

without taking some food along with them. These folks never travel without a cooler of food in the car, and once they reach a destination, they exploit whatever refrigerators, blenders, and kitchen facilities they can find. These athletes pay attention to what they eat and when they eat, and they never risk missing a meal. That meal, they know, may be the one that makes the difference between recovering adequately between workouts and not recovering at all.

You probably aren't a professional athlete, but it doesn't matter. Exciting new research shows how important it is to eat the right foods at the right times to build as much strength and endurance as possible from your workouts. In other words, no matter what you do, the more you focus on nutrition, the better you'll do.

You'll find two meal plans in this chapter. The first is for people who are mostly interested in increasing sports-related strength in the gym. The second is for those who are mostly interested in game-day endurance. (Incidentally, the strength program should also improve your endurance, and vice versa, although to a lesser degree.) I envision these plans being used in one of three ways.

• Some of you will want to follow the strength meal plan exclusively. This plan will help you get stronger without putting on too much bulk.

• Some of you will want to use the endurance meal plan exclusively. Those of you who focus primarily on running long distances year-round, for example, might not be interested in a strength plan.

• A good number of you, especially those who play organized sports, will want to make significant gains in both strength and endurance. For you, I suggest treating the strength meal plan as an off-season cross-training program. When your season arrives, switch to the endurance meal plan.

General Guidelines for Sports Nutrition

Regardless of which meal plan you go with—the strength plan or the endurance plan—there are some general rules to follow.

EAT MORE OFTEN. Eat five meals daily. Better yet, eat six or seven. To eat for high performance, you'll need to chow down every 3 hours or so, and you can't afford to skip meals. If you do, you're liable to run out of fuel when you need it most: mid-workout. What's more, if your meals are spaced too far apart, your body will adapt by slowing down your metabolism, which will promote fat storage. If it's time for one of those five meals and you're not hungry, don't force-feed yourself. However, don't overcompensate by eating excessively at your next meal.

EAT SIMPLE AND NATURAL. It's this simple: If you eat junk, you'll probably turn in junk-worthy performances. The easiest way to avoid processed foods is to focus your shopping on the periphery of the supermarket, avoiding the aisles. On the fringes, you'll find good things like fresh fruits and vegetables, fish, low-fat milk, and fresh farm eggs. In the belly of the beast, you'll find junk foods, TV dinners, and shopping carts stuffed with gossip rags and screaming kids. Steer clear.

Here are some of the foods you should be looking for.

Healthy, energy-packed carbs, including brown rice, buckwheat, whole-wheat pasta and couscous, potatoes with skin, sweet potatoes, winter squashes, beans, peas, and assorted fruits. Keep your bread consumption to a minimum. If you do eat bread, choose a sprouted-grain, high-protein variety, which can be found at most regular grocery stores these days, as well as at health food stores. Also, go for the so-called free fruits and vegetables—tomatoes, bell peppers, celery, jicama, and radishes. These make great snacks because they're completely or nearly calorie free and loaded with fiber.

Assorted lean proteins, with an emphasis on fish that are high in omega-3 fatty acids, eggs, chicken, turkey, dairy, vegetable proteins, protein powders, and red meat, the last eaten sparingly

Selected healthy monounsaturated fats, such as canola oil, olive oil, avocados, nuts, peanut butter, and olives.

Eat meals that smartly combine protein and carbs. If you can, get protein and carbs at every meal. One of your main sports nutrition goals is to get more carbs stored in your muscles, where you can access them fairly easily. I'll get into this more later, but for now, understand that

SUPERMARKET SHOPPING TIPS

Make your life easier: If you have no junk foods in the house, you'll eat the healthy options you buy at the store. Buy the following every time.

- A variety of fresh fruits. Buy three of each of several kinds of portable fruits like apples, bananas, pears, grapes, and oranges.

- Whole-grain breads. Look for 2 grams of fiber or more per slice.

- Lean meats for quick sandwiches. Think turkey, chicken breast, lean roast beef, or lean ham.

- Fresh greens and salad fixings. Buy precut veggies in the produce section.

- Fat-free or low-fat dairy sources. When in doubt, rely on milk and yogurt.

eating a mix of protein and carbs is one of the best ways to make sure this happens. Carb consumption causes your body to secrete insulin, which transports sugar out of the blood and into the muscles. Protein consumption enhances this process, first by making insulin work more efficiently and second by slowing the release of glucose into the bloodstream. If too much glucose is released at once, your insulin won't be able to shuttle it into your muscles fast enough and the glucose will ultimately become fat. Of course, getting more athletic and getting fatter are contradictory goals, so it's best to avoid this.

Steadily eating protein throughout the day has even more advantages, beyond helping with carb utilization.

• The body can absorb only a certain percentage of the protein you eat at each sitting, and no one is entirely sure what that percentage is. Because the body stores only very small pools of protein, it makes sense to replenish it throughout the day.

• Probably most important for the athlete in you is that protein is an important anabolic driver. You want to make sure your body has what it needs to build muscle throughout the day in response to your workouts. Remember that your body breaks down and rebuilds protein in your muscles constantly, and that this process is in overdrive in the 48 hours after a workout.

AIM FOR VARIETY. Different foods within different groups contain different combinations of nutrients. Nutritionists are only now discovering how important that is, mainly due to technology-driven changes in our ability to measure things in smaller and smaller amounts. We can now get a much clearer picture of why foods affect us, often dramatically, in specific ways. That's how we now know why you need a variety of animal products, fruits, vegetables, and other foods in your diet.

To ensure dietary variety, set aside two-thirds to three-quarters of your plate for plant-based foods. That will help you eat enough fruits, veggies, grains, beans, nuts, and seeds at every meal. Then put differently colored plant foods on your plate, aiming for at least one green food, one yellow, one red, one orange, one white, and one brown during the course of the day. Stay away from single-color meals. Potatoes, white fish, milk, and a banana aren't bad choices, but too many of them may mean you're not getting enough variety.

STEER CLEAR OF BEER. All it offers is empty calories and more

Give yourself a C

Collagen is abundant in connective tissues, tendons, bones, and muscles. Vitamin C is a key component of your body's collagen recipe, so load up on the vegetables and fruits.

fat storage, along with a short buzz and, perhaps, a long hangover. Obviously, it's hard to play your best when you're nursing a headache, sore limbs, and woozy eyesight. Alcohol consumption in general should be minimized, although an occasional glass of wine or whiskey is fine.

HYDRATE, HYDRATE, HYDRATE.

I saved this one for last because I want to emphasize this: When it comes to athletic performance, no nutrient is more important than water. It will trump carbs and protein in a heartbeat. Loss of just 2 percent of your body weight as fluid will diminish your physical and cognitive performance by 20 percent. Once you become 3 to 4 percent dehydrated, your health is at risk.

How quickly can you lose that much fluid? Contrary to our drive to eat, our drive to drink is not as keen. Our thirst mechanism doesn't kick in until we are already mildly dehydrated. When you're working out moderately in a mild climate, you are probably losing 1 to 2 quarts (2 to 4 pounds) of fluid per hour through perspiration. That means that a 150-pound person can easily lose 2 percent (3 pounds) of his or her body weight in fluid within an hour. If exercise is more intense or the environment is more extreme, fluid losses will be greater. You can see how easily you become dehydrated. If you don't replenish your fluid losses during exercise, you will fatigue early and your performance will diminish.

THE HYDRATION SECRET: KNOW YOUR SWEAT RATE

Seventy-five percent of muscle mass is made up of fluid. If you don't drink enough, your risk of cramps, strains, and sprains rises. Even if you don't pull up lame, a dehydrated performance is never your best. The funny (sad) thing? Every athlete knows how important proper hydration is. And yet at every practice or training run, every big game or race, you always see competitors cramping up or flaking out because they couldn't keep up with their sweat rate. Do you know your sweat rate?

IT'S SIMPLE: weigh yourself before and immediately after your workout. The difference is how much sweat you poured out (temperature and climate will affect this, obviously). In hot weather, some athletes can lose up to a half-gallon of sweat per hour.

HOW TO HYDRATE? Even if you drink plenty of fluids during your activity, any weight loss during an event means lost sweat, so hydrate afterward by drinking 1 to 1 ½ times the amount of ounces lost in fluid ounces.

Example: You lose 2 pounds, which is 32 ounces, so drink at least 32 to 48 ounces to replenish.

Fueling for Strength

Here are the general rules you need to remember if you are eating to build strength for sports.

CONSUME 2 TO 4 GRAMS OF CARBS FOR EVERY POUND OF BODY WEIGHT EACH DAY. When you lift weights, your primary energy source is carbohydrates. You may associate carbs with endurance exercises and protein with strength training, but you can't confuse the building materials with the fuel. Eat a healthy dose of carbs daily and you'll get the energy you need during training cycles, when the intensity and volume of your training are high. The greater your training volume, the more carbs you'll need. If you really are training mainly for fitness and health and not to gain much mass, then keep your carbs in the range of 2 grams per day. Otherwise, you'll start to bulge rather than burn. Our meal plan for strength-building days uses 2.6 grams of carbohydrate per pound as a mid-point, putting a 185-pound guy close to a 55 percent carb diet, which is ideal for starting or maintaining a hard training program.

Something to remember here: Most weight lifting taps the carbs stored in the working muscles. To fuel the short bursts of activity that weight lifting entails, you need good fuel stores

Give yourself another C

Calcium. A study from Brigham and Women's Hospital found that injured athletes typically consumed 25 to 40 percent less calcium than their uninjured counterparts—i.e., the winners.

in the muscles that you're exercising. If you did a heavy upper-body workout 2 days ago and now you're about to train your upper body again, you won't be able to maximize your performance in the gym if you haven't recovered from the preceding workout. And recovering fully requires eating carbs between then and now.

A key replenishment window opens up for the few hours after you train, but the process of replenishing glycogen stores in the liver and muscles will continue, albeit at a less intense rate, from one workout to the next. Assuming an ideal intake of carbs, glycogen stores are replenished at a rate of 5 to 7 percent per hour, meaning that it takes pretty much a full day to restore muscle-glycogen levels to what they were before you started training.

The goal, then, is to keep stoking the glycogen replenishment and tissue building from one training session to the next. That's something you'll want to keep in mind when designing your training routine. It's one of several reasons that heavy lifting sessions for the same muscle groups are best avoided on consecutive days.

CONSUME 0.8 GRAM OF PROTEIN FOR EVERY POUND OF BODY WEIGHT EVERY DAY.

This is the no-brainer. Protein is the key between training sessions for muscle repair, protein synthesis, and maintaining hormone balance. In this plan, you're going for strength, not size, so you'll need a little less.

If you want to see some size gains, bumping up your calories by adding extra protein before and after your exercise sessions, in addition to what you've calculated for the day, is a good strategy.

ALLOW THE REST OF YOUR CALORIES TO COME FROM FAT.

We know quite a bit about how much protein and carbohydrates you need to fuel your exercising body. We know a lot less about fat. Here's a good guideline: After you meet your needs for protein and carbs, you can get the rest of your calories from fat. Choose healthful sources, such as fish, nuts, and olive oil, over unhealthful sources, such as fatty meats and processed foods.

FAVOR WATER OVER SPORTS DRINKS.

As I said before, drinking liquids is important, no matter what your exercise program entails. But different liquids are better for different things. When it comes to training for strength, I suggest water over sports drinks and other sugar-laden liquids.

A weights-based workout usually uses less energy than a cardio workout and causes the body to lose fewer electrolytes. A strength trainer's replenishment needs are therefore less dire than an endurance athlete's. In the end, water should be more than able to keep you hydrated during your workouts, allowing you to get your energy-stoking carbs from more nutritious sources, including grains, fruits, and vegetables.

A Day in the Life of a Strength Eater

Here's how this all works out during a typical day.

IMMEDIATELY BEFORE TRAINING

Begin your workout well nourished but with your stomach pretty much empty. If you're undernourished by having, let's say, skipped breakfast and lunch before an afternoon workout, your body will likely run out of fuel and crash before the workout ends. Conversely, if your stomach is full of food before you lift your first weight, too much blood will be drawn to your stomach rather than to your muscles, where you want it, and an insulin spike will have negative effects on growth-hormone release.

Ideally, you want to consume a high-energy meal 2 to 3 hours before your workout—one loaded with complex carbs, along with some protein. Then, an hour before training, get an added boost from a meal-replacement shake or a formulated energy drink with protein and some carbohydrates, plus 16 ounces of water.

If you're an early morning exerciser and just can't face breakfast before your workout, try to drink a cup of fat-free milk or eat a small carton of low-sugar yogurt. It will make a world of difference.

DURING TRAINING

Fluid replacement should equal fluid loss. The recommended water intake per hour is 20 to 40 ounces. Drink cool or cold water (40° to 50°F) at a rate of 4 to 6 ounces every 15 to 20 minutes while training.

Remember, you probably won't need anything more than good old-fashioned water to rehydrate. If you want an extra dose of electrolytes, find a bottled water that has them added in.

IMMEDIATELY AFTER TRAINING

This meal is really an extension of the workout because the results you get will depend directly on what you eat and drink after training. Secondarily, what you consume afterward will have a direct effect on your next workout, even if it's several days away.

The impact that postworkout nutrition can have on your body is profound. Along with hydration, a major priority is replenishing glycogen stores. (The average Joe stores 1,500 to 2,000 carbohydrate calories, equal to 375 to 500 grams, as glycogen in his muscles and liver.) You need to consume carbs to do that, and how many you take in is largely a function of your training goal (see the upcoming eating plans for details). In all situations, you need some carbs to help maximize increases in muscle mass and provide the fuel needed for your next workout.

Refill your muscles and liver with glycogen, in the form of carbohydrates, ASAP after exercising. Those carbs will raise your blood sugar level, and this is the one time of day when this is a good thing. In fact, now is when simple carbs that score up near 100 on the glycemic index are ideal. What this does postexercise is promote the release of insulin, the "master" hormone, which in turn will stimulate the transport of amino acids into muscle, promoting protein synthesis. What's more, it will blunt the rise of cortisol, a stress hormone that signals your body to store fat. Immediately after exercising, your body begins repairing damaged muscle proteins, so give your body all the help it needs.

Specifically, this is when you need a major slug of protein and carbohydrates—about 250 to 500 calories' worth, combined. Because it's often hard to eat a meal right after training, you might try bringing a premade smoothie with you to the gym for consumption afterward. Depending on your size, the right mix for this drink is 20 to 40 grams of protein and 40 to 90 grams of carbs. By combining blended whole foods (bananas, berries, etc.) with some protein powder, fat-free milk, flaxseed oil and other essential fatty acids, and water or ice chips, you get a great combination that your body will soak up like a sponge.

TWO HOURS AFTER YOUR WORKOUT

Have a real meal. For example, combine protein and carbohydrates this time by eating 6 ounces of grilled salmon with an ear of corn, brown rice pilaf, and sliced tomatoes and mozzarella drizzled with extra-virgin olive oil, all washed down with a big glass of water. For a different feel, go for ground sirloin with a slice of Cheddar on a whole-grain bun with sautéed mushrooms and onions, bean soup, and a big salad with olives and balsamic vinaigrette dressing.

Rapid rehydration is also important here. As a rule of thumb, after exercising, you need to ingest at least 16 to 24 ounces, or 2 to 3 cups, of water for every pound of body weight lost during that session.

Fueling for Endurance

An easy plan for athletes who want to go long.

In 1974, Muhammad Ali and George Foreman fought their famed Rumble in the Jungle, an eight-round pummel fest that, blow for blow, is considered one of the greatest tactical boxing matches ever. The first seven rounds saw Ali take a heroic beating: Unable to stand up to the bigger, stronger Foreman, Ali seemed drawn to the ropes, where he faced one Foreman barrage after the next. By the eighth round, it appeared that Ali was doomed. Instead, Ali rose from his corner relaxed and poised and proceeded to knock Foreman out.

The millions of stunned onlookers who couldn't believe what they saw learned later that Ali had spent those rounds letting Foreman wear himself out, using the ropes to absorb the power from most of Foreman's blows. Meanwhile, Foreman was throwing himself at Ali, assuming he was on the brink of a knockout. That knock-

out never came, and Ali left with the heavyweight title.

The Rumble in the Jungle is a prime example of the need for sports endurance, not so much on Ali's part (who, admittedly, had to endure a lot, ropes or no ropes), but on Foreman's. Foreman was easily the stronger, more vital man, having just won 41 straight bouts. In comparison, Ali, who was 32 years old at the time, was past his prime—a slower, less effective version of his former self. None of that matters when you are not tired and your opponent is. Foreman's body may have been a fantastic machine, but when the parts weren't working, he couldn't do a thing with it.

You probably don't consider boxing a traditional endurance sport. More often, people think of aerobic exercises, like marathon running or swimming. But endurance is a much more general idea. And it applies to nearly all sports. The entire range of athletes, from prototypical triathletes to football linemen, need the physical endurance to avoid weariness and stay focused. That is the subject of this section.

ALL ROADS LEAD TO CARBS

It is next to impossible to endure in sports if you haven't mastered the art of eating carbs. Your body hoards the stuff in its muscles, waiting until you need it—like when you are about to dive into the water to start a triathlon or explode from the starting blocks to begin a track meet. Without carbs, your personal best would be awfully similar to your worst performance. Carbohydrates make the difference.

Having enough carbs is especially important toward the end of a competition. Ideally, you'll have already prepared your body to take advantage of these carbs. With proper training, you can help your body reserve carbs in your muscles for longer and revert to them only when your body has used a significant amount of another fuel source: fat.

Here's how that works: Your body will begin any athletic endeavor by burning carbs. If your body is well trained, it will soon stop burning carbs and move to your stores of body fat for energy. From about 10 to 20 minutes into exercise (depending on your training status) until just before you hit the wall with fatigue,

you'll use that fat. After that, it's back to carbs again.

The logic here is simple. The faster you can access fats for fuel during exercise, the more glycogen (the stored form of carbohydrates in your muscles) you retain, and the more fuel you've got left for those last few moments of exertion at the end of a competition. Over time, the better trained you are, the better your endurance.

None of this matters, though, if you don't have enough carbs in your system. The amount of carbohydrates stored (as glycogen) in muscles is directly related to how many carbohydrates you eat and how well trained you are. In general, a diet with upward of 60 percent of calories from carbohydrates will allow for the greatest storage of glycogen in the muscles on a daily basis. In the meal plan I outline on page 335, that will come to just more than 3 grams of carbohydrates per pound of body weight.

(NOTE: If you are training for more than 2 hours daily, you'll probably need more. I suggest increasing your carbs in that case to about 3.6 to 4.5 grams per pound. This high a level of intake will reduce the common risk of chronic fatigue and overtraining syndrome. But beware the trap in this diet strategy. You must still consume enough protein and fat. The body cannot perform on carbs alone! If you can't eat enough calories to consume adequate protein and fat and still maintain your body weight, then drop your carbs down a notch.)

GOOD CARBS, BAD CARBS

As you realize by now, not all carbs are created equal. If you don't know how certain carbs are processed in your body and how the nutrients they contain aid performance, you cannot effectively use your carbs. There's a right time for whole grains, vegetables, and fruits, and there's even a right time for sugar (especially if you are a long-distance runner). There are also the matters of how they all fit in with proteins and fats and how carbs interplay with them. Knowing how to mix your macronutrients like a pharmacist mixes drugs will help you maximize certain effects.

Here's what you should concentrate on.

CONSISTENCY. The first rule of eating carbs for endurance is consistency. When you're fueling up for endurance performance, you must include carbohydrates every time you eat throughout the day. Each meal and snack should have some whole-grain bread, vegetable, fruit, legume, or milk product.

VARIETY. Notice how pasta is not listed as the only source of carbohydrates for the endurance athlete's diet? I'm certain that some of my clients used to think that the more pasta they ate, the faster and longer they'd run, until almost all they ate all day was pasta. Oh, and of course potatoes.

This way of thinking couldn't be more wrong. Though pasta and potatoes are good carb sources, all the other foods just listed are so much fuller in vitamins, minerals, and phytochemicals, all of which are incredibly important for supporting elite athletic performance. Athletes who focus solely on pasta and spuds consume a diet remarkably devoid of protein and fat. Ultimately, their performance diminishes, and that's why they end up in my office looking for help.

COMBINATION. Carbohydrate-rich foods should always be eaten in combination with protein and/or fat. The goal is to keep your body from absorbing the carbs too fast. The protein and fat act as gatekeepers, allowing carbs to enter the bloodstream at a time-released pace and avoiding a carbohydrate stampede. If carbs aren't controlled, you'll experience the superelevated peaks and valleys of insulin secretion that are associated with high-carbohydrate diets. Your body will not rush to remove sugar from the bloodstream (which leads to fat storage) and instead will use that sugar as energy or put it into muscle storage. Also, you'll minimize the secretion of stress hormones, which negatively impact muscle recovery and performance.

ONE LAST WORD ON CARBS

With all the low-carb hype, you're probably wondering about the sanity of eating a moderately high-carb diet.

A study at the University of Colorado showed that cyclists on a low-carb diet (100 grams per day) performed just as well on a 45-minute endurance test as those eating a high-carb diet (600 grams per day). But the high-carb group had much higher levels of muscle glycogen (carb storage) at the end of the test, and the low-carb group gained no fat-burning advantages, either. If this test had been performed on the same riders over the course of several days, I suspect the results would have been different. If you're planning to do just one bout of exercise and no more—ever—then that low-carb diet is for you. If you plan to exercise day after day, then your exercise will become harder each day as your muscle fuel stores become depleted on a low-carb diet. If you exercise intensely more than 3 days per week, a low-carb diet is not for you.

PROTEIN AND ENDURANCE

Even though you're not training to build muscle, you still need protein to repair your muscles and help them recover and gain strength and endurance. You can't do any of this without adequate protein. You need protein to cover the jobs that only protein can perform throughout your whole body. An endurance athlete needs at least 0.54 to 0.64 gram of protein per pound of body weight per day. If you are a vegetarian, add another 10 percent. If you're eating fewer calories than you need in order to burn more fat, then you need at least 0.72 gram of protein per pound of body weight per day.

Speaking of vegetarians, you will benefit greatly from having a variety of sources of protein in your diet, just as I've been advocating variety in all the other food groups. Though poultry is high in tryptophan and pork is high in thiamine (vitamin B_1), red meat is highest in iron and zinc, two incredibly essential minerals supporting endurance performance.

If you avoid animal products, then you must supplement with fortified foods and dietary supplements to ensure adequate nutrition.

FAT AGAIN

A healthy diet includes healthy dietary fats. Fat should make up between 20 and 25 percent of your calories. Stick with vegetable oils, avocados, nuts, and seeds. Choose lean meats and low-fat and fat-free dairy products. Just because you're active does not mean that you're protected from the health dangers of saturated fats.

When you are looking for great fatty snacks, choose nuts. They are dense in calories, healthy fats, protein, and fiber. They are also high in chromium and magnesium. Chromium, often found to be lacking in the diets of athletes, is essential for the transfer of glucose into cells for energy production. Magnesium helps relax muscles after contraction and plays a role in the conduction of nerve impulses.

PAY EVEN MORE ATTENTION TO HYDRATION

Getting dehydrated when you're working for strength is possible, but not a given. But dehydrating when you're working toward endurance is almost guaranteed if you aren't replenishing your system regularly. Without fluid replenishment after exercise, your performance on successive days will decay, and your long-term health may be at risk. I suggest carrying water and other fluids with you as a constant reminder to drink. Freeze fluids in water bottles to keep them cold during long-distance exercise. Don't forget that fruits and vegetables are great sources of water.

If you're working out for more than an hour (or even working out intensely for less than an hour), you'll probably need more than water to stay appropriately charged. Carbohydrate-electrolyte sports drinks are excellent choices to help you do this. By replacing carbs during exercise, you'll have more fuel available at the end of your training or competition, when you need it most. These drinks contain sodium to help drive your thirst mechanism, and they also enhance carbohydrate absorption by helping to usher glucose across the intestinal lining into the bloodstream. During ultra and extreme events, you'll benefit from the electrolyte replacement, because your body will have lost significant amounts of electrolytes in your sweat, and your performance could suffer without an external source.

DO THE GOO

Long-distance, ultramarathon, and extreme-sport athletes sometimes need special products to keep their bodies from using up all the fuel. That means refueling on the fly, so to speak. There are many ways to do it, but among the most popular are gels and goos. Basically, these products are concentrated sources of carbs in the form of sugar, allowing athletes to consume far more carbs than they would if they simply drank a bottle of Gatorade during competition. Also, many people's bodies cannot handle more complex, dense foods (like bread or fruits) when they are in the middle of an event. Eating these can make an active body nauseated, which isn't a wonderful feeling when you're standing still, but it's even more burdensome when you're running 25 miles. Of course, some people get nauseated from goos and gels—it's all about figuring out what works for you.

Two words of advice on using gels and goos: First, try them out on training days before using them in competition. You never want to try a new product—especially a goo or gel—on the day of a competition. Second, make sure you drink water with them. Although these products are designed to provide carbs without the extra liquid from a liter of sports drink, you'll still need a cup or two of water to regulate your body's fluid levels. Forget to drink, and your body will go looking for more liquid to dilute the carbs in your intestines. This will come from other cells, which will lead to dehydration.

AVOID OVERHYDRATION

On the flip side of dehydration, you must also guard against overhydration. Hydration is a delicate balance between fluids and minerals in your body. The concentrations of sodium and other minerals (collectively known as electrolytes) in your bloodstream must fall within a very narrow range, or it can affect your muscle contractions. That includes the most important muscle: your heart.

When you take in too much water relative to the amount of electrolytes in your body, the result will eventually be a condition called hyperhydration, or hyponatremia. The problem is that your blood has become too diluted, which is just as dangerous as dehydration, in which you have high levels of electrolytes without enough fluids.

Hyperhydration occurs more frequently than you might think, particularly in endurance and ultra-endurance sports like marathons. You can avoid hyponatremia by taking a few simple precautions.

• If you're training for your first marathon or triathlon, don't cut all the salt out of your diet (even though, as a general rule, most of us could get away with a lot less than we currently take in).

• If the day is cooler or less humid than you expected, compensate by drinking less than you'd planned during the event.

• Go for sports drinks over pure water.

• Don't think you have to match the better-trained competitors drink for drink. Their sweat is literally different from yours, containing more water and fewer electrolytes. Your body is leaking sodium, while theirs are holding on to it.

• If you find yourself slowing down toward the end of the race, don't take this as a sign that you should drink more. If you're running slower, you're also sweating less.

• If you see pretzels being handed out along the course of a distance race, help yourself, as long as you're not sodium sensitive and you don't have high blood pressure.

Surprisingly, the symptoms of dehydration and hyperhydration are basically the same. If you collapse and require medical attention, that doctor or paramedic may not be able to tell if you've had too little or too much to drink. If you're in a condition to answer his or her questions, one of the first will concern your fluid intake.

A Day in the Life of an Athlete Who Endures

Here's how this all works out during a typical day.

BEFORE YOUR SESSION

How you eat before your session will contribute greatly to your overall athletic development.

If you work out first thing in the morning: Replace the fluid and carbs lost during sleep by eating or drinking carbs in some form. Cereal and milk, a bagel and cream cheese, plain yogurt and fruit, even a cold slice of last night's pizza will all fit the bill. Going into your workout feeling good will enable you to work even harder and burn even more calories, and your ability to burn fat is going to be enhanced when you end a great workout still energetic. The food before exercise will improve endurance on a long-distance workout, decrease the muscle-damaging effects of exercise, and enhance your recovery afterward. Eat or drink just enough before your workout to feel good—but not so much that you feel sluggish and tired.

If you do cardio at any other time of day: Consume your carbs long enough before exercise that they will have been assimilated into your body to some extent.

If you want to burn body fat, the best approach is to consume 60 calories of protein and 150 calories of low to moderate glycemic index carbs an hour and a half before exercise. Lower GI foods won't spike your insulin, as you want to avoid an insulin response preworkout. Manage insulin by keeping it within as narrow a range as possible. That way, the food you consume will be burned as fuel rather than stored.

Combining protein and carbohydrates not only offers your body a good source of fuel before exercise, but also appears to decrease the catabolic (tissue breakdown) effects that naturally result from the exercise to come. As you exercise, you work your muscles, and that work inflicts damage. By repairing it, your body builds itself up. It's just the natural way the body works. By minimizing that damage, you'll be less sore, allowing you to work out harder on successive days, but you'll still provide enough stimulus to produce an adaptive response.

DURING YOUR SESSION

Now that your session has started, your goal is to maximize your performance. That may not be possible, though, if you didn't take in carbohydrates beforehand. Fatigue will come sooner without those carbs.

That's why it's a good idea to sip liquid carbs from a sports drink throughout your session. Once you begin to fatigue, your body is less capable of making available the enzymes that are required to transport oxygen from your lungs to your working muscles. As your body is less and less able to get oxygen into the cells, fat will be less available as an energy source, and carbohydrates will come back into the picture with a vengeance as your primary fuel source. Remember, you've got to have oxygen around to burn fat, but not to burn carbs. Even though your muscles are nearly out of carbs at this point, you'll get an extra burst of energy from that external fuel source toward the end of your session, and it will take you longer to reach fatigue.

AFTER YOUR SESSION

Immediately after cardiovascular work, you have to replace the fuel stores you just tapped in your muscles. As soon as possible after your foot leaves the pedal or rubber, begin maximizing the muscle-recovery process by consuming a little more than ½ gram of carbohydrates per pound of body weight, along with about ¼ gram per pound of protein. The sooner, the better: This is the time when these nutrients are entering back into your cells the most rapidly. Repeat this strategy again within 2 hours of the workout. For the average 190-pounder, that would amount to 95 grams of carbohydrates and 47 grams of protein for the first meal immediately after exercise. If you are smaller, cut those numbers in half. You can eat slightly less for the meal 2 hours later. As you can see, a pretty big slug of your day's nutrition will come at these two times. Don't, however, neglect the rest of the day, because you will continue to recover all day long.

If your cardio session lasted for more than 1 hour—or much longer than 1 hour, if you're training for, say, a marathon—you really need to consume not only enough water, but also enough electrolytes such as sodium, potassium, and magnesium. The best way to do that is by draining any one of the numerous sports drinks on the market that are formulated to include those electrolytes. They speed up the absorption of fluids and help your body retain them. Remember, if you are looking for an edge, try a sports drink with added protein.

EATING-FOR-STRENGTH MEAL PLAN

This is the diet to help you tone up, improve strength, and support all your sporting endeavors. It is the ideal program for a cross-trainer. There are enough carbohydrates to fuel your training but avoid fat gain. Proteins are carefully selected and timed for strength gain and muscle recovery. The "Daily Breakdown" below shows your allotted portions of certain types of food per day.

DAILY BREAKDOWN*†

14 bread
8 fruit
4 milk
23 teaspoons added sugar
6 vegetable
9 very lean protein
5 lean protein
1 medium-fat protein
7 fat

* Use every day.
† Based on a 185-pound man

DAILY ASSUMPTIONS*†

3,434 calories
489 grams of carbohydrates
185 grams of protein
82 grams of fat

NOTE: Occasionally, a fat-free product, like mustard or cooking spray, is included on the menus. These do not count toward your daily breakdown but should not be overused.

THE MENU

DAY 1

Preworkout

SMOOTHIE
Blend until smooth.

1 milk	1 cup fat-free milk
2 fruit	1 cup orange juice
2 very lean protein	14 grams whey protein powder
	Ice cubes

Workout

8 teaspoons added sugar	16-ounce sports drink
	Water

Breakfast

3 bread	3 slices whole-grain bread
1 milk	1 cup fat-free milk
2 fruit	1 cup cubed cantaloupe
	1 cup fresh raspberries
9 teaspoons added sugar	3 tablespoons 100 percent fruit spread
1 medium-fat protein	1 egg, scrambled in a nonstick pan
3 very lean protein	6 egg whites, scrambled with whole egg
2 fat	⅛ avocado, chopped into cooked egg
	1½ tablespoons ground flaxseed
	Water
	Fat-free cooking spray (for eggs)

Snack

2 bread	8 whole-wheat crackers
1 vegetable	1 cup celery sticks
2 fat	2 tablespoons natural peanut butter

Lunch

5 bread	Footlong Subway sandwich (from their "6 grams of fat or less" list)
2 vegetable	Lettuce, tomato, bell pepper, onion
2 fruit	1 small banana
	1 apple
1 milk	1 cup fat-free milk
4 very lean protein	Included (in sandwich)
1 fat	1 teaspoon olive oil or 1 tablespoon salad dressing

Snack

1 fruit	¾ cup blueberries
1 bread	¼ cup Grape-Nuts cereal
1 milk	1 cup plain fat-free yogurt
3 teaspoons added sugar	1 tablespoon honey

Dinner

3 bread	1 sweet potato, baked
	1 small ear corn on the cob
1 fruit	1 slice watermelon
3 teaspoons added sugar	½ cup frozen yogurt
3 vegetable	Salad with 2 cups romaine lettuce, ½ cup tomato, ½ cup cucumber, ½ cup cooked broccoli
5 lean protein	5 ounces salmon, grilled
2 fat	2 tablespoons olive oil (for dressing)
	Vinegar (for dressing)

DAY 2

Preworkout

SMOOTHIE
Blend until smooth.

1 milk	1 cup fat-free milk
2 fruit	1 cup orange juice
2 very lean protein	14 grams whey protein powder
	Ice cubes

Workout

8 teaspoons added sugar	16-ounce sports drink
	Water

Breakfast

YOGURT PLUS
Combine yogurt, fruit, and honey.

1 milk	1 cup fat-free unsweetened yogurt
2 fruit	2½ cups fresh strawberries
9 teaspoons added sugar	3 tablespoons honey
3 very lean protein	6 eggs, hard cooked (discard yolks)
2 fat	1½ tablespoons ground flaxseed
	Water

CALIFORNIA EGG SANDWICH
Combine muffin, avocado, and egg for sandwich.

3 bread	1½ whole-wheat English muffins
1 medium-fat protein	1 egg, hard cooked
	⅛ avocado, sliced

Snack

2 bread	4 rice cakes
1 vegetable	1 cup vegetable sticks
2 fat	2 tablespoons salad dressing (for dipping)

Lunch	5 bread	2 slices whole-grain bread
		1 ounce croutons
		1 cup brown rice
	2 vegetable	Large salad with romaine lettuce, tomato, grilled eggplant, roasted red bell pepper
	2 fruit	2 kiwifruits, sliced
	1 milk	1 cup fat-free milk
	4 very lean protein	4 ounces skinless white-meat chicken, grilled with lime juice
	1 fat	2 tablespoons fat-free dressing
		1 teaspoon olive oil (for roasted vegetables)

Snack	1 fruit	8 dried apricot halves
	1 bread	¾ ounce pretzels
	1 milk	1 flavored latte, tall
	3 teaspoons added sugar	1 tablespoon syrup (for latte)

Dinner	3 bread	1 cup cooked pasta
		1 slice garlic bread
	1 fruit	1½ cups whole strawberries
	3 teaspoons added sugar	½ cup flavored gelatin dessert
	3 vegetable	2 cups ratatouille (over pasta)
		Salad with 1 cup lettuce, ¼ cup tomato, ¼ cup cucumber
	5 lean protein	5 ounces lean ground beef (add to ratatouille)
	2 fat	2 tablespoons fat-free dressing

DAY 3

Preworkout	**SMOOTHIE**	
	Blend until smooth.	
	1 milk	1 cup fat-free milk
	2 fruit	1 cup orange juice
	2 very lean protein	14 grams whey protein powder
		Ice cubes

Workout	8 teaspoons added sugar	16-ounce sports drink
		Water

Breakfast	3 bread	3 slices whole-wheat bread
	1 milk	1 cup fat-free cottage cheese (put on bread; sprinkle with sugar and cinnamon)
	2 fruit	4 ounces freshly squeezed orange juice (with pulp)
		½ cup sliced pineapple
	9 teaspoons added sugar	3 tablespoons sugar
	1 medium-fat protein	1 egg, cooked sunny-side up in a nonstick pan
	3 very lean protein	6 egg whites, cooked with sunny-side-up egg
	2 fat	1½ tablespoons ground flaxseed
		1 teaspoon oil (for egg)
		Water

Snack	2 bread	1 bagel
	1 vegetable	Tomato, sprouts
	2 fat	2 tablespoons cream cheese

Lunch	5 bread	2½ cups rice
	2 vegetable	1 cup Chinese vegetables, stir-fried with garlic, onions, fresh ginger
	2 fruit	1 cup any citrus fruit sections
	1 milk	1 cup fat-free milk
	4 very lean protein	4 ounces scallops, stir-fried
	1 fat	1 teaspoon oil (for stir-frying)

Snack	1 fruit	1¼ cups sliced strawberries
	1 bread	1 slice 8-grain bread
	1 milk	1 cup fat-free plain yogurt
	3 teaspoons added sugar	1 tablespoon honey

Dinner	3 bread	2" square of corn bread
		1 cup kidney beans (for chili)
	1 fruit	1 pear
	3 teaspoons added sugar	½ cup frozen yogurt
	3 vegetable	1 cup chopped cooked tomatoes with chili seasoning (for chili)
		½ onion, garlic (for seasoning)
		Salad with 1 cup lettuce, ¼ cup tomato, ¼ cup cucumber
	5 lean protein	Included (in beans)
		3 ounces soy crumbles (for chili)
	2 fat	2 slices bacon, cooked very crisp (crumble into chili)
		Included (in corn bread)

DAY 4

Preworkout	**SMOOTHIE**	
	Blend until smooth.	
	1 milk	1 cup fat-free milk
	2 fruit	1 cup orange juice
	2 very lean protein	14 grams whey protein powder
		Ice cubes

| Workout | 8 teaspoons added sugar | 16-ounce sports drink |
| | | Water |

Breakfast	2 fruit	2 cups raspberries
	1 milk	1 cup fat-free milk (½ cup for making French toast)
	FRENCH TOAST	
	3 bread	3 slices whole-wheat bread
	9 teaspoons added sugar	3 tablespoons maple syrup
	1 medium-fat protein	1 egg
	3 very lean protein	6 egg whites
	1 fat	1½ tablespoons ground flaxseed
		1 teaspoon oil (for frying)
		Water

Snack	2 bread	24 small whole-wheat crackers
	1 vegetable	1 cup sliced bell pepper
	2 fat	4 tablespoons reduced-fat salad dressing (for dipping)

Lunch

2 fruit	1½ cups blueberries
1 milk	1 cup fat-free milk

FAJITAS
Combine ingredients.

5 bread	1½ cups Spanish rice
	2 tortillas
2 vegetable	1 cup sautéed onion, bell pepper
	2 tablespoons salsa
4 very lean protein	4 ounces skinless white-meat chicken, grilled with lime juice
1 fat	1 teaspoon olive oil (for cooking)

Snack

1 bread	¾ ounce pretzels

SMOOTHIE
Blend until smooth.

1 fruit	½ large frozen banana
1 milk	1 cup fat-free milk
3 teaspoons added sugar	1 tablespoon chocolate syrup
	Ice cubes

Dinner

3 bread	1 ounce croutons (for salad)
	1 cup chicken noodle soup
	4 crackers
1 fruit	1 nectarine
3 teaspoons added sugar	1 cup reduced-calorie cranberry juice cocktail
3 vegetable	3 cups salad with lettuce, tomato, cucumber, bell pepper
5 lean protein	5 ounces swordfish, grilled with ginger and scallions
2 fat	4 tablespoons reduced-fat salad dressing

DAY 5

Preworkout

SMOOTHIE
Blend until smooth.

1 milk	1 cup fat-free milk
2 fruit	1 cup orange juice
2 very lean protein	14 grams whey protein powder
	Ice cubes

Workout

8 teaspoons added sugar	16-ounce sports drink
	Water

Breakfast

3 bread	1½ cups quick oats (not instant)
1 milk	1 cup fat-free milk
2 fruit	1 apple, diced
	1¼ cups sliced strawberries
9 teaspoons added sugar	3 tablespoons brown sugar
1 medium-fat protein	1 egg, hard cooked
3 very lean protein	6 eggs, hard cooked (discard yolks)
2 fat	1½ tablespoons ground flaxseed
	6 slivered almonds (for oatmeal)
	Water

Snack

2 bread	1½ ounces baked tortilla chips
1 vegetable	½ cup salsa
2 fat	8 black olives
	⅛ avocado, cubed

Lunch

5 bread	1½ cups minestrone soup
	1½ cups cooked linguini
2 vegetable	1 cup marinara sauce
2 fruit	1 whole grapefruit, sectioned
1 milk	1 cup fat-free milk
4 very lean protein	4 ounces shrimp, grilled
1 fat	1 teaspoon olive oil (for cooking)

Snack

1 fruit	½ cup canned pineapple
1 bread	¼ cup Grape-Nuts cereal
1 milk	1 cup plain fat-free yogurt
3 teaspoons added sugar	1 tablespoon honey

Dinner

3 bread	1 large pita
	1 ounce croutons
1 fruit	2 large figs
3 teaspoons added sugar	10 ounces apricot nectar
3 vegetable	3 cups salad with lettuce, tomato, cucumber, bell pepper
5 lean protein	5 ounces lean lamb, grilled with lime juice
2 fat	2 tablespoons vinaigrette

DAY 6

Preworkout

SMOOTHIE
Blend until smooth.

1 milk	1 cup fat-free milk
2 fruit	1 cup orange juice
2 very lean protein	14 grams whey protein powder
	Ice cubes

Workout

8 teaspoons added sugar	16-ounce sports drink
	Water

Breakfast

3 bread	3 slices multigrain toast
1 medium-fat protein	1 egg, scrambled in a nonstick pan
3 very lean protein	6 egg whites, scrambled with whole egg
	Fat-free cooking spray (for eggs)

SMOOTHIE
Blend until smooth.

1 milk	1 cup fat-free milk
2 fruit	½ cup orange juice
	1 fresh peach
9 teaspoons added sugar	3 tablespoons honey
2 fat	2 teaspoons flaxseed oil
	Water

Snack

2 bread	2 slices whole-wheat bread
1 vegetable	Tomato, lettuce
2 fat	2 slices bacon
	Fat-free mayonnaise

Lunch	5 bread	1 whole-wheat bagel
		1 cup potato salad (made with reduced-fat mayonnaise)
		¾ cup vegetable noodle soup
	2 vegetable	1 cup carrot sticks
		Onion, tomato
	2 fruit	2 cups honeydew melon
	1 milk	1 cup fat-free milk
	4 very lean protein	4 ounces smoked salmon
	1 fat	1 tablespoon reduced-fat cream cheese

Snack	1 bread	5 reduced-fat whole-wheat crackers

SMOOTHIE
Blend until smooth.

	1 fruit	1 cup frozen raspberries
	1 milk	1 cup fat-free milk
	3 teaspoons added sugar	1 tablespoon vanilla syrup

Dinner	3 bread	2 slices rye bread
		½ cup pasta salad
	1 fruit	17 grapes
	3 teaspoons added sugar	½ cup frozen yogurt
	3 vegetable	1 cup coleslaw
		½ cup chopped vegetables (cucumbers, carrots, onions; mix into tuna)
	5 lean protein	5 ounces tuna in olive oil, drained
	2 fat	2 tablespoons reduced-fat mayonnaise

DAY 7

Preworkout

SMOOTHIE
Blend until smooth.

1 milk	1 cup fat-free milk
2 fruit	1 cup orange juice
2 very lean protein	14 grams whey protein powder
	Ice cubes

Workout

8 teaspoons added sugar	Sports drink, 16 ounces
	Water

Breakfast

3 bread	1½ cups shredded wheat cereal
1 milk	1 cup fat-free milk
2 fruit	2 cups raspberries
9 teaspoons added sugar	3 tablespoons sugar
1 medium-fat protein	1 egg, hard cooked
3 very lean protein	6 eggs, hard cooked (discard yolks)
2 fat	1½ tablespoons ground flaxseed
	6 almonds
	Water

Snack

2 bread	2 tortillas
1 vegetable	½ cup sliced vegetables
	½ cup salsa
2 fat	8 black olives, chopped
	⅛ avocado, chopped

Lunch	5 bread	1 large multigrain roll
		6 ounces baked yam
	2 vegetable	Sliced tomato, lettuce (for sandwich)
		1 cup whole radishes, celery, carrots (for dipping in dressing)
	2 fruit	2 nectarines
	1 milk	1 cup fat-free milk
	4 very lean protein	4 ounces skinless white-meat chicken, grilled with lime juice
	1 fat	2 tablespoons low-fat ranch dressing (for dipping)

Snack	1 fruit	2 tablespoons dried sweetened cranberries
	1 bread	¾ ounce pretzels
	1 milk	1 fat-free latte, tall
	3 teaspoons added sugar	Included (in cranberries)

Dinner	3 bread	3" square of corn bread
		1 ounce croutons
	1 fruit	1 large tangerine
	3 teaspoons added sugar	½ cup flavored gelatin dessert
	3 vegetable	3 cups salad with lettuce, tomato, cucumber, bell pepper
	5 lean protein	4 ounces salmon, poached
		1 ounce shredded cheese
	2 fat	2 tablespoons low-fat Caesar dressing
		Included (in corn bread)

EATING-FOR-ENDURANCE MEAL PLAN

T he goal for this diet is to keep you well fueled so you can go the distance. It's got the right carbs at the right times to power your body and your mind. The combinations of protein and fat with carbohydrates are timed to maximize performance, minimize muscle damage, and allow for maximum recovery so you can go long and strong at your next training session. The plan is packed with vitamins, minerals, antioxidants, and phytochemicals to catalyze energy production and keep you healthy throughout your training and competitive seasons.

DAILY BREAKDOWN*†

14 bread
10 fruit
3 milk
31 teaspoons added sugar
6 vegetable
4 very lean protein
4 lean protein
1 medium-fat protein
9 fat

* Use every day.
† Based on a 185-pound man

DAILY ASSUMPTIONS*†

3,500 calories
550 grams of carbohydrates
141 grams of protein
80 grams of fat

NOTE: Occasionally, a fat-free product, like mustard or cooking spray, is included on the menus. These do not count toward your daily breakdown but should not be overused.

THE MENU

DAY 1

Preworkout

SMOOTHIE
Blend until smooth.

1 milk	1 cup fat-free milk
4 fruit	1 cup orange juice
	1 large banana
	Ice cubes

Workout

16 teaspoons added sugar	Sports drink (32 ounces)
	Water

Breakfast

3 bread	3 slices whole-grain bread
1 milk	1 cup fat-free milk
2 fruit	1 cup cubed cantaloupe
	1 cup fresh raspberries
9 teaspoons added sugar	3 tablespoons 100 percent fruit spread
1 medium-fat protein	1 egg, scrambled in a nonstick pan
2 fat	⅛ avocado (chopped into cooked egg)
	1½ tablespoons ground flaxseed
	Water

Snack

2 bread	1½ ounces whole-wheat pretzels
1 vegetable	1 cup celery sticks
3 fat	30 peanuts

Lunch	5 bread	Footlong Subway sandwich, with extra meat (from their "6 grams of fat or less" list)
	2 vegetable	Lettuce, tomato
	2 fruit	1 small banana
		1 apple
	4 very lean protein	Included (in sandwich)
	2 fat	2 teaspoons olive oil or 2 tablespoons salad dressing

Snack	1 bread	½ cup Grape-Nuts cereal
	1 milk	1 cup fat-free plain yogurt
	3 teaspoons added sugar	1 tablespoon honey
	1 fruit	¾ cup blueberries

Dinner	3 bread	1 large sweet potato, baked
	1 fruit	1 slice watermelon
	3 teaspoons added sugar	½ cup frozen yogurt
	3 vegetable	Salad with 2 cups romaine lettuce, ½ cup tomato, ½ cup cucumber
		½ cup cooked broccoli
	4 lean protein	4 ounces salmon, grilled
	2 fat	2 tablespoons olive oil (for dressing)
		Vinegar (for dressing)

DAY 2

Preworkout	**SMOOTHIE**	
	Blend until smooth.	
	1 milk	1 cup fat-free milk
	4 fruit	1 cup orange juice
		1 large banana
		Ice cubes

Workout	16 teaspoons added sugar	Sports drink (32 ounces)
		Water

Breakfast	**YOGURT PLUS**	
	Combine yogurt, fruit, and honey.	
	1 milk	1 cup fat-free, unsweetened yogurt
	2 fruit	1½ cups fresh strawberries
	9 teaspoons added sugar	3 tablespoons honey
		½ cup graham cereal (for yogurt)
	CALIFORNIA EGG SANDWICH	
	Combine muffin, avocado, and egg for sandwich.	
	3 bread	1 whole-wheat English muffin
	1 medium-fat protein	1 egg, hard cooked
	2 fat	1½ tablespoons ground flaxseed
		6 almonds, sliced
		Water

Snack	2 bread	2 rice cakes
	1 vegetable	1 cup vegetable sticks
	3 fat	3 tablespoons salad dressing (for dipping)

Lunch	5 bread	2 slices whole-grain bread
		1 ounce croutons
		1 cup brown rice
	2 vegetable	Large salad with romaine lettuce, tomato, grilled eggplant, roasted red bell pepper
	2 fruit	2 kiwifruits, sliced
	4 very lean protein	4 ounces skinless white-meat chicken, grilled with lime juice
	2 fat	2 tablespoons fat-free dressing
		2 teaspoons olive oil (for roasted vegetables)

Snack	1 bread	¾ ounce pretzels
	1 milk	1 cup fat-free milk
	3 teaspoons added sugar	1 tablespoon chocolate syrup
	1 fruit	15 grapes

Dinner	3 bread	1 cup cooked pasta
		1 slice garlic bread
	1 fruit	1 cup strawberries
	3 teaspoons added sugar	½ cup flavored gelatin dessert
	3 vegetable	2 cups ratatouille (over pasta)
		Salad with 1 cup lettuce, ¼ cup tomato, ¼ cup cucumber
	4 lean protein	4 ounces lean ground beef (add to ratatouille)
	2 fat	2 tablespoons reduced-fat dressing
		1 teaspoon butter (for garlic bread)

DAY 3

Preworkout

SMOOTHIE
Blend until smooth.

1 milk	1 cup fat-free milk
4 fruit	1 cup orange juice
	1 large banana
	Ice cubes

Workout

16 teaspoons added sugar	Sports drink (32 ounces)
	Water

Breakfast

3 bread	3 slices whole-wheat bread
1 milk	1 cup low-fat cottage cheese (put on bread; sprinkle with brown sugar and cinnamon)
2 fruit	4 ounces freshly squeezed orange juice (with pulp) ½ cup sliced pineapple
9 teaspoons added sugar	3 tablespoons brown sugar
1 medium-fat protein	1 egg, cooked sunny-side up in a nonstick pan
2 fat	3 tablespoons ground flaxseed
	Water
	Fat-free cooking spray (for egg)

Snack

2 bread	1 bagel
1 vegetable	Tomato, sprouts
3 fat	3 tablespoons cream cheese

Lunch	5 bread	2½ cups rice
	2 vegetable	1 cup Chinese vegetables, stir-fried with garlic, onions, and fresh ginger
	2 fruit	1 cup citrus fruit sections
	4 very lean protein	4 ounces scallops, stir-fried
	2 fat	2 teaspoons oil (for stir-frying)

Snack	1 bread	½ cup puffed rice cereal
	1 milk	1 cup fat-free milk
	3 teaspoons added sugar	1 tablespoon honey (drizzle on berries)
	1 fruit	1 cup strawberries

Dinner	3 bread	2" square of corn bread
		1 cup kidney beans (add to chili)
	1 fruit	1 pear
	3 teaspoons added sugar	½ cup frozen yogurt
	3 vegetable	1 cup chopped cooked tomatoes with chili seasoning
		½ onion, garlic for seasoning
		Salad with 1 cup lettuce, ¼ cup tomato, ¼ cup cucumber
	4 lean protein	Included (in beans)
		2 ounces soy crumbles (for chili)
	2 fat	2 slices bacon, cooked very crisp (crumble into chili)
		Included (in corn bread)

DAY 4

Preworkout	**SMOOTHIE**	
	Blend until smooth.	
	1 milk	1 cup fat-free milk
	4 fruit	1 cup orange juice
		1 large banana
		Ice cubes

Workout	16 teaspoons added sugar	Sports drink (32 ounces)
		Water

Breakfast	2 fruit	1 cup raspberries
		½ cup orange juice
	1 milk	1 cup fat-free milk (½ cup for French toast)
	FRENCH TOAST WITH WALNUTS	
	3 bread	3 slices whole-wheat bread
	9 teaspoons added sugar	3 tablespoons maple syrup
	1 medium-fat protein	1 egg
	2 fat	3 tablespoons ground flaxseed
		4 walnut halves, chopped
		Water

Snack	2 bread	24 small whole-wheat crackers
	1 vegetable	1 cup sliced bell pepper
	3 fat	3 tablespoons salad dressing (for dipping)

Lunch	2 fruit	1½ cups blueberries
	FAJITAS	
	Combine ingredients.	
	5 bread	1 cup Spanish rice
		2 tortillas
	2 vegetable	1 cup sautéed onions, bell peppers
		2 tablespoons salsa
	4 very lean protein	4 ounces skinless white-meat chicken, grilled with lime juice
	2 fat	1 teaspoon olive oil (for cooking)
Snack	1 bread	2 rice cakes
	1 milk	1 cup fat-free milk
	3 teaspoons added sugar	1 tablespoon 100 percent fruit spread (for rice cakes)
	1 fruit	½ large banana
Dinner	3 bread	1 ounce croutons for salad
		1 cup chicken noodle soup
		4 crackers
	1 fruit	1 nectarine
	3 teaspoons added sugar	1 cup reduced-calorie cranberry juice cocktail
	3 vegetable	3 cups salad with lettuce, tomato, cucumber, bell pepper
	4 lean protein	4 ounces swordfish, grilled with ginger and scallions
	2 fat	2 tablespoons dressing

DAY 5

Preworkout

SMOOTHIE
Blend until smooth.

1 milk	1 cup fat-free milk
4 fruit	1 cup orange juice
	1 large banana
	Ice cubes

Workout

16 teaspoons added sugar	Sports drink (32 ounces)
	Water

Breakfast

3 bread	1½ cups quick oats (not instant)
1 milk	1 cup fat-free milk
2 fruit	½ cup chopped apples
	1 cup sliced strawberries
9 teaspoons added sugar	3 tablespoons maple syrup
1 medium-fat protein	1 egg, hard cooked
2 fat	1½ tablespoons ground flaxseed
	6 almonds, sliced (for oats)
	Water

Snack

2 bread	1½ ounces baked tortilla chips
1 vegetable	½ cup salsa
3 fat	8 black olives
	¼ avocado, cubed

Lunch

5 bread	1½ cups minestrone soup
	1½ cups cooked linguini
2 vegetable	1 cup marinara sauce
2 fruit	1 grapefruit, sectioned
4 very lean protein	4 ounces shrimp, grilled
2 fat	1 teaspoon olive oil (for cooking)

Snack

1 bread	10 Melba toast rounds
1 fruit	1 cup pineapple tidbits in natural juice
1 milk	½ cup fat-free cottage cheese
3 teaspoons added sugar	Included (in pineapple)

Dinner

3 bread	1 large pita
	1 ounce croutons
1 fruit	2 figs, large
3 teaspoons added sugar	½ cup apricot nectar
3 vegetable	3 cups salad with lettuce, tomato, cucumber, bell pepper
4 lean protein	4 ounces lean lamb, grilled with lime juice
2 fat	2 tablespoons vinaigrette

DAY 6

Preworkout	**SMOOTHIE**	
	Blend until smooth.	
	1 milk	1 cup fat-free milk
	4 fruit	1 cup orange juice
		1 large banana
		Ice cubes

Workout	16 teaspoons added sugar	Sports drink (32 ounces)
		Water

Breakfast	3 bread	3 slices multigrain toast
	1 medium-fat protein	1 egg, scrambled in a nonstick pan
		Fat-free cooking spray (for egg)
	SMOOTHIE	
	Blend until smooth.	
	1 milk	1 cup fat-free milk
	2 fruit	½ cup orange juice
		1 fresh peach
	9 teaspoons added sugar	3 tablespoons honey
	2 fat	2 teaspoons flaxseed oil
		Water

Snack	2 bread	2 slices whole-wheat bread
	1 vegetable	Tomato, lettuce
	3 fat	2 slices bacon
		1 tablespoon reduced-fat mayonnaise

Lunch

5 bread	1 whole-wheat bagel
	1 cup potato salad, made with reduced-fat mayonnaise
	½ cup vegetable noodle soup
2 vegetable	½ cup carrot sticks
	Onion, tomato
2 fruit	¼ honeydew melon
4 very lean protein	4 ounces smoked salmon
2 fat	2 tablespoons low-fat cream cheese

Snack

1 bread	4 crispy rye crackers
1 milk	1 cup fat-free milk
3 teaspoons added sugar	1 tablespoon 100 percent fruit spread
1 fruit	2 tablespoons raisins

Dinner

3 bread	2 slices rye bread
	½ cup pasta salad
1 fruit	24 grapes
3 teaspoons added sugar	1 tablespoon sugar (sprinkled on fruit)
3 vegetable	1 cup coleslaw
	½ cup chopped vegetables (cucumber, carrot, onion; mix into tuna)
4 lean protein	4 ounces tuna in olive oil, drained
2 fat	2 tablespoons reduced-fat mayonnaise
	Tea

DAY 7

Preworkout

SMOOTHIE
Blend until smooth.

1 milk	1 cup fat-free milk
4 fruit	1 cup orange juice
	1 large banana
	Ice cubes

Workout

16 teaspoons added sugar	Sports drink (32 ounces)
	Water

Breakfast

3 bread	1½ cups shredded wheat cereal
1 milk	1 cup fat-free milk
2 fruit	1 cup raspberries
	½ cup grapefruit juice
9 teaspoons added sugar	3 tablespoons sugar
1 medium-fat protein	1 egg, hard cooked
2 fat	1½ tablespoons ground flaxseed
	10 peanuts
	Water

Snack

2 bread	2 tortillas
1 vegetable	½ cup sliced vegetables
	½ cup salsa
3 fat	8 black olives, chopped
	¼ avocado, chopped

Lunch	5 bread	1 large multigrain roll
		6 ounces baked yam
	2 vegetable	Sliced tomato, lettuce (for sandwich)
		½ cup whole radishes, celery, carrot (for dipping in dressing)
	2 fruit	2 nectarines
	4 very lean protein	4 ounces skinless white-meat chicken, grilled with lime juice
	2 fat	4 tablespoons low-fat ranch dressing (for dipping)

Snack	1 bread	3 cups popcorn (air popped)
	1 milk	1 cup fat-free milk
	3 teaspoons added sugar	¼ cup chopped dried fruit
	1 fruit	Included (in dried fruit)

Dinner	3 bread	3" square of corn bread
		1 ounce croutons
	1 fruit	2 large tangerines
	3 teaspoons added sugar	Sprinkle sugar on fruit
	3 vegetable	3 cups salad with lettuce, tomato, cucumber, bell pepper
	4 lean protein	4 ounces salmon, poached
	2 fat	2 tablespoons low-fat Caesar dressing
		Included (in corn bread)

INDEX

Underscored page references indicate sidebars.
Boldface references indicate illustrations and photographs.

Index

Index